WORKING VIRTUE

In Working Virtue: Virtue Ethics and Contemporary Moral Problems, leading figures in the fields of virtue ethics and ethics come together to present the first substantial and comprehensive collection of essays dealing with practical moral issues from a virtue-ethical standpoint. Articles are written by leading figures in the fields of virtue ethics and ethics generally and cover topics in bioethics, professional ethics, ethics of the family, law, interpersonal ethics, and the emotions.

Virtue ethics is centrally concerned with character traits or virtues and vices such as courage (cowardice), kindness (heartlessness), and generosity (stinginess). These character traits must be looked to in any attempt to understand which particular actions are right or wrong and how we ought to live our lives. As a theoretical approach, virtue ethics has made an impressive comeback in relatively recent history, both posing an alternative to, and, in some ways, complementing well-known theoretical stances such as utilitarianism and deontology. Yet there is still very little material available that presents virtue-ethical approaches to practical contemporary moral problems, such as what we owe distant strangers, our parents, or even non-human animals. This book volume fills the gap by dealing with these and other pressing moral problems in a clear and theoretically nuanced manner.

The contributors embrace a variety of stances, including pluralistic, eudaimonistic, care-theoretical, Chinese, comparative, and stoic. This variety allows the reader to appreciate not only the wide range of topics for which a virtue-ethical approach may be fitting, but also the distinctive ways in which such an approach may be manifested.

Rebecca Walker is Assistant Professor of Social Medicine and Adjunct Assistant Professor of Philosophy at the University of North Carolina at Chapel Hill

Philip Ivanhoe is Professor of Philosophy at the City University of Hong Kong

Working Virtue

Virtue Ethics and Contemporary Moral Problems

Edited by
REBECCA L. WALKER
PHILIP J. IVANHOE

CLARENDON PRESS · OXFORD

OXFORD
UNIVERSITY PRESS

Great Clarendon Street, Oxford OX2 6DP

Oxford University Press is a department of the University of Oxford.
It furthers the University's objective of excellence in research, scholarship,
and education by publishing worldwide in

Oxford New York

Auckland Cape Town Dar es Salaam Hong Kong Karachi
Kuala Lumpur Madrid Melbourne Mexico City Nairobi
New Delhi Shanghai Taipei Toronto

With offices in

Argentina Austria Brazil Chile Czech Republic France Greece
Guatemala Hungary Italy Japan Poland Portugal Singapore
South Korea Switzerland Thailand Turkey Ukraine Vietnam

Oxford is a registered trade mark of Oxford University Press
in the UK and in certain other countries

Published in the United States
by Oxford University Press Inc., New York

British Library Cataloguing in Publication Data

Data available

Library of Congress Cataloging in Publication Data

Data available

Typeset by Laserwords Private Limited, Chennai, India
Printed in Great Britain
on acid-free paper by the
MPG Books Group, Bodmin and King's Lynn

ISBN 978–0–19–927165–8 (Hbk.)
ISBN 978–0–19–957086–7 (Pbk.)

1 3 5 7 9 10 8 6 4 2

For George Dearborn Spindler, anthropologist, great-grandfather, and an inspiration.

Acknowledgements

We would like to thank the Oxford University Press external reviewers for their detailed and helpful comments, our respective institutions for their support, and Amber Raynor and Ida Ballard for their extensive assistance in preparing this volume.

Contents

Notes on Contributors

Annette Baier (B.Phil., University of Oxford) taught at the University of Pittsburgh before retiring to her native country, New Zealand. She has published widely in ethics, and wrote a book and two encyclopedia entries about David Hume.

Lawrence Blum (Ph.D., Harvard University) is Professor of Philosophy and Distinguished Professor of Liberal Arts and Education at University of Massachusetts, Boston. He is the author of four books (the most recent being *'I'm Not a Racist, But. . .' The Moral Quandary of Race*) and many articles on race, multicultural education, moral philosophy, and moral education.

Jeffrey Blustein (Ph.D., Harvard University) is Professor of Bioethics at Albert Einstein College of Medicine and Adjunct Associate Professor of Philosophy at Barnard College. He has published extensively in leading scholarly journals and anthologies in the fields of ethics and bioethics. He is co-author or co-editor of two books and is the sole author of two books, one on parents and children and the other on care and commitment.

Rosalind Hursthouse (D.Phil., University of Oxford) is Professor of Philosophy at the University of Auckland, New Zealand. She is the author of *On Virtue Ethics* (2000, OUP) and numerous associated articles, and also works on Aristotle's ethics.

Philip J. Ivanhoe (Ph.D., Stanford University) specializes in the history of East Asian philosophy and religion and its potential for contemporary ethics. Professor Ivanhoe has written, edited, or co-edited more than a dozen books and published more than thirty articles, as well as numerous dictionary and encyclopedia entries, on Chinese and Western religious and ethical thought.

Peter Koller (Dr.jur., Dr.phil., University of Graz) is Professor of Law at the University of Graz, Austria. His main research interests are in the areas of systematic political philosophy and legal theory. His publications include two monographs, a dozen edited volumes, and more than a hundred articles on various subjects in these areas.

Nel Noddings (Ph.D., Stanford University) is Lee Jacks Professor of Education Emerita, Stanford University and Adjunct Professor of Philosophy and Education at Teachers College, Columbia University. She has published fifteen books and more than 200 articles and chapters. Her latest book is *Critical Lessons: What Our Schools Should Teach*.

Edmund Pellegrino (M.D., New York University) is Professor Emeritus of Medicine and Medical Ethics at the Center for Clinical Medical Ethics at Georgetown University Medical Center. Author of more than 500 publications, he is best known for his discussions of Christian virtue and medical ethics in the treatment of patients, humanism and the physician, and the philosophical basis of medical treatment.

Jennifer Radden (D.Phil., University of Oxford) is professor and chair of the Philosophy Department at the University of Massachusetts, Boston. Her published research explores ethical and philosophical issues arising out of psychiatric practice, mental health concepts, and mental health policy.

Nancy Sherman, (Ph.D., Harvard University) is University Professor of Philosophy at Georgetown University. Professor Sherman has written widely in the areas of ancient moral philosophy, Kantian ethics, moral psychology, emotions, military ethics, and psychoanalysis. She is the author of three books, the editor of another, and has written over thirty scholarly articles, including several encyclopedia entries, in the above areas.

Michael Slote (Ph.D., Harvard University) is UST Professor of Ethics at the University of Miami. The author of several books and many articles in ethics, he is currently writing a book on the ethics of caring.

Christine Swanton (B.Phil., D.Phil., University of Oxford) is a professor in the Philosophy Department at the University of Auckland, New Zealand. She specializes in virtue ethics, and her paperback version of *Virtue Ethics: A Pluralistic View* (OUP) appeared in 1995.

Rebecca L. Walker (Ph.D., Stanford University) is Assistant Professor of Social Medicine and Adjunct Assistant Professor of Philosophy at the University of North Carolina at Chapel Hill. Her research interests and published work are in the areas of bioethics and moral theory.

1

Introduction

Rebecca L. Walker and Philip J. Ivanhoe

In contemporary society, talk about virtue and vice may sound hopelessly old-fashioned. To some, an exhortation to 'be virtuous' is on par with 'just saying no' to sex, drugs, and rock and roll. Yet when the discussion turns serious and focuses on the virtues themselves, these initial impressions fade quickly. Everyone who cares about being a good person can see that this involves being courageous and generous. Adults with children of their own hope that those children will grow into young adults with a strong sense of kindness and justice. They harbor such hopes not only because that is a good way for their children to be but also because being that way is good for them.

Any action that is cruel, stingy, cowardly, or unjust is of a type that, other things being equal, would be wrong to do. No one seriously doubts this. Moreover, when asked what kinds of actions fit these descriptions no one with a basic sense of morality has any trouble giving examples. It may be a bit surprising then that at the theoretical level a common critique of virtue ethics has been its lack of ability to guide moral action (Louden 1997). This type of objection has already prompted substantial and powerful rebuttals (Solomon 1988; Hursthouse 1997, 1998). Yet there is still a relative paucity of writings that offer clear examples of virtue ethics actually *at work* in various practical fields. To our knowledge there is no available collection of virtue ethical views that engages and explores a substantial range of issues in contemporary practical ethics.[1] The present volume fills this need. Our hope is that it will provide insight and unique perspectives on the topics covered by focusing on the role of the virtues or a virtue ethical approach to these topics, present sustained practical examples of virtue analyses at work engaging practical moral problems, and promote a wider understanding of the virtues and virtue ethics by offering a variety of theoretical perspectives under the umbrella of virtue-based analyses.

---

[1] There are, however, excellent works focused on more specific topics in applied ethics. See for example Oakley and Cocking (2001) on virtue ethics and professional roles and Sandler and Cafaro (2005) on environmental virtue ethics.

WHAT IS VIRTUE ETHICS?

By most accounts, the current revival of virtue ethics as a theoretical approach to moral theory began with the 1958 publication of G. E. M. Anscombe's 'Modern Moral Philosophy'. Anscombe argued that both deontological and utilitarian approaches to ethics relied upon theologically derived notions of obligation, which many people no longer found compelling, and that the only alternative to such theories was virtue ethics. But while Anscombe argued that traditional virtue ethicists such as Plato and Aristotle were appropriate models for this general approach, she insisted that on their own they were inadequate. Classical virtue ethics did not offer a plausible conception of the virtues themselves, for these theories did not provide an adequate moral psychology. This, she argued, is where modern moral philosophy should turn its attention. Virtue ethical approaches to moral theory and to contemporary moral problems now present a widely recognized third type of approach, along with deontological (duty based) views and those concerned primarily with the consequences of actions. Like deontological and consequentialist views, virtue ethics is not really a single kind of approach to ethics but rather a family of approaches held together by a focus on the virtues as a core method of ethical analysis.

David Solomon has made a useful distinction between two claims associated with the revival of virtue ethics. He notes that 'any developed ethical theory must include a component that deals with virtue,' but also that in order for a normative theory to be an example of virtue ethics, it 'must have a structure such that assessment of human character is, in some suitably strong sense, more fundamental than either the assessment of the rightness of action or the assessment of the value of the consequences of action' (1988: 428–9). The second claim aims to distinguish virtue ethics from its competition—deontological and consequentialist views. Deontology frequently is characterized as focusing on the rightness and wrongness of acts and intentions to act while consequentialism focuses on the good-and-bad making consequences of actions.

In the contemporary literature, the issue of how to understand and explain the second, or a related, claim about the unique character of virtue ethics has received careful attention (Trianosky 1990; Watson 1990). Quite clearly, a rights-based view of morality that also attends to the development of virtues of character consistent with or supporting respect for rights is not thereby a virtue ethical view. So it seems we can distinguish, with Solomon, between views of morality with virtue components and views that are virtue ethical. But if that is clear, it is far from obvious what makes a view virtue ethical. Should we start by picking out views that focus fundamentally on assessment of character in opposition to right action or consequences of action? Or does this characterization draw the lines either too widely or too narrowly both for virtue ethics and for the other ethical views in consideration? One might have thought that it is not assessment of human character per se that makes a theory virtue ethical but rather its focus on the virtues. But 'focus on the virtues' is far too broad, since our rights theorist above may use up most of her theoretical energy talking about the virtues yet present a theoretical structure in which being virtuous is simply the best social expression of mutual respect for human rights.

The issue of how to characterize virtue ethics has become even more complicated in the current theoretical climate in which proponents of various strains of deontology and consequentialism have turned to careful and thorough investigations of the role of the virtues in morality (Railton 1988; O'Neill 1993; Korsgaard 1996; Herman 1996; Driver 1998; Hursthouse 1999). For virtue ethicists, this is a positive turn since the revival of virtue ethics as a theoretical option is also the impetus for the revival of interest in the virtues under other theoretical rubrics. Indeed, many theorists will now agree with the claim, heralded above as part of the revival of virtue ethics, that any developed moral theory must include an account of the role of the virtues. However, since many theorists other than virtue ethicists now also pay careful attention to the virtues, it is that much more difficult to say neatly what it is that makes a theory uniquely virtue ethical. In this regard, however, virtue ethics is in a relatively good position vis-à-vis the other theories—or rather families of theories. It is little noted but nonetheless true that any easy characterization of other approaches to moral theory, for example deontology, is also elusive.[2] In this respect, we think that virtue ethics suffers in the modern context from a 'new kid on the block' effect. She has somehow to establish a clear and easily recognizable identity in order to be accepted.

In fact, of course, virtue ethics is one of the oldest kids on the block, with ancient roots, both Eastern and Western. Perhaps it is not surprising that so many approaches to virtue ethics are available when one considers the variety of authors from whom contemporary virtue ethicists get their inspiration. While it is common to think of Plato and Aristotle when one thinks about the origins of virtue ethics, we cannot ignore or forget classical Confucians such as Kongzi ('Confucius'), Mengzi ('Mencius'), and Xunzi (Hsün-tzu), or the Stoics, Aquinas, Hutcheson, Hume, and yes, even Nietzsche.

The variety of available approaches to virtue ethics runs the gamut: virtue ethical views may be monistic or pluralistic in their theoretical structure, eudaimonistic or non-eudaimonistic (regarding the relationship between the virtues and the good life), foundationalist with respect to justification or non-foundationalist, and they may embrace or reject modern approaches to moral theory generally. The authors writing for this volume differ from one another along many of the axes mentioned. Yet all share something in common by offering virtue-based analyses of contemporary moral issues.

For the purposes of this volume, we embrace a pluralistic approach toward virtue ethics as a general category of ethical investigation and will not take a particular stand on what makes a view virtue ethical. Instead we present 'virtue ethics' as an umbrella term covering a plurality of theoretical and even anti-theoretical (with respect to modern moral theory at least)[3] approaches to ethics. Many of the contributors to this

---

[2] Rosalind Hursthouse makes the same point (1999: 4).

[3] For example, Annette Baier (1989) does not think that modern moral theory has offered a productive approach to philosophical ethics, but she offers a virtue ethical analysis in this volume and generally approves of a Humean approach to ethics.

volume would accept the label 'virtue ethical' as a proper description of the analyses they present, and yet the approaches offered both here and in their theoretical work elsewhere are quite varied. We think it is part of the appeal of this volume that we have gathered together such an interesting range of authors to write under the rubric 'Working Virtue'.[4]

Does this mean that 'anything goes' in virtue ethics? We think not. Although we cannot, and would argue that we should not, offer necessary and sufficient conditions for labeling a view 'virtue ethical', there are significant generalities marking the family resemblances that virtue ethical views share with one another. In general, virtue ethical views assess human character as a primary mode of understanding the rightness or wrongness of actions and the goodness or badness of lives lived, view traits of character as stable dispositions to act and feel in contextually appropriate or inappropriate ways, and understand the virtues and vices as the primary mode of assessing character. As discussed above, we also accept that there is an important distinction to be made between views that incorporate accounts of virtue and those that are virtue ethical. Julia Driver has noted a distinction between virtue theory—giving an account of what virtues are—and virtue ethics—basing ethics on virtue evaluation (1998: 111). We think a distinction like this is helpful in sorting out the difference between theories that merely incorporate an account of the virtues and theories that are virtue ethical. Consequentialist and deontological theories can include a virtue theoretical account while failing to be virtue ethical views. While this volume is in large part dedicated to practical applications of virtue ethics, not all of our authors would identify their work as 'virtue ethical' in the sense that Driver indicates.[5] A second aspect of the volume is to describe virtue 'at work' regardless of whether it is part of a larger virtue ethical theory.

THE SIGNIFICANCE OF VIRTUE ETHICS

The influence of virtue ethics extends far beyond its contribution as a third type of moral theory. As has already been noted, the renewed interest in virtue ethics has led to a greater focus on the virtues by proponents of other theoretical viewpoints. The study of the virtues has also resulted in a general broadening of the range of issues examined within contemporary ethics. For example, it has focused attention

---

[4] While the authors' different theoretical approaches obviously influence the analyses offered in this volume, many of the theoretical choices that our authors make in their other works are not always as apparent in their work for this volume. This is appropriate since these differences are not always relevant to the practical implications of a virtue ethical approach. Indeed, the practical nature of the work in this volume gives additional reason for not identifying particular necessary or sufficient conditions for 'virtue ethics'. In the descriptions of the essays below we will indicate, where appropriate, differences in theoretical structure.

[5] Peter Koller, for example, does not think that virtue ethics offers a stand-alone theory. He would no doubt accept the label 'virtue theoretical' as distinguished by Driver to describe his contribution. Edmund Pellegrino also notes in passing that he does not think virtue theory is a stand-alone theory, yet it is not clear whether he is referring to 'virtue theory' in the sense distinguished or making a general claim about 'virtue ethics' as a theoretical approach to morality. Nel Noddings offers a virtue ethical approach combined with a care theory approach.

on educational theory, returning to Aristotle's early concern with becoming good as opposed to merely understanding what the good might be. Such concerns have led some philosophers to explore developmental moral psychology and the role that practices or role models play in moral education. It has also given rise to questions about the nature and role of virtue for educators themselves. Aside from the goal of teaching virtue to others is the broader question whether certain virtues enable one to be a better teacher—regardless of topic.[6]

In recent years, a number of philosophers have used both virtue ethics and virtue theory as resources to explore non-Western ethical views.[7] This has proven to be a powerful conceptual tool for understanding other ethical traditions. Unlike the cases of deontology or utilitarianism, sophisticated theories about the virtues and related views about human nature, self-cultivation, and human flourishing are found in many non-Western traditions. At the same time, the study of other traditions of virtue raises important issues for virtue ethics, virtue theory, and ethics in general. For example, the fact that different cultures emphasize different sets of virtues poses a challenge to traditional versions of virtue ethics, which assume that there is a single ideal set of virtues.[8]

The revival of virtue ethics has also led several important and influential philosophers to offer new accounts about moral epistemology and the ontological status of moral values. For example, John McDowell has likened moral values to secondary qualities and argued that the acquired sensibilities associated with the virtues are necessary for detecting, appreciating, and judging the relative worth of such values.[9] McDowell's work has led other philosophers, notably R. Jay Wallace (1991), to analyze and develop various models of moral connoisseurship in an effort to make sense of how one could acquire a moral sensibility that still renders judgments that are objective, in some robust sense.[10]

OBJECTIONS TO VIRTUE ETHICS

Virtue ethics continues to exert a widening influence within contemporary ethics. Nevertheless, the re-emergence of virtue ethics has generated a variety of objections.

---

[6] For advocates of a virtue approach in education, see Jacobs (2001), Lickona (2004), and Ryan and Bohlin (2003). For criticisms of the virtue approach and an argument for an alternative, see Noddings (1992, 2003).

[7] David S. Nivison (1996) was one of the first to use Western virtue theory as a way to explore classical Chinese philosophy. See also the authors and works listed below in our discussion of Doris's work.

[8] For a response to this critique see Martha Nussbaum (1993).

[9] See his 'Values and Secondary Qualities' and 'Virtue and Reason' both reprinted in 1998. Jonathan Dancy (1993) advocates a distinct but related particularist account of moral qualities and moral perception.

[10] Eric L. Hutton (2001, 2002a) proposes a further refinement of Wallace's view by suggesting a distinction between elemental and constitutive forms of moral connoisseurship. Peter Railton (1998) also draws a strong analogy between our sense of moral values and the ability of connoisseurs, specifically wine connoisseurs, and argues that this way of thinking about moral values offers us a way to naturalize moral discourse.

One can group the bulk of these objections into three principal types. Our volume is focused primarily on the third of these three types. Nevertheless, it will help to have a good sense of the full range of criticisms as references to these appear in some of the contributions and often are somewhere in the background of others. First are those who seek to deploy psychological studies to undermine the traditional notion of virtue as a strong and stable disposition or trait of character. Gilbert Harman (1998–9, 1999–2000, 2001, 2003) and John Doris (2002) both contend that psychological studies prove that the stable and reliable traits of character that lie at the heart of virtue ethical theory simply do not exist. While such objections allow a place for virtue theory, they purport to offer severe challenges to most forms of virtue ethics.[11] Such objections have already elicited responses from those who wish to defend more traditional conceptions of virtue (Kupperman 2001; Kamtekar 2004).

Within this emerging literature, there is considerable disagreement over how to interpret the psychological studies that have been offered by the critics of virtue and whether they offer a solid basis for the implications these critics draw. For example, some of the studies that Harman cites as offering evidence *against* the traditional notion of character appear to endorse the very notion he seeks to deny.[12] Doris seeks further to discredit virtue ethical appeals to character by claiming that the conception of character employed in traditional forms of virtue ethics is 'substantially a cultural peculiarity, one considerably more prominent in Western cultures than in East Asian ones' (2002: 7). But this is clearly inaccurate, as is obvious from reading any of the core texts of Confucianism or a wide range of prominent and influential studies of Chinese ethics that employ and defend a virtue ethics interpretation (Hutton 2002b; Ivanhoe 2000, 2002; Kline 1998, 2000; Kupperman 1999; Shun 2001; Van Norden 1997, 2003; Wong 1998; Yearley 1990). Another pressing question for such critics is the selective nature of their appeal to psychological literature. For example, there is a highly developed and widely employed use of virtue theoretic approaches in the study of vices by law enforcement agencies in this and other countries around the world. At every echelon, these agencies employ 'character profiling' to predict the behavior of criminals across *a wide variety* of contexts. The well-documented success of such an approach seems to offer good evidence for the kind of stable traits of character that Harman and Doris disavow.[13] In summary, this first type of objection to virtue ethics raises important and interesting questions, but the debate appears to be in its very

---

[11] Harman sees merit in some forms of virtue ethics that do not require character traits in the ordinary sense, for example, that described by Judith Jarvis-Thomson in Harman and Thomson (1996).

[12] For example, in his 1998–9 essay, Harman quotes with approval Ross and Nisbett (1991), 'individuals may behave in consistent ways that distinguish them from their peers not because of their enduring predispositions to be friendly, dependent, aggressive, or the like, but rather because they are pursuing consistent goals using consistent strategies, in the light of consistent ways of interpreting their social world.' But, first of all, traits like 'friendliness' or 'aggressiveness' are not even candidates for being virtues, while settled dispositions that resulted from *choosing* to pursue 'consistent goals using consistent strategies, in the light of consistent ways of interpreting their social world' is all a virtue ethicist would require for identifying a virtue.

[13] The virtue ethics approach also enjoys wide use as a tool for the assessment, management, and training of police officers in the United States. See the seminal work by Edward Delattre (2002).

early stages. While we acknowledge the importance that these issues have for the field and future of virtue ethics, our volume will not engage this particular set of problems.

J. B. Schneewind (1997) has advanced a second type of objection based upon the study of the modern history of virtue ethics. He contends that a careful examination of the history of Western ethics reveals a string of theoretical failures on the part of virtue ethics. Since many advocates of virtue ethics look back to earlier stages of the Western ethical tradition for inspiration, an understanding of precisely how virtue fell out of favor is a reasonable place to begin looking for criticisms of virtue ethics.[14] Schneewind describes how the defenders of virtue did not adequately respond to certain past challenges as the history of Western ethics unfolded; this purportedly shows that virtue ethics is no longer a viable theoretical player. Nevertheless, regardless of how one views Schneewind's impressive reconstruction of the history of Western ethics and the 'misfortunes of virtue', the fact that traditional forms of virtue ethics failed to respond in compelling ways to certain *historical* challenges provides no *philosophical* reason for rejecting this theory. After all, deontology, in the form of divine command theory, did not fare well during fairly long periods in the history of Western ethics. Yet now it enjoys great popularity, owing to the particular formulation of it given by Kant. Whether contemporary or future defenders of virtue ethics can develop a more robust and defensible version of their favored theory remains an open question. Our volume will not explicitly explore this second type of criticism beyond what we have said here.

While the psychological critique finds virtue ethics at odds with purported truths about human nature, and the historical challenge faults virtue ethics for historical failures to respond to theoretical challenges, the final type of objection faults the theoretical philosophical resources presently available to an ethics of virtue.[15] A number of challenges fall into this camp, including the claim that virtue ethics problematically emphasizes the goodness of the agent's own life and character, that virtue ethics cannot adequately account for the requirements of justice, and that virtue ethics fails to provide clear guidance for moral action. While some of the contributions to this volume also address others of these theoretical critiques, the point about action-guidance is of interest for the volume as a whole. Despite accounts already cited which respond to the critique of impracticability, it is difficult to shake this criticism without a variety of worked out examples of virtue ethics at work. Such variety is presented in the present volume.

The main title for this volume, 'Working Virtue', indicates three general themes we hope it will exemplify in addition to the specific goals stated in the opening section of this introduction. As with the familiar sign 'Men at Work' — or more properly 'Men and Women at Work' — virtue is put to work in this volume in various practical areas

---

[14] For example, G. E. M. Anscombe's 1958 essay calls for a return to the Aristotelian and Thomistic traditions. Alasdair MacIntyre's highly influential 1981 volume purports to trace the modern history of Western ethics in a way that both explains why philosophical ethics has reached a state of irreconcilable disagreement and shows the way to a form of virtue ethics that can remedy this malaise.

[15] Using a somewhat similar schema, Solomon (1988: 431) characterizes these kinds of critiques as 'internal' because they 'come from within ethical reflection itself'.

of ethical inquiry. In this way the contributors 'work virtue' and virtue in turn shows its practical merit. Virtue also works for us. Being virtuous is a necessary component of leading a good life. We do not presuppose the eudaimonistic picture in which being virtuous leads to our own flourishing, but all virtue ethicists would agree that a good life requires virtue. For us, then, as ethical beings, 'virtue works'. Finally, in this volume we see the details of how virtue analyses work. That is, how they lead us to substantive and useful methods of approaching practical ethical situations and contexts. In other words we hope that in this volume, the reader will see that 'virtue analyses work.'

THE CONTRIBUTIONS

Nel Noddings, 'Caring as Relation and Virtue in Teaching'

In her essay, Noddings explores caring as an important constituent of good teaching. She argues that her particular conception of caring is consistent with and shares certain similarities to virtue ethical approaches but differs from them in seeing a relational sense of caring as 'underlying' and 'giving reliable meaning' to caring as a virtue. According to Noddings, virtue ethical conceptions of caring describe only attitudes or feelings, while the relational model that she prefers makes clear how the virtue of caring works, that is to say, what people must *do* and what effects they must *produce*, in order genuinely to care.

Noddings begins by sketching her well-known and highly influential account of caring as a moral relation. One of the critical features of her conception is that in any caring encounter between carer and cared-for both must 'contribute something' to the relation. The carer must bracket her own projects and values and attend to and seek to understand and appreciate the needs of the cared-for. In some sense the carer must absorb the perspective, desires, values, and aspirations of the cared-for and allow these to inform, direct, and inspire a response, and she must work to respond in a way that preserves and enhances her relationship with the cared-for. But the cared-for must also contribute to the caring relation. She must respond to the carer's response in a way that acknowledges that she has received the caring response and recognizes it as an expression of care.

Noddings goes on to explain how her conception of relational caring differs from more common conceptions of 'caring'. For example, her description of caring clearly is different from and avoids some of the obvious shortcomings of what she calls 'Case 2 caring'. In the latter, the carer does not work to bracket her own projects and values and gain a sympathetic understanding of the cared-for's needs, desires, and values. Instead, she infers what the cared-for needs by projecting her own ideals and aspirations onto the cared-for, and acts in light of such inferences. While such an agent may be motivated by a desire to care for another, Noddings argues that often such people do not succeed in caring for the would-be cared-for. By not putting the interests and perspective of the other ahead of their own and by failing to focus adequately upon maintaining and enhancing the relation of caring, they often fail in their attempts to care.

This points to the importance of the response to caring on the part of the cared-for, and Noddings gives a sensitive and revealing account of how this functions not only to guide and confirm the success of the carer's efforts, but to constitute and sustain the relation. She offers a rich and careful discussion of an apparent problem for her view: cases in which the person cared-for simply is incapable of responding. For example, this seems to be the case with comatose patients. Noddings though argues first that those who actually care for such individuals are able to detect subtle responses to care. Secondly, she insists that those caring for such patients act and must act *as if* their patients can respond, both in order to avoid the defects described above in 'Case 2 caring' and to sustain their own emotional capacity to care. The need for a response from the cared-for, even when this exists only as a counterfactual, reveals the primacy of caring as a relation. As Nodding herself notes, the greatest challenge to her account lies in cases where the carer actually is acting in the best interests of the cared-for but the latter can but does not acknowledge this. For in such cases, care apparently would be expressed without the mutual relation that she has described. Perhaps though there are reasons to believe that such examples are best understood as genuine but incomplete efforts to care.

Noddings goes on to elucidate the differences between cases of 'natural caring' and 'ethical caring'. The former, roughly, involve spontaneous inclinations to care for others in the right way, at the right times, and to the right extent. Such actions are motivated by love and concern. In contrast, ethical caring requires recourse to principles, intentions, and will. Ethical care is called for when we are too tired to care or when the one cared-for proves difficult, recalcitrant, or even mean. In such cases, we must rely on what Noddings calls our 'ethical self—the image of ourselves at our caring best'. She notes how similar this is to the way certain virtue ethicists rely upon conceptions of the virtues and one might add real or ideal ethical exemplars as both a guide and inspiration for action. From the perspective of care theory, natural care is the preferred or ideal state. We resort to ethical caring in order to 'restore the conditions characteristic of natural caring.' Noddings goes on to say that in cases where one must fall back on ethical caring, 'we might say with Bernard Williams that the carer had "one thought too many." ' Here is another example of a similarity between care theory and classical forms of virtue ethics. Noddings's ethical hierarchy of care resembles the distinction commonly made by virtue ethicists between continent and fully virtuous agents.

Noddings begins her application of care theory to teaching by noting that teachers are responsible both for 'the direct person-to-person caring that contributes to the growth of individual students and for the establishment of conditions under which caring can flourish'. Her discussion of care theory in education focuses on its use to motivate students to learn, its implications for pedagogy and the shape of the curriculum, and how it might inform and give shape to the teaching and evaluation of teachers. In general, relational caring is committed to bringing the interests, abilities, and general perspective of individual students—whatever their level and future goals—fully into the project of learning. One clear implication of this view is that it calls for the most broadly educated teachers possible. Only such teachers have the resources needed to respond to the diverse needs, abilities, and desires of their various students, and only such 'renaissance thinkers' offer their students an ideal model of a properly educated human being. This highly demanding practical implication is best understood as an expression of something we all understand: real caring is as difficult to achieve as it is attractive to behold.

Noddings shows that relational caring shares a number of important features with the general approach of virtue ethics. She highlights their common 'rejection of fixed principles in favor of reliance on the good character of moral agents to guide moral life'. Her analysis notes or implies additional similarities as well. Both relational caring and virtue ethics place great importance on the development of sensibilities and moral discernment, endorse the ideal of spontaneously and joyfully acting well, and see the moral life diachronically—in terms of a course of development for the self and others. One might also argue that both require people to educate themselves broadly in order to live well, as individuals and in community with others. Traditional virtue ethicists such as Aristotle can even be seen as sharing Noddings's central concern with the critical role of interpersonal relations as fundamental to our moral lives. For Aristotle insisted that no one could live well apart from a good *polis*, and more than one-fifth of the *Nicomachean Ethics* is dedicated to an analysis of *philia*. Nevertheless, Noddings's arguments about the primacy of relation in caring and particularly the role of the one cared-for raises an important challenge to many forms of virtue ethics and contributes a crucial and productive insight into the complex nature of our lives together.

Edmund D. Pellegrino, 'Professing Medicine, Virtue Based Ethics, and the Retrieval of Professionalism'

While Noddings discusses a relational sense of caring as a virtue in teaching, Pellegrino's essay provides a virtue-based approach to professional ethics for the helping professions generally (medicine, law, teaching, and ministry). However, Pellegrino focuses his analysis on the case of clinical medicine and appeals to his highly influential earlier work establishing the goal of medicine as the good of the patient with respect to the following elements: medical good, perception of the good, human good, and the spiritual good. However, in this essay, Pellegrino presents these categories with new insights and also generalizes the paradigm to incorporate other helping professions. He sees the professional in all cases as one who, through the act of profession, promises specialized knowledge and skills and in addition willingness to use these to the good of others. The four ends of medicine are also seen as the ends of the other three helping professions where the first good is simply understood as the technical good appropriate to the profession. Interestingly, as Pellegrino discusses, the relationship of these various goods to one another can vary with the profession and with the individual patient, client, student, or parishioner.

A classical teleological view of virtue ethics, based on the views of Aristotle and Aquinas, grounds Pellegrino's approach to the good of the patient. The good of the patient is then what is aimed at with the particular virtues of the physician. Pellegrino believes a teleological approach to the good of the patient is necessary to avoid a circular definition of the virtues of the physician; however, he also recognizes that it is difficult to support a general teleological view of human ends. As a way of avoiding the difficulties associated with such a view, he limits his teleology to the specific human goods with which professions are concerned. For medicine the good that is aimed at is the good of the patient where fulfillment of this good is not a purely technical art, but also a moral end. However, in so far as the good of the patient is broader than fulfillment of the technical ends of medicine (i.e. physiological health), the clinician must also take into account the good of the patient as a human and spiritual being. One issue that arises at this point is whether the need to support a teleological approach to the human end as such has re-emerged.

Specifically with regard to clinical medicine, Pellegrino understands the good aimed at as a composite of four goods: medical-physiological, personal as perceived by the patient, patient as human being, patients' perception of spiritual good. The individual definitions and orderings (hierarchy) of these goods is left to the individual patients' understanding, although Pellegrino gives general definitions. Leaving the hierarchy and specific understanding of the fulfillment of these goods to the patient solves the classical tensions between spiritual beliefs (and other personal ends) and the ends of medicine as proper physiological functioning by leaving the choices to the patient him- or herself. If the Jehovah's Witness chooses to avoid blood transfusion, abiding by this is behaving in a way that serves the patient's good since for her, the spiritual beliefs trump the physical need. We then avoid the standard dilemma of a conflict between 'autonomy' and 'beneficence' since doing what is good for the patient just means abiding by her autonomous choices in this way.

Indeed, Pellegrino's approach offers a highly significant alternative to a widely accepted principles-based approach to medical ethics.[16] According to the principles approach to biomedical ethics the moral elements of medicine stem from adherence to four different prima facie principles found in common morality: beneficence, respect for autonomy, non-maleficence, and justice.[17] If one tried to squeeze Pellegrino's approach into this model, one might conclude that his view falls entirely under the principle of beneficence as he thinks it is the goal of medicine to serve the good of the patient. However, his understanding of beneficence is very different from that of the principlists since for him, for example, respecting patient autonomy just is acting for the good of the patient. The principles-based view sees beneficence more in line with the strictly medical understanding of the patient's good. Of course, Pellegrino's approach also differs in that his is concerned with virtues and so takes on an entirely different methodology, including teleological discussion of the ends appropriate to medicine. As Pellegrino himself notes, his approach is concerned only at one level with human good per se, whereas he understands the principles-based approach as occurring at that level entirely.

Pellegrino's essay serves as an excellent companion and comparison piece to Nel Noddings's essay on 'Caring as Relation and Virtue in Teaching'. Pellegrino focuses primarily on the helping profession of clinical medicine but also applies his model to teaching as a profession. Noddings does not present her concern as primarily one of professional ethics per se, but as an extension of the ethics of care to the

---

[16] The principles-based approach to medical ethics purports to account for biomedical ethics broadly while Pellegrino aims to account for the helping professions in general, so the area of overlap is really just in the area of health professional–patient relationships. However, since this is a significant portion of biomedical ethical concerns, it is important to recognize the important differences between these two approaches.

[17] For a detailed account of these four principles in the context of biomedical ethics see Beauchamp and Childress (2001).

case of the student–teacher relationship. The essays are thus complimentary in focus since Pellegrino's consideration of professional ethics can be furthered by a more in depth account of the caring that takes place in the relationship between the helping professional and the 'helped', while Noddings's focus on the caring aspect of the relationship between the teacher and student may be complimented by an account of the purely professional ethical role of the teacher. Whereas Pellegrino grounds his approach in a classical teleological model of virtue ethics, Noddings grounds her approach to the virtues in a relational sense of caring. Despite this foundational difference there are many complementary ideas in the two pieces. For example, it is a key aspect of both pieces that the values and perspective of the cared-for play a central role in the relationship. For Noddings this contribution is fundamental to a virtuous caring relationship; for Pellegrino it is only acting out of concern for the patient's (parishioner's, client's, student's) own values and interests that one can truly achieve the ends of the helping profession at issue. We see, then, that despite significant foundational differences, these virtue ethical approaches actually *at work* have major points of agreement.

Jeffrey Blustein, 'Doctoring and Self-Forgiveness'

Blustein's contribution fills two substantial gaps in the virtue ethics literature. First, he discusses the constitutive elements of self-forgiveness as a virtue. In this discussion he also points out differences and similarities to well-known discussions of other-forgiveness. Secondly, Blustein applies this discussion to an ignored but essential aspect of medical ethics, namely physician self-forgiveness. As Blustein points out, an account of self-forgiveness is especially important in a professional culture of high perfectionism in which the consequence of error can be devastating. For example, in a widely cited Institute of Medicine report on medical error (Kohn, Corrigan, and Donaldson 2000), as many as 98,000 deaths per year are due to medical error. However, Blustein focuses not only on cases of error, but also on unreasonable physician self-expectation in the face of death and incurable disease. With respect to the second gap in the literature, this piece serves as an important compliment to Pellegrino's account of professional ethics. While Pellegrino's work in general has focused on standard virtues such as compassion, benevolence, honesty, fidelity to promises, and courage, an account of self-forgiveness enriches the understanding of characteristic motivational structures required for the good physician.

At first blush the idea of self-forgiveness might seem philosophically suspect. After all, isn't it necessary that the person forgiving is also the one wronged or harmed? Yet in the case of self-forgiveness the self is both the wrongdoer and the forgiver. A number of aspects of Blustein's account help to make sense of the notion of self-forgiveness, however. First, according to Blustein we need not assume that there is one kind of thing 'forgiveness' which is manifested in both self- and other-forgiveness, and his account of self-forgiveness points to ways in which this phenomenon is both alike and different from other-forgiveness. For example, in cases of self-forgiveness, the thing that is forgiven may be something that never harms or even wrongs any other person, such as malicious desires or thoughts.[18] Secondly, the notion of self-forgiveness is a common-sense notion that is widely accepted and it is from this idea, not some philosophically technical sense, which Blustein starts. Thirdly, there are ways in which the self can be both the harmer and the harmed, such as in a failure to develop talents or in the case of personal vices such as over-indulgence, and Blustein acknowledges these as part of the proper subject matter of self-forgiveness.

However, Blustein does not limit self-forgiveness to the more obvious cases in which the self is both the harmer and the harmed. Yet in all cases of self-forgiveness, according to Blustein, there is some harm to the self; that harm is to one's sense of self-worth. Indeed, self-forgiveness is only applicable in cases of harm to one's sense of self-worth. In the case of physician self-forgiveness, the two most relevant sources of self-worth are the holding of a professional set of standards where these may or may not involve moral norms, and the moral commitments of morally serious persons in general. In Blustein's account, the focus on self-worth serves as an interesting contrast to other-forgiveness, since in other-forgiveness overcoming harm to self worth is not necessary (we may forgive others for harms done to ourselves that do not undermine our self-worth). This divergence results from the fact that in the case of self-forgiveness it is the self that is also the wrongdoer. Presumably, then, for those with the virtue of self-forgiveness acting, feeling, or thinking in certain kinds of ways necessarily and properly undermines self-worth. The process of self-forgiveness is then one of reconciliation with the self in a manner addressing that harm.

Blustein also discusses the ways in which self- and other-forgiveness are parallel. In general he views the act of forgiveness as a process of changing one's emotional stance toward and assessment of a person who has acted wrongly or is somehow deficient, whether that person is oneself or some other. In the case of the self this is through a process of overcoming of self-reproach. Self-reproach is used as a term for a wide variety of emotions carrying with them negative self-assessment and so an undermining of self-worth, such as guilt and shame. Importantly, however, while painful self-regarding feelings may motivate a start to the process of self-forgiveness, this process is not simply a way of lessening self-reproach. Rather, it is a process involving difficult recognition of one's actual wrongdoing and the taking on of tasks specific to the situation which make one the proper subject of forgiveness both by the self and by others.

So far then we have a view of some of the ways in which the concept of self-forgiveness is both made sense of and also enriched by Blustein's insightful account. However, we may still wonder why self-forgiveness is a virtue on his view and in particular why it is a virtue for physicians. We should take these issues in turn. The first question that might arise is why self-forgiveness which is not itself a character trait, but rather a self-regarding activity, should be a virtue. In truth, the labeling of the character trait in question as 'self-forgiveness' seems to be something of a convenience in this case, since the trait at issue has no simple name. That trait is to be properly disposed with respect to self-reproach including knowing when it is appropriate (being neither too lenient nor too stern) and going through the tasks included in being worthy of forgiveness by others as well as the self.

---

[18] On some accounts, such 'sins of the mind' are also ways of wronging others.

Blustein gives substance to his discussion of self-forgiveness as a virtue by describing it within an Aristotelian framework. In particular, he addresses the virtue as a mean and the ways in which it benefits the possessor. Blustein explains that self-forgiveness benefits the possessor of this virtue with psychological health, reclaiming of effective agency, and restoring of self-respect where this has been undermined. A similarity between self- and other-forgiveness arises at this point since one of the aims of other-forgiveness is reconciliation in the sense of an establishment or repair of mutual respect. While self-forgiveness is compatible with remaining self-reproach, it is incompatible with remaining lack of self-respect.

Blustein also deals with the question whether self-forgiveness can be a virtue because virtues are about what is difficult, but self-forgiveness may seem to be too easy. He rejects this characterization of self-forgiveness, however, since for him self-forgiveness is not merely a corrective to an emotional state of self-reproach, but rather a corrective to this state that involves a particular process including an honest handling of one's wrongs or shortcomings and an addressing of the harm to others where appropriate. In other words self-forgiveness properly requires a number of 'tasks'. Exactly which ones are no doubt settled contextually by persons with the proper virtue. Rather than being easily achieved, then, self-forgiveness is the corrective to indulgent self-generosity. This point connects to the sense in which self-forgiveness represents a mean between being overly self-indulgent and overly strict with oneself.

As already noted, traditional medical education and practice hasn't left much room for self-forgiveness as a virtue. However, Blustein makes a compelling case for the significance of self-forgiveness for physicians; in particular he argues that it is necessary for them to perform well in their role as physicians. In order to make this point he focuses on two difficult areas of medicine, namely, caring for the incurable and disclosing medical error.

Physicians are sometimes accused of distancing themselves from situations that reveal their lack of power over processes of disease and the inevitability of death. This may involve emotionally abandoning patients who are incurable or attempting to exert control over death processes in a way that undermines the autonomy of the patients and values of the family. Much of the time the reason that a disease process is irreversible is not something for which the physician is actually responsible; however, the culture of medicine reinforces the emotional sense of responsibility in the sense of blameworthiness nonetheless. Though physicians may recognize the limitations of their powers theoretically in 'fighting' death, they may still feel personally blameworthy when such is not possible. Physicians who blame themselves, though, when a result is actually due to an incompleteness in medical technology or knowledge or simply due to natural courses of events lack the proper virtue of self-forgiveness since they fail to discern where self-blame is appropriate. According to Blustein, then, part of the virtue of self-forgiveness is the ability to perceive when such is necessary.

It is also difficult for physicians to admit error in the context of a culture that encourages the ideal of physician infallibility. There are also legal fears, financial risks, and fears about damages to reputation. The approach to errors suggested at the health care policy level stresses system problems, but this further enforces an avoidance of admission of error by individuals. As Blustein points out, patients and families are owed (at minimum) an explanation and apology for medical errors. These are tasks that individual physicians should take on as part of the 'tasks' involved in the process of proper self-forgiveness. When the physician making an error has the virtue of self-forgiveness, she will neither evade responsibility nor hold herself to a standard of infallibility, but will admit error and make amends as appropriate. Where the risk of error is high in day-to-day care of patients and the results sometimes disastrous, such a virtue is highly significant for the physician to perform properly in her role.

Jennifer Radden, 'Virtue Ethics as Professional Ethics: The Case of Psychiatry'

Radden discusses the virtues relevant to psychiatry as a professional practice. She argues that being virtuous is of the utmost importance for the psychiatrist because of the nature of the therapeutic relationship and the particular vulnerabilities of psychiatric patients. At the same time, special challenges to virtue arise for the psychiatrist, such as the temptation to feign virtue. Radden focuses her analysis of the virtuous psychiatrist on traits of character that are moral virtues only within the context of the mental health care setting. These virtues are specific examples of role-constituted virtues. On Radden's view, role-constituted virtues are those traits that further the goals of some particular profession and are moral virtues only in the context of that role. Nevertheless, some role-constituted virtues are also connected in various ways to general moral virtues.

Radden's contribution thus provides an in depth analysis of a particular area of clinical medical practice and serves as an excellent companion to Pellegrino's and Blustein's contributions. While Radden discusses traits of character that are moral virtues only in the context of the mental health care setting, Pellegrino discusses more easily recognizable moral virtues (benevolence, some degree of effacement of self-interest, intellectual honesty, compassion, courage, and humility) for the clinician generally. In comparison with Pellegrino's approach, Blustein's focus on self-forgiveness broadens the virtues at issue for clinical medicine; however, he also views self-forgiveness as a general moral virtue that is particularly salient in the clinical context. Like Blustein, Radden specifically addresses non-conventional moral virtues but claims that these are moral virtues only in the professional setting at issue.

Since Radden argues that in general some traits of character that are morally neutral outside the professional role are morally salient within that role, she also argues for a robust sense of role morality in the virtue ethics context. Indeed, it appears that it is precisely the relationship to the goals of some particular profession that underlies the transition from a non-virtue, or at least non-moral virtue, to a moral virtue in the professional context. However, Radden distinguishes her approach from what she calls 'strong role morality' according to which there may be fundamental conflicts between what morality permits, requires, and prohibits in general versus within a particular role context. She claims instead that her view requires only a weaker form of role morality under which roles may only require more stringent moral obligations.

Radden begins by describing some of the particular challenges for the virtuous psychiatrist. An interesting point here is that there are two general kinds of reasons that psychiatrists might act in accordance with particular virtues. The first kind of reason refers to the virtues required by the context, including patient vulnerabilities, issues of power difference, the particularly high demands of treatment, and the difficulty of achieving these goals. The second kind of reason is therapeutic and involves, for example, modeling particular kinds of virtues in the hopes of inculcating these in the patient. In her analysis, Radden focuses on the role-constituted virtues of self-knowledge, self-unity, unselfing, and realism. As we saw with the virtue of self-forgiveness, a question arises about the extent to which these role-constituted virtues can truly be considered traits of character. However, addressing that question here would take us too far afield.

Radden points to close ties between self-unity and self-knowledge, since the former is often sought through the latter. She portrays self-knowledge as 'understanding of one's own subjectivity, psychic states and traits, life, and character [while] Self-unity or integration is a condition of psychological coherence and consistency'. Self-unity in addition bears a close relationship to a more recognizable overarching moral virtue, namely integrity. Radden suggests that self-unity may actually be a precondition for moral integrity. The particular context of the mental health care profession, moreover, Radden suggests, requires particularly strong moral integrity in its practitioners since the patients are especially vulnerable and the potential for exploitation, for example, especially high. Self-unity also gains significance in the mental health care setting under the second kind of reason for being virtuous: the therapeutic reason. This is because of the particularly high value placed on self-unity as a goal for psychiatric patients.

Radden uses the term 'unselfing' to denote the 'personally effaced yet acutely attentive attitude adopted by the effective practitioner toward the patient'. As she notes, this is necessary to maintain the ethical and effective psychiatrist's professional role. Interestingly, unlike self-knowledge and self-unity, which are valued in everyday life although not moral virtues in those contexts, Radden claims that 'unselfing' is not even particularly valued outside the therapeutic context, although there is a parallel virtue of all professionals in so far as their roles require attentiveness solely to the needs of their clients. Thus, for Radden, unselfing is a role-constituted virtue furthering the goals of the profession but not underlying the development of a general moral virtue.

Realism, as Radden explains, is at best a prudential virtue outside the psychiatric context. However, because mental disability and disease often cause a loss of a sense of commonly accepted reality and a favoring of a kind of personal reality, realism becomes a special virtue in the context of psychological treatment. Radden likens the value of realism in psychiatry to that of the realism required in raising children. One wonders at this point whether realism in those involved in raising children would also be a role-constituted moral virtue on Radden's schema. An answer to this question might promote the introduction of an interesting distinction between role-constituted virtues and professional virtues, since presumably the parent, for example, is not a professional but does occupy a specific social role.

The virtuous psychiatrist, on Radden's view, must not only develop the variety of special role-constituted virtues discussed here, but also faces specific challenges to the maintenance of virtue in the mental health care setting. One example of this type of challenge is the temptation to feign virtue. While the mere appearance of virtue can be effective in many areas of life, Radden points out that in psychiatric practice the appearance of character traits of particular types in the practitioner are absolutely essential. In this sense, the character traits of the practitioner, or at least the appearance to the patient of particular character traits, is part of the healing process. An example Radden discusses is trustworthiness. The patient must believe that the practitioner is a trusted confidant if the psychiatrist–patient alliance is to achieve the desired healing effects. Thus it is essential that the psychiatrist appear to be trustworthy. But is the appearance of trustworthiness all that is needed? If so, is it possible to feign such a virtue? Would doing so be compatible with ethical practice and effective in healing?

Because of the artificiality of the therapeutic context and the mental state of the psychiatric patient, he or she may have a more difficult time than other patients in discerning accurately whether a psychiatrist is feigning virtue. One might think initially that any feigning of virtue is morally suspect; however, as Radden points out there are at least two morally distinct modes of feigning virtue. The first is to do so for some personal gain, which she thinks is clearly wrong in any context. The second, however, is to undertake a semblance of virtue for some good end. This end may be the end of inculcating the virtue in oneself, as when one educates oneself to be virtuous through habituation (relevant to psychiatrist practitioners in training). Or, in the developed practitioner's case, also includes undertaking the semblance of virtue for therapeutic reasons. Radden argues that only the goal of inculcating actual virtue is an acceptable reason for feigning virtue. Feigning virtue for therapeutic reasons, Radden worries, will in fact be unsuccessful and exhibits a kind of problematic disrespect of the patient.

In the context of her discussion of feigned virtue, Radden also addresses the challenge to virtue ethics brought by John Doris and others stressing the highly contextual nature of so-called virtuous behavior. As discussed in an earlier section of the introduction dealing with general objections to virtue ethics, this critique might be interpreted as undermining the very existence of the virtues since they are uniformly thought of as settled traits of character. However, as Radden interprets the challenge, it is consistent with the maintenance of compartmentalized traits of character. Thus the psychiatrist might be trustworthy when it comes to keeping patients' secrets, but not when it comes to keeping the secrets of colleagues. For Radden, the relevant issue is whether virtues manifested only in particular situations are feigned or whether they are real virtues that are compartmentalized. By way of response, Radden points out that professional roles are identity conferring and so it is likely that virtues in the professional context will carry over to other aspects of the professional's life. Furthermore, she points out that it is a moral flaw to exhibit compartmentalized virtues since the life aspects in which the professional is not virtuous in the relevant respect are still aspects of her life. Interestingly, neither response really answers the question whether compartmentalized, but real, virtues might nevertheless be sufficient in the role context. However, Radden's response to the question whether feigned virtues are therapeutically effective answers that question if the virtues at issue are merely feigned.

Annette C. Baier, 'Trust, Suffering, and the Aesculapian Virtues'

Baier opens her essay with a portrayal of Aesculapius, the Zeus-designated god of healing, asking what virtues we want in healers. What, that is, are the Aesculapian virtues? Among other virtues, she points to calm communicativeness and right timing but much focus is on compassion toward the suffering of others. Baier argues, in the latter sections of the chapter, that compassion is a fully realizable virtue only if euthanasia is legally permissible. This particular claim follows from a nuanced and detailed account of the situations people face toward the end of life and the ethical significance of both respect and compassion in those contexts. However, it also follows from the theoretical scaffold of trust, relationships, power, and virtue that Baier builds at the start of the essay.

A central beam of that scaffold runs between trust and the virtues. In earlier works, Baier has developed an influential set of views on the nature of trust and the elements of power within relationships. In this essay she explicitly ties her framework to a virtue ethical one writing, 'Virtues, on my analysis, are personal traits that contribute to a good climate of trust between people, when trust is taken to be acceptance of being, to some degree and in some respects, in another's power.' As Baier describes, the Aesculapian virtues are exactly those found in trustworthy healers. Hence it is not blind trust that she endorses. Rather it is trust that is deserved by trustworthy individuals (and institutions).

The distinctions that Baier makes between a good climate of trust and one that is not good (for example when the trusted person abuses her power) is a significant contribution to the literature on trust in the health care context. Much of the current focus on trust in the health care context is on the importance of establishing the trust of patients, family members, and research subjects in health care professionals, institutions, and researchers and on methods of furthering this trust. Baier's framework reminds us that trust is only a proper attitude under circumstances in which the recipient is trustworthy but at a deeper level reminds us of the delicate balance of trusting relationships by locating the (ideally reciprocal) power of individuals over one another as a central element.

Baier discusses not merely the trustworthy physician (and other health care workers), but also what is necessary for institutional trustworthiness. The rights of patients play a key role here since the recognition of such rights in the health care context helps to empower patients. Further, such empowerment ameliorates some of the imbalance of power in the relationship between the patient and health care workers.

In addition to asking what doctors and institutions owe patients in the way of trustworthiness, Baier asks what patients can contribute to the trusting relationship. Because of her model in which virtue builds a climate of proper trust within relationships, which are essentially reciprocal, such a question is natural. Baier's analysis reminds us, then, that part of what it is for patients to be empowered is also to allow that they may either contribute to or detract from a good climate of trust. By focusing on the institutional elements of trust as well as what patients can add to the development of a good climate of trust, Baier's essay adds a highly complementary element to the chapters by Pellegrino, Blustein, and Radden. Those authors, while diverse in their approaches as has been discussed, focused primarily on the virtues of professionals as individuals.

As Baier points out, it is common to assume that a central goal of healing is the relief of suffering where such relief is not merely tied to the restoration of physical health. However, such relief may not be readily available when the time-honored goal of medicine is the extension of life, which sometimes conflicts with the relief of suffering. A significant aspect of Baier's portrayal of the failure to relieve the suffering of patients and the related failure to uphold or develop trusting relationships comes in the form of personal stories. While the stories she tells are crucial elements for building on her core themes, it also seems that she delves into her own perspective to relieve in advance the idea that she might be writing from a neutral point of view.[19]

In either case, these stories are enlightening. For example, one way in which her own trust in her physician was undermined was not from incompetence or even bad bedside manner, but a lack of communication about what was happening with her case that may have been the fault of unreflective administrative practices. This matches with the fact that many of the ways in which patients suffer in hospitals or other care centers have to do with the details of their care. Is there a mere curtain between beds while intimate questions are asked? Does the physician introduce herself when she comes in the room and state the purpose of her visit? Are medical students with little experience readily introduced as such or does this become evident only when a painful procedure is botched? Problems in day-to-day aspects of care which for some may cause great distress and even suffering are only sometimes due to any readily identifiable individual fault. However, these aspects of institutional care may undermine trust in individuals even when the real problem may be administrative or institutional.

For Baier, the failure to relieve suffering reaches its most extreme form in denial of assistance in dying to patients. This denial, she argues is a highly significant source of mistrust in health care professionals and institutions. One way in which such a denial leads to mistrust is in the sense of abandonment that a patient may feel at the end of life. But other mechanisms are also discussed. For example, if expressions of a desire to end one's life due to suffering are taken only as signs of depression, then the patient's suffering may not be taken seriously. This failure to respect the patient by taking her requests seriously further undermines the patient's relative power in the relationship and thus properly erodes a sense of trust.

Baier's analysis is backed up by some evidence that simply possessing the knowledge that assistance in dying is available may be enough to allow one not actually to follow through with the final request for such assistance. This evidence comes from the few places in the world in which euthanasia and/or physician-assisted

---

[19] Baier's concern to avoid the misleading perception that particular ethical positions, especially particular ethical theories, can be developed and defended from a neutral point of view is clear in her essay 'Doing Without Moral Theory?' (1989).

suicide are legal. The idea, then, is that the availability of such assistance also provides the grounds for trust. That trust comes from the recognition of the validity of the patient's request and in the practical support, should it be necessary, of death. This empowerment removes the kind of desperate fear of dying a horrible death that itself causes great suffering at the end of life.

Rosalind Hursthouse, 'Environmental Virtue Ethics'

Hursthouse's chapter begins from a particular assumption about environmental ethics, namely, that it is primarily concerned with articulating and defending the view that we must radically change our relationship to and interactions with the environment. She calls this view the 'green belief'. Starting from this normative framework, Hursthouse then goes on to formulate a much needed virtue ethical articulation and defense of the green belief. In so doing, she considers two quite different approaches. The first starts with traditional virtues and vices and reinterprets these in light of the green belief. The second approach creates new virtues (at least one such) to account for what is truly a radical new way of being in the world.

Starting from the traditional virtue of practical wisdom and the vices of greed, self-indulgence, and short-sightedness, Hursthouse shows how much of what we might want out of the green belief can be articulated in these, and related, traditional virtue and vice terms. The vice of short-sightedness is perhaps the easiest to illustrate. In so far as pollution, for example, is harmful to us eventually, appeal to the vice of short-sightedness works to condemn polluting activities. Of course, some pollution will not harm us (currently living human beings), but rather our descendants. Concern about those future people highlights one reason to appeal to the vices of greed and self-indulgence. It is greedy for me not to cut back on my own consumption (and corresponding pollution) when I know that others will suffer from my indulgence later on. Since it is safe to assume that virtuous people care about future generations as well as current ones, a failure to protect the interests of those future persons is also short-sighted.

As Hursthouse explains, a virtue ethical account relying on traditional virtues and vices also brings in a host of complex explanatory elements to account for the sometimes subtle ways in which activities harming the environment are vicious. A virtue ethical account can make sense of the way that vices aggravate one another. An overly proud person is less likely to acknowledge that her actions are self-indulgent, for example. Furthermore, a virtue ethical perspective can draw a distinction between those people who directly participate in cruelty to animals and those who benefit from such cruelty. For example, people who eat meat 'processed' under cruel conditions are not themselves cruel, yet they are also not compassionate. That is because they knowingly endorse that cruelty by partaking of its products. Those who prefer to turn a blind eye to such practices may instead be self-deceived, which is also a kind of vice.

It appears then that much of what is wrong with our current ways of interacting with nature may be attributed to familiar vices understood in the context of environmentalism. However, Hursthouse worries that the view that virtue ethics offers so far seems problematically human centered. This problem is addressed in part by a discussion of the familiar but somewhat outdated notion of humility. As Hursthouse explains, humility is often invoked in environmental ethics literature in the course of establishing the intrinsic value of non-human, but biological, entities and communities. In contrast, however, for virtue ethics, the strategy is to focus on humility as a virtue and thus on what actions proper humility requires in the context of our interactions with the environment as opposed to the vice of arrogance. Unlike the vices of greed, self-indulgence, and short-sightedness, arrogance is not centered on negative effects on human beings stemming from problematic treatment of the environment. Rather, humility requires recognizing the relative greatness and wonder of nature and seeing ourselves as part of, rather than dominant in relationship to, the natural world.

Hursthouse's general strategy for applying traditional virtues and vices to environmental virtue ethics is simply a matter of reinterpreting the virtues in light of this new context. Since the virtues and vices are usually interpreted and constructed to deal with human relationships, this new consideration gives the virtue or vice a somewhat new interpretation and gives us a new perception of what they require. Hursthouse then asks whether virtue ethics reconsidered in light of environmental values is still human centered in a way that might be objectionable to those espousing the green belief. She considers the idea that such a virtue ethics could still be problematically human centered in that it embraces *eudaimonia* as a 'top' value. However, she rejects any interpretation of *eudaimonia* that would make virtue ethics problematically human centered. One important aspect of this rejection is Hursthouse's view that there is no need for any foundation for virtue ethics other than the virtues and vices themselves. The claim that something is right because virtuous relies on no more foundational claim about its right making features. At the same time, however, Hursthouse embraces the view that the virtues benefit their possessor and are part of living well. She simply disagrees with the view that this makes *eudaimonia* a value that is somehow more foundational than the virtues.

Having established a fairly promising strategy for an environmental virtue ethics relying on the traditional virtues and vices, Hursthouse then considers whether a more clearly new way of thinking about, feeling about, and relating to nature may be required. Such a possibility she thinks may be available through the creation of a new virtue to deal with our interactions with nature. She notes from the start how difficult a truly new virtue is to come by since virtues involve acting in the proper way for the right kinds of reasons, being disposed in certain kinds of ways in the emotions, and perceiving in a particular kind of way relevant happenings. Further it needs a preliminary version for children to emulate—to be on the right track though not yet having the virtue.

Hursthouse settles on respect for nature, or as she comes to prefer, being rightly oriented to nature, as the best option for such a new virtue. This comes by way of a consideration of Taylor's notion of respect for nature. While she agrees with much of his practical view about what respect for nature entails, Hursthouse disagrees with the justification that Taylor gives in so far as it relies on foundational premises about the inherent worth of living things and on the idea that one can simply take up an efficacious attitude of respect for nature by a rational process.

Hursthouse's rejection of the idea that we must locate foundational intrinsic worth in the environment is closely related to her rejection of a foundational value for virtue ethics in general. As she points out, the idea of intrinsic worth brings with it a prob-lematic issue about degrees of such worth as well as requiring that the source of such value be located in some one or few characteristics. For example, Taylor associates such value with 'living things', but what about the non-living aspects of the envir-onment? According to Hursthouse, what is needed is the affirmation that action in accordance with the good of the environment provides non-instrumental reasons, but that this does not require the location of intrinsic value as a foundational premise. The kinds of reasons are exactly those that we provide to children when inculcating a virtue of right action to nature. Such as, 'don't squash it, you will harm it' or 'be sure to give it plenty of water, it is good for it.' A colloquial sense of inherent worth is attached to such notions, but not a foundational one. Hursthouse recommends that we appeal to the unity of the practice of providing such reasons rather than to some foundational premise about inherent worth by virtue of which such reasons can be derived.

Hursthouse thinks that the substantial and radical new attitude that one would have to take toward nature in order to be consistent with Taylor's own notion of respect for nature would actually require the development of a new virtue. Respect on that view would not merely be a requirement of rationality, but would involve a radical change of one's emotions and perceptions of one's reasons for action. While respect for nature cannot be garnered simply by deciding to take it up or by becoming convinced of the need for such respect, it can be had through the kind of habituation and proper education associated with virtue.

Hursthouse's essay constitutes a major contribution to the literature on practical virtue ethics in her groundbreaking discussion of what it takes to provide a *working* virtue ethical support of the green belief. In so doing she shows how the traditional virtues and vices work when reinterpreted in light of the green belief but also how the development of an entirely non-human centered virtue might work better if prop-erly formulated, inculcated, and developed in the deep and sustained ways required of virtue. In the end, Hursthouse indicates that, practically speaking, which approach we take is not that important; what is important is that we *put virtue to work* for the environment.

Rebecca L. Walker, 'The Good Life for Non-Human Animals: What Virtue Requires of Humans

At the start of her chapter, Walker directs us to the concern that a satisfying account of the ethically proper treatment of animals is not sufficiently available from either a rights-based or utilitarian perspective. To motivate this point, she uses the example of the seemingly contented zoo animal, about which the primary ethical worry seems to be not so much that the animal is suffering or even that its rights are violated, but that it is not flourishing in a way characteristic of its kind. Yet Walker does not aim in this paper to support the intuition that it is characteristic flourishing rather than rights or utility that we care about, but rather to develop a scaffold for a type of eudaimonistic virtue ethical view of how we ought to treat non-human animals. Such a scaffold, she thinks, is necessary to make a virtue ethical account of the ethics of how we ought to treat animals a serious contender to these other theoretical approaches.

On any eudaimonistic virtue ethics it is our own good that is in some sense the end of our actions. Leaving aside for the moment the worry that such an ethic is problematically agent centered, it might seem that a view like this is at least too focused on *human* good to account properly for how we ought to treat non-human animals. Walker intends her view to avoid any such problem by focusing not simply on how treating animals well is good for us as part of virtue, but also by incorporating a focus on the flourishing of the animals at issue into an account of why this is so. Her description of what it means for non-human animals to flourish in comparison to humans also serves as a step in her argument for why we should care about the flourishing of non-human animals.

Walker appeals to a roughly Aristotelian view of human flourishing in so far as this is 'mixed' in requiring both virtue (as excellence in characteristic functioning) and other external elements. Walker then widens the elements involved in human flourishing such that there is a broad scope of external goods and, unlike on Aristotle's view, characteristic functions, that are shared between humans and animals. Walker maintains that flourishing even on this inclusive account is the highest human end since she takes this to be a foundational claim of eudaimonism. Hence our highest end is not achievable by excellence in activity expressing reason (or virtue) alone and is shared in some parts (though not in the capacity for moral virtue per se) with other animals.

Walker does not think that her account of animal flourishing alone substantially justifies the position that care for animal flourishing is required by virtue. In order to show that is the case one must know something about why we ought to care about the flourishing of other humans and then see whether this same rationale applies to the case of animals. While theorists like Kant and Mill clearly thought the question why we should extend care to others was a significant question for ethics,[20] ancient eudaimonistic virtue ethicists were not so worried about this question as such. Rather they simply incorporated concern for others in one way or another in their theories as an obvious element of virtue.[21]

Yet in the modern context it is hard to take concern about others as simply a given. It is hard in particular since eudaimonistic virtue ethics is so often criticized for being precisely focused on the good of the agent him- or herself. Now clearly that good is only achievable through virtue which itself requires concern about and actions in accordance with the good of others. Yet the nagging question why this is so does not get answered so easily. To answer this question, Walker appeals to an argument closer in kind to those offered by Kant and Mill, yet, she hopes, avoids some of the problematic elements involved in their arguments. In part she aims to avoid these problems by offering a much less ambitious claim. She means to show only that if we manage to latch on properly to virtue, we will care about the good of others.

Walker's contribution to the present volume is closest in topic to Hursthouse's contribution, 'Environmental Virtue Ethics'. Clearly there are close connections

---

[20] See, e.g. Mill, *Utilitarianism*, ch. IV and Kant, *Groundwork*, 66 (AK 429).
[21] For an excellent discussion of how ancient virtue ethical views dealt with concern for others see Annas (1993), chs. 10–13.

between a focus on the environment and a focus on animals and both contributors are interested, for example, to give an account of virtue ethics that is not problematically human centered (though they accomplish this task in very different ways). On the other hand tensions arise between an environmental ethics and a focus on animals since concern for individual animals can be in tension with concern for animals as members of species or of ecosystems. While it seems both authors would agree that such tensions *may* arise in some cases, neither makes much of this potential conflict. It is in fact reasonable that a virtue ethical account hold that the good of an individual animal does not *characteristically* conflict with its good as a member of a particular species.

As with Hursthouse's chapter, Walker's chapter may be considered a contribution to the 'bioethics' literature when that term is broadly understood. An understanding of bioethics as incorporating the ethics of how we treat non-human animals as well as aspects of environmental ethics is much closer to the original meaning of the term as coined by Van Renneslaer Potter (1970) than is the narrow focus on medical ethics that is currently fashionable (Walker 2005). The contributions by Pellegrino, Radden, Baier, Blustein, Walker, and Hursthouse thus can be taken together to form this volume's substantial contribution to the field of bioethics. This is significant since virtue ethical approaches to bioethics topics are otherwise significantly under-represented.

Peter Koller, 'Law, Morality, and Virtue'

Koller argues for the importance of virtues in ethical *practice* and uses the specific examples of their relationship to morality and law in order to make his case. He begins by offering an account of virtue and morality, focusing on the role of the former in the latter, and then seeks to answer two related questions concerning virtue and the law. First, to what degree, if at all, may the law be used as a legitimate means for enforcing or fostering moral virtues? Secondly, to what extent does a well-functioning legal order depend upon the possession of moral virtues on the part of its citizens and officials?

Koller begins by drawing a distinction between intellectual and practical virtues and divides the latter into the two fairly distinct categories of non-moral and moral virtues. Non-moral virtues are 'instrumental to the pursuit of particular interests of certain individuals or collectives' while moral virtues concern 'conduct that seems desirable from a general and impartial point of view'. Throughout his essay, Koller insists that the virtues cannot provide a fundamental or complete account of morality. He maintains that we need an independent theory of morality in order to identify what traits of character count as virtues and to understand the content of what such conceptions might be. While some have argued that virtue ethics is indeed capable of meeting these specific challenges (Hursthouse 1997), Koller proceeds on this assumption and explores the question of what role virtues can play within and against the background of a more 'fundamental' theory of morality. He shares Kant's general point of view and sees virtues as important because of their ability to motivate agents to comply with and in special cases to exceed moral norms. Koller does not discuss their possible function in regard to moral epistemology, nor does he consider whether there may be moral value simply in possessing certain feelings, attitudes, or sensibilities. On these issues, his view is quite different from the position of some of our other contributors, for example, Blum, Noddings, and Slote, et al. Nevertheless, Koller argues that virtues do a great deal of *work* in supporting the rational moral standards that he believes they always must serve.

Despite certain significant functional differences, the law is connected to morality in that the former, at some level, requires moral justification. Nevertheless, the primary aim of the law is to establish and maintain a reasonable social order; its aim is to protect the basic common interests of all citizens. The law is not charged with enforcing moral standards that go beyond these core goods, for example, in regard to what Koller calls 'eccentric' moral ideals. Nor should the law be concerned with *enforcing* widely endorsed types of laudable behavior—for example, supererogatory actions—or supervising the inner thoughts, feelings, and beliefs of individuals. All such activities exceed the law's primary charge and tend to undermine its purpose. But, despite what these limitations on the legitimate scope of the law might seem to imply, Koller argues that the law still has an important and in fact essential role to play in the inculcation of virtue. The law can and must offer *indirect support* for rather than direct enforcement of the virtues. This should happen in two distinct ways.

First, a legal system must provide social conditions that make moral conduct clearly in the best interests of individual citizens. Koller claims that this is absolutely essential for the flourishing of virtue. Even though a proper legal system has no business enforcing the practice of the virtues, it provides 'a necessary precondition' for their cultivation and preservation. Secondly, a legal order may support and encourage the practice of moral virtues by providing appropriate *positive incentives*. Through proper education, appropriate social services, and special commendations and awards, the law can not only support but also should encourage the practice of moral virtues. By so doing, it remains true to its distinctive mission of seeking to benefit all of its citizens without requiring any of them to perform in particular ways or intruding directly into their thoughts, feelings, and aspirations.

Koller then turns his attention to the rational choice model that underlies much legal theory and practice. The basic idea in play here is that in designing the rules and institutions of law, one should not count on the virtuous nature of citizens but rather should plan with the worst case in mind. While approving of this general principle, Koller points out that it does not entail what he calls the 'strong position', namely, 'that a well-functioning legal order could emerge and persist even when all people concerned were mere egoists without any moral motivation'. Koller rejects this jaundiced reading of the principle underlying legal systems and offers five good reasons for believing that, in addition to sanctions and other disincentives, any legitimate legal system requires the support of reasonably virtuous citizens and officials. Without the support of such members, he contends, it is hard to see how the legal system could be regarded as legitimate or how it could function effectively.

Koller's essay begins with what many virtue ethicists would regard as a quite modest conception of the virtues and focuses on an area—the law—that many contemporary thinkers regard as cool if not hostile to discussions of virtue. One of the great strengths of his contribution is to demonstrate that even such a conception of the virtues at work in this area of our shared moral lives not only allows for but also depends upon a broad and robust role for the moral virtues.

Christine Swanton, 'Virtue Ethics, Role Ethics, and Business Ethics'

Swanton develops a novel and ingenious approach to role ethics with particular application to the case of business ethics. She approaches role ethics from her pluralistic theory of virtue ethics developed in *Virtue Ethics: A Pluralistic View* (2003). On her view, and as expressed in her contribution to this volume, a virtue is a disposition to respond to items in its field(s) in an excellent or good enough way, where the 'items' at issue may be such things as people or objects or even situations, inner states, or actions (2003: 1). Swanton's view is pluralistic in a variety of ways, but particularly salient for her contribution to this volume is her pluralism with respect to the standards for virtue and with respect to the modes of moral responsiveness.

First, the attainment of virtue is not judged only by the standards of the ideal human being as such, but also by what is excellent or good enough responsiveness within the various roles that we occupy. Hence, Swanton's view allows for both a threshold notion of virtue and a robust conception of role virtues. Secondly, Swanton endorses plural modes of responsiveness to the items in a virtue's field including promoting good, appreciating, loving, respecting, and creating—among others. Hence many of our role constituted goals and activities, which might not otherwise appear to be *moral* goals and activities, are counted as morally salient. A final feature of her view, though not a feature that by itself implies pluralism, is that virtues need not characteristically contribute to or be constitutive of *eudaimonia*. The proper responsiveness of a virtue may or may not hook up with the flourishing of the agent.

Swanton's approach to business ethics, and to role ethics generally, focuses on alleviating a core problem for role ethics. That problem may be illustrated by a dilemma. Either role ethical requirements conflict with general moral requirements or they do not. If they do conflict, then we are stuck with deep moral dilemmas in which actors are torn between their ethical duties in their identified roles (as soldiers, teachers, lawyers, physicians, mothers, etc.) and their ethical requirements as human beings. If they do not conflict, then there is no distinctive ethical arena for roles—all ethical responses are merely those of a good human being. In this case, either roles are so watered down that the distinctive institutional goals which they serve are construed merely in terms of the general human good, or any distinctive institutional goals and corresponding roles are considered to be outside the arena of morality.

Business ethics serves as an excellent example of this dilemma since common perceptions are that business goals as such are non-moral or that if one is a good businesswoman or- man, one risks becoming a bad human being. In this way, Swanton's focus on business ethics does for business what Koller's contribution does for the law by making room for a core dependency on virtue in an arena that otherwise may seem divorced from virtue and vice talk. Swanton solves the role problem generally by showing that role ethics and human ethics do not characteristically conflict (although she leaves open the possibility that there might be conflict in some cases). Despite this lack of conflict, Swanton carves out a robust arena for roles in the moral life. She does so by incorporating role virtues into the very fabric of her explanation of how virtues function and can be understood. On her view, role virtues are not an addition to an already complete account of how to be a good human being, but a necessary part of any such account.

As Swanton points out, virtue ethics is actually well poised to offer a solution to the role ethics problem since virtues are usually thought of as best understood contextually. Part of that context is that standards of goodness vary by social and institutional role. So, to use one of Swanton's examples, the virtue of friendship will look quite different depending on whether it is friendship between peers, between a student and teacher, or between a lawyer and client. While friendship in the first instance includes mutual affection, intimacy, and shared interests, 'friendship' as a role virtue of lawyers towards their clients is closer to loyalty. Swanton also points to contextual cultural factors (in the determination of politeness for example) and the narrative structure of a life (in the determination of generosity for example) that further contribute to the contouring of virtues in context.

The standard Aristotelian view of such differentiated roles is that they aim overall at a standard of the good human being as such. On Swanton's pluralistic view, roles are good in themselves with no hierarchy such that the human good per se is at the top. However, Swanton understands role virtues themselves as contoured prototype virtues, where prototype virtues are the characteristically human virtues. While it is role (and other) contextual contouring that gives much of the specificity of the virtue in terms of action guidance, prototype virtues already provide some more vague action guidance. They do this through their 'thick' manifestation in 'mother's knees' rules like 'be kind' or 'don't lie.' While these rules do not hold categorically, prototype virtues will nevertheless hold a person up short of meanness or dishonesty, which may seem (mistakenly) to be required in the context of being good in one's role. So, for example, the role of a salesperson may allow for some exaggeration of the benefits of her product or for a minimization of the shortcomings of the product, but it will not allow for any actual misrepresentation of the product that could lead to harm to the consumer.

Swanton's view of role ethics in general and business ethics in particular avoids an incorporation of prototype virtues into institutional goals in a way that undermines the distinctive function of a business (or other institution). On her account, for example, stakeholder theories of business ethics that appeal to a duty to consider equally the good of all affected by particular business practices are problematic. This is because such an appeal undermines the distinctive goals of any particular business (such as competitively creating profit). As she points out, however, a rejection of the stakeholder view thus characterized is consistent with the claim that business as a whole (i.e. as a general form of human activity) may be guided by appeals to the human good per se. At the other extreme, Swanton's view avoids the claim that institutional goals as such must be maximized by role virtues. On that view, for example, if the goal of a business is to make a profit, then individuals must aim at maximum profit for the business. Rather, Swanton points out, the aim of the role is to realize the institutional goals in an excellent or good enough way. This will not require a maximization of profit in those cases where such maximization is contrary to prototype human virtues such as honesty, justice, and kindness.

Swanton's focus on role ethics and business ethics through the lens of her virtue ethical pluralism greatly enhances the virtue ethics literature on this topic. Topically,

Swanton's chapter may be grouped with other contributions in this volume focusing specifically on some aspect of role ethics including those by Pellegrino, Blustein, Noddings, Baier, and Radden. Swanton's essay is unique in providing a general account of role ethics as such and in focusing on business ethics rather than the helping professions. A kind of side bonus of Swanton's chapter is that her view of role ethics responds to the common critique of virtue ethics that it does not give practical action guidance. In effect, Swanton agrees that prototypical virtues do not give the kind of detailed practical action guidance expected by those who look to ethics to solve the truly hard moral cases. On the other hand, prototype virtues do give enough guidance to avoid those actions that are inconsistent with being a good human being. Furthermore, role differentiated virtues provide robust action guidance in context. Thus Swanton shows that both prototype virtues and role virtues work, in different ways, to give practical moral guidance.

Lawrence Blum, 'Racial Virtues'

Blum explores the ethical dimensions of race. He argues that contemporary ethical theory ignores a range of rich and complex values associated with race and racial identity, and that it tends to restrict discussions of race to issues like discrimination and affirmative action. In this respect, Blum contends that 'moral philosophy has not kept pace with public concern', which is the site of lively and passionate debates about the broader ethical importance of race. Blum goes on to argue that virtue theory offers excellent theoretical resources for helping us to gain a more complete and nuanced understanding and appreciation of the range of values associated with race and racial identity because of its characteristic concern with the complex phenomena of moral psychology. Moreover, virtue theory has important things to say not only about what can go morally wrong or badly in regard to race but also about positive values associated with race that one can discover, appreciate, and work to realize, in one's own life as well as in the lives of those within one's community and beyond.

In pursuing his analysis, Blum criticizes and rejects as disabling two common approaches that he believes constrict our understanding of race and racial identity. The first is 'that we should endeavor to ignore people's race as much as possible'. The focus of this first concern is the idea that a color- or race-blind perspective is the most adequate way to address the value—and here the issue is the disvalue—of race. To the contrary, Blum insists that often *race matters* in positive and indispensable ways in the course of an ethical life. The second approach he criticizes and rejects is 'to focus only on "racism" as the general form of all disvalue in the racial domain'. While no reasonable person would deny or should ignore the various and profound harms caused by beliefs, attitudes, or behaviors of racial superiority, exclusion, or discrimination, Blum insists that there are a range of more subtle but deeply reprehensible beliefs, attitudes, and behaviors that fall outside the common conception of 'racism'. Failing to recognize these forms of moral failure leaves us with an incomplete and inadequate account of the moral features of race.

Blum builds much of his analysis around a critique and criticism of Jorge Garcia's valuable and influential work, which presents an analysis of racism as a kind of vice. He contends that Garcia's account suffers from three shortcomings. First, it does not offer an adequate psychological description of even its own account of racism. Secondly, it does not offer a comprehensive analysis of the various values and disvalues associated with race. Thirdly, it does not explore the distinctive and complex ways in which virtues and vices operate in the realm of race. Blum argues that a general form of this last point is a common weakness of many virtue theoretic accounts and that it points toward the discovery of new forms of virtues and vice. In this respect, like the contribution by Rosalind Hursthouse, Blum's essay adds to the ongoing evolution of virtue theory; at the same time, it provides an application of virtue theory to the particular challenges involved in the ethics of race.

Blum's essay offers a rich and revealing account of the ethical dimensions of race and racial identity. His analysis engages not only Garcia's seminal writings but also the larger context of philosophical work on the moral aspects of race. He shows how racism has as much to do with feelings, attitudes, and motives as it does with will and action, and how virtue ethics, which holds us responsible for managing and cultivating these aspects of ourselves as constitutive aspects of virtue and vice, offers an indispensable resource for philosophical study. His analysis not only deepens and extends our understanding and appreciation of this critical part of human life but also illustrates in a decisive and compelling way the particular and distinctive strengths of virtue ethics.

Nancy Sherman, 'Virtue and a Warrior's Anger'

Sherman plumbs the depths of anger, the 'runaway emotion' that often serves soldiers so well in combat but almost always badly when they return to civilian life. She begins by tracing the history of philosophical accounts of anger, noting the movement from Plato, who described anger as a distinctive property of warriors, which lives in the core of the spirited part of such men's souls, to Aristotle, who denied that courage, as a virtue, could be understood as an animal-like rage, but who nonetheless allowed for a kind of moral outrage that could propel a warrior in combat. Sherman points out the dramatic and distinctive change introduced by the Stoics and in particular Seneca, who renounced anger altogether, seeing it as an expression of defensiveness and vulnerability rather than strength.

Sherman begins by exploring what she calls 'the traditional view of warrior anger' that is found in the *Iliad*. She then moves on to examine Aristotle's account, according to which anger can play a normative role in both military and civic virtue, and the Stoic renunciation of anger as yet another irrational emotion that must be eliminated. Sherman argues against the Stoic view by examining a range of concrete, contemporary cases of what she calls 'rational warrior anger' and ends her essay with an account of various Stoic recommendations for treating anger.

Sherman provides a vivid and concise account of Achilles' famous rage as described in the *Iliad*. She notes that this is a case of 'warrior anger gone amok', but claims that implicit in Homer is the view that properly constrained anger and specifically revenge is a viable and important source of a warrior's motivation. She then turns to Aristotle who argues that emotions have specific cognitive contents, which are important constitutive elements of the emotion itself. On such an 'appraisal theory', emotions involve judgments or evaluations about the goodness or badness of some perceived or imagined action or state of affairs and often are accompanied by an 'action tendency' that guides and motivates a particular kind of response. Applying this idea to anger, Aristotle claims that it is constituted by a sense of a 'wrongful slight to self or those near to one' which is 'accompanied by pain' and which typically results in a 'desire for revenge'. Aristotle's account tends to focus on anger directed toward specific individuals, rather than groups or apparently objectless emotional states such as angst, and he rejects the idea that we ever properly feel anger against inanimate objects, such as a malfunctioning Xerox or soda machine. Such feelings are misplaced, for only people can wrong us and set in motion the psychological mechanisms that generate anger. Aristotle's powerful account offers rich resources that can be used to explain a wide range of intriguing psychological phenomena. For example, his theory provides a way to explain why my admission that I have wronged you, along with my apology and promise of restitution, have the power to mitigate your anger and restore a more civil, less emotionally charged relationship between us.

For the Stoics, anger is like a potent form of alcohol, something we all would do well to avoid. It is a disease that requires lifelong vigilance in order to cure. Even the even-tempered can fall off the wagon and overindulge this dangerous and unruly emotion. Many of the worst actions of human beings can be traced to anger. Seneca describes it as a 'departure from sanity' and according to the Stoics this is true of all emotions. But anger and our other emotions also are subtle and nefarious; rather than emotions being separate forces opposed to reason, Stoics defend the more radical view that emotions in fact are perverted but fully cognitive constructs: fundamentally mistaken or false judgments. Emotions are reason at war with itself. Given this potentially debilitating internal struggle, we must make great efforts to reform our selves. As with the first stages in an emotional nine-step program, we must recognize our problem and our need for a sustained and powerful therapy to cure us of this malignancy.

Stoics insist that our emotions not only are within our control but that they can only arise with our complicity and assent. Contrary to how our experience of emotions often feels, they do not come over us but arise out of our own appraisals and approvals. More importantly, emotions typically express attachments to 'indifferents'—things that lie beyond the genuine good of inner virtue. As a result, they tend to corrupt our ability to judge the value of different ends and pull us away from the true source of happiness. This is why freedom from emotions is the only way of preserving our rational ability to judge what is truly good and bad, which sets us upon the royal road to happiness. These insights lead the Stoic sage to live a life untouched by the emotions. Though he may feel tinges of emotion in highly charged circumstances, these will strike him more as echoes or shadows, than as sounds or shapes. In such moments, he quickly withholds his assent and therefore is never taken in by these false appearances of value.

This though seems to leave the Stoic sage without what many regard as important insights about the way the world is, at least the way it is for creatures like us, and vital resources for negotiating his way through it. As Sherman puts it, the genuine Stoic 'seems remote to our lives'. Emotions such as anger can misfire and even well-aimed anger can leave residues that are profoundly disruptive and even dangerous to both self and others, if not channeled and mitigated. Nevertheless, in many cases, anger seems like an appropriate and perhaps even necessary response. Sherman does not explicitly make this point, but it is strongly implied in her moving account of the My Lai massacre. Hugh Thompson, the recon helicopter pilot who stepped in at great risk to his own life and the life of his crew and stopped the atrocity at My Lai was *outraged* by what he had observed from the air. His anger came with a feeling familiar to many combat veterans—*not on my watch*—and this feeling guided and motivated his heroic actions. In such cases, anger seems indispensable and well worth its present dangers and lingering scars.

Sherman concludes her essay by comparing the Stoic solution of extirpating emotions with Harry Frankfurt's recommendation that we 'dissociate' or 'separate' some core of the self from those parts of us with which we choose not to 'identify'. She contrasts both of these views with Freud's approach to emotional conflict and specifically his worries about the fragmentation and disintegration of the self. As Sherman points out, the very therapies that Seneca and Frankfurt prescribe as cures, Freud diagnoses as a disease. While less clean and straightforward than either of these cures, perhaps the only way to respond to powerful, persistent, and potentially dangerous emotions such as anger is the crooked and convoluted path that seeks to tame and integrate these parts of the self into a unified and more harmonious whole.

Michael Slote, 'Famine, Affluence, and Virtue'

Slote offers a sentimentalist virtue ethics response to the central claims made by Peter Singer in his classic paper, 'Famine, Affluence, and Morality'. In particular, Slote replies to Singer's claim that our moral obligation to relieve human suffering in distant parts of the world is just as great as our obligation to save a child drowning in a shallow pool of water right in front of us.[22] Slote begins by sketching the general features of sentimentalist virtue ethics. The defining characteristic of this approach is to see fundamental moral value in motives such as benevolence, compassion, public-spiritedness, or gratitude. Two of its clearest and most widely recognized representatives in the West are Hutcheson and Hume, but Slote argues that contemporary defenders of 'caring' such as Carol Gilligan and Nel Noddings are best understood as members of this tradition as well. All of these thinkers evaluate actions in terms of how much of some valued inner *sentiment* is expressed, as opposed say to whether they are expressions of moral duty or maximize some non-moral consequence. The focus on sentiment distinguishes this type of virtue ethics from traditional forms of Aristotelianism, which link moral evaluation to a conception of human flourishing.

Slote sets an ambitious goal for himself and his theory. His ultimate aim is to defend a version of an ethics of caring that can explain and justify our attitudes and

---

[22] Singer's example of a child drowning in a shallow pool of water was preceded by two millennia by Mengzi's thought experiment describing how one would react to suddenly seeing a child on the verge of falling into a well. Mengzi's example is analyzed and discussed by Darwall (1998). Aside from historical interest, this is worth noting because Mengzi comes to a conclusion that is very similar to Slote's. Mengzi believes that care should be graded and that it must be augmented or 'extended' to all within the four seas.

actions toward not only those who are near and dear but toward distant others as well. Moreover, contrary to what Singer claims, Slote's theory will show that while the ideal caring individual will be 'substantially concerned' about distant others and non-human animals as well, they will not only be more concerned about those who are near and dear to them, but they will have good reasons for this hierarchy of concern. Slote argues that the key to providing such an account is to look back to earlier, eighteenth-century views about 'sympathy' or what today we would call 'empathy'.[23] The idea is that empathy can provide not only an explanation but also a justification for the kind of graded concern described above.

Slote draws upon recent work in psychology, which seems to show that the development of empathy is necessary in order to cultivate altruistic concern for others—a view referred to as the 'empathy-altruism hypothesis'. He describes how he was first drawn to the potential power of this idea when he realized that the very fact that most human beings find it much easier to empathize with born humans (even neonates) than with a developing fetus, might provide us with good reasons for thinking that it is 'morally worse to neglect or hurt a born human than to do the same to a fetus or embryo'. The crucial insight here is the idea that *empathy* 'has moral force or relevance'. Rather than looking to intuitions about where our obligations lie, we can look more directly to a conception of developed human caring shaped and informed by empathy. An empathy-based ethics of caring might well provide a way to respond to Singer's challenge by showing that we have more good reasons to save the life of a child right in front of us than to work to save the lives of children more distant and beyond our immediate perception.

Singer famously argues that physical proximity to suffering is not morally relevant in determining our obligations to offer aid to those in need. This leads him to conclude that we are under equal obligation to aid those in far-off lands as we are to save the drowning child who is right in front of us. Building out from this conclusion, Singer insists that 'most of us are morally obligated to make enormous sacrifices of our time, money, comfort, etc., in order to help distant (or nearby) others who are much worse off than we are'. Before showing how empathy might help us to understand such cases, Slote explores some of the best literature concerning our common intuitions about physical distance and moral obligations. He then goes on to argue that the psychological force of cases like Singer's drowning child engages normal human empathy in ways that more distant cases simply do not. If, as Slote suggests, morality is seen in terms of empathy-based caring, we can explain the widely held intuition that we are more obligated to rush to the aid of the child drowning before our eyes than to work for the relief of those whose suffering is only something about which we know. But this is not all his theory has to offer. Slote shows how empathy-based caring also can be used to explain our intuitions about cases where the distance that distinguishes

---

[23] Slote explains that 'by "sympathy" . . . we mean a kind of favorable attitude toward someone. One feels sympathy for someone in pain, for example, if one feels *for* them (or their pain), wishes they didn't have the pain, wants their pain to end. By "empathy", on the other hand, we mean a state or process in which someone takes on the feelings of another: one empathizes for another who is in pain, if one "feels their pain" (as opposed to feeling *for* their pain).'

instances of suffering is temporal. Consider an example discussed with great care by Charles Fried. Most people feel that we have a much more pressing moral obligation to save miners who right now are trapped and will die than we do to save perhaps unspecified miners who will likely suffer a similar fate in the future. This is why most feel compelled to use available resources to save those who are suffering such a fate right now than to invest the same resources in systems and equipment that might save even more miners in the future.

Slote goes on to show that his proposed theory may also have the resources to account for deontological prohibitions, which at first glance seem beyond the reach of the 'mere' sentiment of human concern for others. He argues that the right kind of sentimentalism can provide a direct and plausible explanation for our different intuitions concerning the relative moral wrong involved in killing versus letting die. The thought is that if we are directly responsible for killing someone, we are more strongly connected in terms of our causal role, than if we simply allow someone to die. This connection leads us to empathize more vividly and powerfully with the other. In this way, an empathy-based ethics of care can be used to explain our intuitions concerning the moral difference between doing versus allowing; it therefore seems capable of accounting for important moral judgments that most believe can only be defended on deontological grounds.

It is important to keep in mind that Slote does not claim that he has offered a complete defense of moral sentimentalism. He is careful to note that certain substantial problems remain for the approach that he advocates, for example, in the area of meta-ethics. His aim is to describe a new version of sentimentalist theory that 'allows us to make some important intuitive moral distinctions in a principled way' and which 'helps us to account for many facets of the moral life'. He argues that moral agents are more empathically concerned with what they directly perceive than with what they don't perceive, that they are more sensitive to what they know is happening at the same time as they engage in moral deliberations than what might happen in the future, and that they feel more responsible for actions in which they play a direct causal role. He has shown how these diverse examples of empathy-based care can be used to explain a range of deep and powerful intuitions about moral value and responsibility. In these respects, his virtue ethical sentimentalism *works* and works in ways that are confirmed by intuitions that in some cases are shared and defended by competing ethical theories as well.

There is much more that might be said in defense of the kind of sentimentalism that Slote proposes. In addition to offering us a systematic way to link a diverse range of moral intuitions, a life guided by developed empathy may play a critical role in helping us to become more reliable moral agents. It does not seem implausible to suggest that those who 'turn away' from people who are suffering before their eyes in order to help someone far away and unseen not only manifest an unsavory coldness but also are developing attitudes, perceptions, and habits of behavior that may harm both themselves and others more extensively and severely in the future. One must also consider the impression and effect upon those suffering, who watch as such agents turn away, and third parties—involved or not—who observe such actions. How would the trapped miners, their families, and their fellow miners feel when they are told that there is no more reason to help those dieing in the mine than to invest in precautions to alleviate future harm to others? Considering such concerns would make clear and help forge additional connections between Slote's view and traditional forms of virtue ethics, which are concerned with the development of character. Such concerns also point to an issue at the heart of the present volume regarding the practical value of virtue ethics.

Like all consequentialists, Singer is concerned with the practical effects of his view. His major and most representative work is entitled *Practical Ethics* (1993) and toward the end of 'Famine, Affluence, and Morality', he explicitly addresses the worry that his proposed theory is simply beyond the psychological resources of most human beings. Of course all moral theories ask us, or at least most of us, to change *something* about the way we currently behave. As Slote points out, his theory is demanding in this way; it insists that we all must work to cultivate a robust and stable level of empathetic concern for others. But Singer seeks to blunt a commonly encountered criticism of his view: that it demands an extraordinary and implausible level of sacrifice. He argues that he and his theory ask no more than did Thomas Aquinas, 'a writer not normally thought of as a way out radical'. Singer's example makes a strong point, but not the one that he intends. For Aquinas made an extraordinary commitment to live a life of chastity, poverty, and loving concern and called on others to act likewise, to devote themselves to emulating Christ. Like most religious figures, Aquinas' life and values illustrate what Joel Kupperman calls a 'super-moral' level of ethical commitment.[24] After all, within his home tradition he is considered a *saint*. If we take Singer's analogy seriously, he is asking us to join him in a religious form of life that takes as its ideal the life of a utilitarian saint.[25] In contrast, one of many attractive features of Slote's proposal is that it builds upon feelings, beliefs, and a style of reasoning about ethical issues that most people already share. It still insists that they develop their present ethical resources and inclinations and shape them in light of an explicit theory, but it works with a number of strong, standing intuitions as it works for a greater and more systematic understanding of ourselves and the lives we should lead. In this way, like many of the contributions in this volume, it shows virtue at work.

Philip J. Ivanhoe, 'Filial Piety as a Virtue'

In his exploration of traditional Chinese notions of filial piety, Ivanhoe makes significant contributions both to modern virtue ethics and to traditional Chinese notions of virtue. First, he seeks to show that there are valuable resources within the Chinese Confucian tradition that should be of interest to contemporary virtue ethicists. At the same time, he hopes to show the power of contemporary virtue ethical theory as a tool for understanding and appreciating a variety of features of traditional Chinese thought. By bringing the Chinese tradition and contemporary ethics into productive

---

[24] See 'The Supra-moral in Religious Ethics: The Case of Buddhism' in Kupperman (1999).
[25] Derek Parfit (1992) is one of the few advocates of utilitarianism who recognizes and defends its radical implications for a conception of the self. It is interesting that he notes the close similarities between his views on ethics and the self and those of another religious tradition, early Buddhism.

dialogue, he further seeks to sketch an account of filial piety as a virtue that will prove compelling to reflective modern individuals.

Since virtues are commonly thought of as dispositions or traits of character that help individuals and those around them to live well, Ivanhoe argues that filial piety ought to be of interest to anyone concerned with reflecting upon and working toward a good life. Nevertheless, certain aspects of traditional accounts of filial piety rely on discredited metaphysical beliefs or conceptual confusions and cannot contribute to a modern conception of filial piety as a virtue. Ivanhoe argues that many traditional views about what children owe their parents for begetting them do not offer an adequate basis for filial piety. Rather, the source of filial piety lies in the wide range of distinctive goods that parents provide for their children and the loving way in which they care for, support, and nurture them throughout the critical early periods of life. Reflective children realize that parents have willingly sacrificed many goods, time, and energy in order to provide for them and that they offered these benefits out of love for their children. Contemplating these facts, most children feel a natural response that combines feelings of gratitude with reverence and love for their parents. A distinctive strength of Ivanhoe's account is that such feelings are equally warranted on the part of adopted as biological children. While biological parents do provide special goods, the main ground of filial piety lies in the broad range of nurture, support, and loving concern that any proper parent seeks to provide.

In the concluding sections of his essay, Ivanhoe applies his account of filial piety to illuminate additional features of traditional Chinese ethical thought. For example, he shows how his analysis enables us to see clearly important similarities between traditional ideals regarding parents and those described for rulers and teachers. This in turn enables us to understand and appreciate why many Chinese have and continue to feel that those who rule and those who teach also can be appropriate objects of filial piety.

Ivanhoe argues that his modern account of filial piety would reject some distinctive features of the traditional Chinese conception of filial piety. For example, according to Chinese tradition, filial obligation represents an overriding or trumping moral imperative for children, calling upon them to ignore clear cases of injustice and to subordinate absolutely their own well-being in serving their parents. Such ideals lack not only appeal but justification, once the traditional metaphysical foundations mentioned above have been left behind. Nevertheless, Ivanhoe argues that one can still find good reasons to stand by one's parents even in the face of severe wrongdoing on their part, and such fidelity remains an important feature of his conception of filial piety as a virtue.

Ivanhoe's contribution puts virtue theory to work and shows how it works not only to understand but also to fashion and defend an ethical point of view. His essay illustrates the value of cross-cultural study of the virtues as part of a much-needed though still widely ignored or resisted effort to broaden our understanding and appreciation of ethics. At the same time, his essay demonstrates how powerful and revealing modern virtue ethical theory can be in the study of other systems of ethics. Beyond helping us to understand and appreciate Chinese conceptions of filial piety, virtue ethical theory provides a way to engage in a critical and constructive assessment of such traditional views, enriching both our own understanding and perhaps that of other traditions as well.

CONCLUSION

The opening sections of this Introduction describe the general state of the field for virtue ethics—both advocates and critics, their views and their debates. It also ties together a range of contemporary philosophical concerns that often are not recognized as parts of the larger revival of virtue ethics. As we have seen, the contemporary re-emergence of virtue ethics is very much a work in progress. Many questions remain and many debates are emerging as this new theoretical area unfolds, gains ground, and is modified and refined. This is an exciting and challenging period in the history of a venerable theory. Virtue ethics, once counted out, is now widely considered by the philosophical community to be the main contender among the available approaches to normative moral theory. The sophistication and richness of what is now a substantial body of literature on this topic proves that this is where it belongs and likely will remain.

Our presentation of the individual contributions offers a general sense of the contents of these essays, how they relate to one another, and our own thoughts on how they can be located in the bigger picture of virtue ethics as practical ethics. We also have endeavored to show how these essays relate to some of the broader themes discussed in the opening sections of the Introduction. In our descriptions of the individual essays, we have bucked convention somewhat by offering substantially longer discussions than one might usually find in an introduction to a collection of essays. Beyond our sheer enthusiasm for the contributions, our choice was made in part because the essays relate to one another in a variety of ways. So much so that no single set of topical divisions for the volume is adequate. Hence our descriptions of the various essays include discussions of how they relate to one another where appropriate, but more importantly are substantial enough for the reader to be able to tell in advance of reading all the particular essays how they might best be grouped for the reader's own purposes.

As is the case with the opening sections of the Introduction, in the course of our presentation of the various contributions, we have included our own impressions and thoughts regarding these contributions in the hope that these may add in some small way to the arguments and ideas these authors have described. We are confident that readers will find much more to think about and much more to say in response to the essays we have collected. If this expectation proves true, it will testify to the value of this volume and offer further examples of virtue at work.

REFERENCES

Annas, Julia. 1993. *The Morality of Happiness.* New York: Oxford University Press.
Anscombe, G. E. M. 1958. 'Modern Moral Philosophy.' *Philosophy* 33.
Baier, Annette. 1989. 'Doing Without Moral Theory?' in Stanley Clarke and Evan Simpson. Eds. *Anti-Theory in Ethics and Moral Conservatism.* New York: SUNY Press. 29–48.
Beauchamp, Tom L. and James F. Childress. 2001. *Principles of Biomedical Ethics*, Fifth Edition. Oxford: Oxford University Press.

Dancy, Jonathan. 1993. *Moral Reasons*. Cambridge, MA: Blackwell.

Darwall, Stephen. 1998. 'Empathy, Sympathy, Care.' *Philosophical Studies*, 89: 261–82.

Delattre, Edwin. 2002. *Character and Cops: Ethics in Policing*. American Enterprise Institute Press.

Doris, John M. 2002. *Lack of Character: Personality and Moral Behavior*. Cambridge: Cambridge University Press.

Driver, Julia. 1998. 'The Virtues and Human Nature' in Roger Crisp. Ed. *How Should One Live? Essays on the Virtues*. Oxford: Clarendon Press.

Harman, Gilbert. 1998–9. 'Moral Philosophy Meets Social Psychology: Virtue Ethics and the Fundamental Attribution Error.' *Proceedings of the Aristotelian Society*, 99.

_____ 1999–2000. 'The Nonexistence of Character Traits.' *Proceedings of the Aristotelian Society*, 100.

_____ 2001. 'Virtue Ethics without Character Traits' in Alex Byrne, Robert Stalnaker, and Ralph Wedgewood. Eds. *Fact and Value: Essays on Ethics and Metaphysics for Judith Jarvis Thomson*. Cambridge, MA: MIT Press.

_____ 2003. 'No Character or Personality.' *Business Ethics Quarterly*, 13.

Harman, Gilbert and J. J. Thomson. 1996. *Moral Relativism and Moral Objectivity*. Oxford: Blackwell.

Herman, Barbara. 1996. 'Making Room for Character' in Stephen Engstrom and Jennifer Whiting. Eds. *Aristotle, Kant and the Stoics: Rethinking Happiness and Duty*. Cambridge: Cambridge University Press.

Hursthouse, Rosalind. 1997. 'Virtue Ethics and Abortion' in Roger Crisp and Michael Slote. Eds. *Virtue Ethics*. Oxford: Oxford University Press.

_____ 1998. 'Normative Virtue Ethics' in Roger Crisp. Ed. *How Should One Live? Essays on the Virtues*. Oxford: Clarendon Press.

_____ 1999. *On Virtue Ethics*. Oxford: Oxford University Press.

Hutton, Eric L. 2001. *Virtue and Reason in Xunzi*. Ph.D. Dissertation. Stanford University.

_____ 2002a. 'Moral Connoisseurship in Mengzi' in Liu Xiusheng and Philip J. Ivanhoe. Eds. *Essays on the Moral Philosophy of Mengzi*. Indianapolis, IN: Hackett.

_____ 2002b. 'Moral Reasoning in Aristotle and Xunzi.' *Journal of Chinese Philosophy*, 29: 3.

Ivanhoe, Philip J. 2000. *Confucian Moral Self Cultivation*. Revised Second Edition. Indianapolis, IN: Hackett.

_____ 2002. *Ethics in the Confucian Tradition: The Thought of Mengzi and Wang Yangming*. Revised Second Edition. Indianapolis, IN: Hackett.

Jacobs, Don Trent. 2001. *Teaching Virtues: Building Character Across the Curriculum*. Lanham, MD: Scarecrow Education.

Kamtekar, Rachana. 2004. 'Situationism and Virtue Ethics on the Content of Our Character.' *Ethics*, 114.3.

Kant, Immanuel. 1964. *Groundwork of the Metaphysics of Morals*. H.J. Paton. Trans. New York: Harper and Row.

Kline, T. C. III. 1998. *Ethics and Tradition in the Xunzi*. Ph.D. Dissertation. Stanford University.

_____ 2000. 'Moral Agency and Motivation in the *Xunzi*' in T. C. Kline, III and Philip J. Ivanhoe. Eds. *Virtue, Nature, and Moral Agency in the Xunzi*. Indianapolis, IN: Hackett.

Kohn, Linda T., Janet M. Corrigan, and Molla S. Donaldson. Eds. 2000. *To Err is Human: Building a Safer Health System*. Committee on Quality of Health Care in America, Institute of Medicine. National Academy Press: Washington, DC.

Korsgaard, Christine. 1996. 'From Duty and for the Sake of the Noble: Kant and Aristotle on Morally Good Action' in Stephen Engstrom and Jennifer Whiting. Eds. *Aristotle, Kant and the Stoics: Rethinking Happiness and Duty*. Cambridge: Cambridge University Press.

Kupperman, Joel J. 1999. *Learning from Asian Philosophy*. New York: Oxford University Press.

—— 2001. 'The Indispensability of Character.' *Philosophy*, 76.

Lickona, Thomas. 2004. *Character Matters: How to Help Our Children Develop Good Judgment, Integrity, and Other Essential Virtues*. New York: Simon and Schuster.

Louden, Larry. 1997. 'On Some Vices of Virtue Ethics' in Roger Crisp and Michael Slote. Eds. *Virtue Ethics*. Oxford: Oxford University Press.

McDowell, John. 1998. *Mind, Value, and Reality*. Cambridge, MA: Harvard University Press.

MacIntyre, Alasdair. 1981. *After Virtue*. Notre Dame, IN: University of Notre Dame Press.

Mill, J. S. 1998. *Utilitarianism*. Roger Crisp. Ed. New York: Oxford University Press.

Nivison, David S. 1996. *The Ways of Confucianism: Investigations in Chinese Philosophy*. Bryan W. Van Norden. Ed. LaSalle, IL: Open Court Press.

Noddings, Nel. 1992. *The Challenge to Care in Schools: An Alternative Approach to Education*. New York: Teacher's College Press.

—— 2003. *Caring: A Feminine Approach to Ethics and Moral Education*. Second Edition. Berkeley University of California Press.

Nussbaum, Martha. 1993. 'Non-Relative Virtues: An Aristotelian Approach' in Amartya Sen and Martha Nussbaum. Eds. *Quality of Life*. Oxford: Oxford University Press.

Oakley, Justin and Dean Cocking. Eds. 2001. *Virtue Ethics and Professional Roles*. Cambridge: Cambridge University Press.

O'Neill, Onora. 1993. 'Duties and Virtures'. *Philosophy*, 35, Supplement.

Parfit, Derek. 1992. *Reasons and Persons*. Reprint. Oxford: Oxford University Press.

Potter, Van Rensselaer. 1970. 'Bioethics: The Science of Survival'. *Perspectives in Biology and Medicine*, 14.

Railton, Peter. 1988. 'How Thinking about Character and Utilitarianism Might Lead to Rethinking the Character of Utilitarianism' in Peter A. French, Theodore E. Uehling Jr., and Howard K. Wettstein. Eds. *Midwest Studies in Philosophy Volume XIII Ethical Theory: Character and Virtue*. Notre Dame, IN: University of Notre Dame Press.

—— 1998. 'Aesthetic Value, Moral Value, and the Ambitions of Naturalism' in Jerrold Levinson. Ed. *Aesthetics and Ethics*. New York: Cambridge University Press.

Ross, Lee and Richard E. Nisbett. 1991. *The Person and the Situation: Perspectives of Social Psychology*. New York: McGraw-Hill.

Ryan, Kevin and Karen E. Bohlin. 2003. Reprint. *Building Character in Schools: Practical Ways to Bring Moral Instruction to Life*. San Francisco, CA: Jossey-Bass.

Sandler, Ronald and Philip Cafaro. Eds. 2005. *Environmental Virtue Ethics*. Rowman and Littlefield.

Schneewind, J. B. 1997. 'The Misfortunes of Virtue' in Roger Crisp and Michael Slote. Eds. *Virtue Ethics*. Oxford: Oxford University Press.

Shun, Kwong-loi. 2001. 'Self and Self-Cultivation in Early Confucian Thought' in Bo Mou. Ed. *Two Roads to Wisdom? Chinese and Analytic Philosophical Traditions*. LaSalle, IL: Open Court Press.

Singer, Peter. 1993. *Practical Ethics*. Cambridge: Cambridge University Press.

Solomon, David. 1988. 'Internal Objections to Virtue Ethics' in Peter A. French, Theodore E. Uehling Jr., and Howard K. Wettstein. Eds. *Midwest Studies in Philosophy Volume XIII Ethical Theory: Character and Virtue*, Notre Dame, IN: University of Notre Dame Press.

Swanton, Christine. 2003. *Virtue Ethics: A Pluralistic View*. Oxford: Oxford University Press.

Trianosky, Gary. 1990. 'What is Virtue Ethics All About?' *American Philosophical Quarterly*, 27.

Van Norden, Bryan W. 1997. 'Mencius on Courage' in Peter A. French, Theodore E. Uehling Jr., and Howard K. Wettstein. Eds. *Midwest Studies in Philosophy Volume XXI The Philosophy of Religion*. Notre Dame, IN: University of Notre Dame Press.

_____ 2003. 'Virtue Ethics and Confucianism' in Bo Mou. Ed. *Comparative Approaches to Chinese Philosophy*. London: Ashgate.

Walker, Rebecca. 2005. 'Bioethics' in Donald M. Borchert. Ed. *Encyclopedia of Philosophy*, Second Edition. Macmillan Reference USA.

Wallace, R. Jay. 1991. 'Virtue, Reason, and Principle.' *Canadian Journal of Philosophy*, 21:4.

Watson, Gary. 1990. 'On the Primacy of Character' in Owen J. Flanagan and Amélie Rorty. Eds. *Identity, Character, and Morality: Essays in Moral Psychology*. Cambridge, MA: MIT Press.

Wong, David. 1998. 'On Flourishing and Finding One's Identity in Community' in Peter A. French, Theodore E. Uehling Jr., and Howard K. Wettstein. Eds. *Midwest Studies in Philosophy Volume XIII Ethical Theory: Character and Virtue*. Notre Dame, IN: University of Notre Dame Press.

Yearley, Lee H. 1990. *Mencius and Aquinas: Theories of Virtue and Conceptions of Courage*. Albany, NY: SUNY Press.

2

Caring as Relation and Virtue in Teaching

Nel Noddings

Caring may refer to a desirable attribute of relations or to a virtue possessed by a moral agent. As a virtue, it seems to be more difficult to describe than other virtues. Under what conditions should we credit a person with the virtue of caring? Surely, it is not sufficient for a person to claim—however sincerely—that she or he cares. We have to know something about what he or she does and with what effect. Indeed, when people say, 'Caring is not enough,' it is usually because they construe caring as an attitude or expression of concern, and they quite rightly regard this as insufficient.

I have argued, and will argue here, that a relational definition of *caring* underlies the virtue sense and gives it reliable meaning (Noddings 2002b). Moreover, the relational view may complement the virtue view and make it more powerful in describing human interaction and pointing the way to a satisfying moral life. If I can give a persuasive argument for these claims, it should be clear that care theory is not exactly a type of virtue ethics, although it displays many similar features. However, the two theories are not incompatible and may be considered complementary. The relational sense is of considerable importance for the analysis of caring in the so-called caring professions and in parenting and helps to avoid some of the difficulties traditionally found in virtue ethics.

I'll start my argument with an analysis of the relational sense and then turn to an examination of the virtue sense. The stage will then be set for an exploration of teaching as a relational practice.

THE RELATIONAL SENSE OF CARING

Consider an encounter or set of encounters in which the first party is called the carer (or one-caring) and the second the cared-for. Such encounters may be represented as a mathematical relation: $\{(A_1, B_1), (A_2, B_2) \ldots (A_n, B_n)\}$ in which A (the carer) and B (the cared-for) appear in successive transformations, each at least minimally affected by the encounters. In the simplest case, that of the single caring encounter, there is but one entry in the relation. In practical terms, this is a case in which carer and cared-for meet just once and briefly.

To justify the label 'caring' for the relation, both A and B must contribute something. If we study our consciousness in a wide variety of situations in which we find ourselves caring (taking the place of A), we can see that two features stand out:

1) A is attentive to B in a non-selective way; that is, A puts aside (temporarily) her own projects and, as nearly as possible, her own evaluative structures and listens to B. Through language or bodily signs, B expresses a need, and A's attention (an almost passive receptivity) is directed at receiving what-is-there in B.

2) A experiences motivational displacement. Her motive energy begins to flow toward B's needs. Many things can block this flow. A may disapprove of the need B has expressed; B's need may be too great for A to handle; A may not yet fully understand what is being expressed. However, so long as A is attentive, the flow of energy is toward some form of positive response to B.

Then, of course, A must act, must respond in some way to B. The desire to meet B's need is primary in shaping A's response, but a host of factors influence what is actually done, among them A's approval or disapproval of the need expressed by B, A's competence in meeting such needs, and the resources available. Not only does A try to meet B's need (or one revised in a direction morally acceptable to A), but also A is committed to maintaining or improving the caring relation itself. This second commitment is crucial because, while the first describes the act as motivated by A's immediate desire to respond in a way that is good for B, the second refers to A's concern for a particular outcome—maintenance or enhancement of the caring relation.

Anthropologists and psychologists are agreed that the desire to be cared for (to receive some form of positive response—ranging from actual help, to respect, to refraining from the infliction of harm) is universal. It makes sense, given this universal feature of human life, to make caring—the establishment of relations in which carers respond to cared-fors—a basic good of moral life. This sounds very like the start one would make in agent-based virtue ethics (Slote 2001: 9). But we cannot simply take *caring* as an intuited and unanalyzed good. We have to describe it, and our description will make clear that both motive and outcome are important. Without this description, as we'll see, we could be forced to accept instances of claims to care that should be rejected.

Let's continue our description of the caring relation. To complete the relation, B must also make a contribution. As cared-for, B must signal in some way that the caring is received and recognized as caring. B's contribution, so apparently effortless, is significant in all caring relations but especially in unequal relations such as parent–child, physician–patient, and teacher–student. In mature, equal relations, we expect A and B to exchange places regularly. A is at one time carer, at another cared-for. But in inherently unequal relations, A (our original carer) bears the major responsibility for caring.

What I have outlined is a sketchy phenomenology of caring. (For a fuller description, see Noddings 2002b.) Is there an alternative description? Suppose we start again with the encounter between A and B. In this version, A does not listen to B or only half-listens; that is, she hears B's words or recognizes bodily signs, but she reads these through a preselected cognitive scheme. She assesses or evaluates or diagnoses B's condition and infers a need, and she then acts to satisfy the inferred need—one which may be entirely different from the one expressed by B. In all that follows, I'll refer to this form of caring as Case 2 caring.

We may suppose that A in Case 2 is motivated by concern for B. Should we not credit A with caring? There may be no objection to crediting A with wanting to care or trying to care, but if the cared-for responds with, 'You just don't care!' we have to admit that there may be incoherence in our position. Should A be credited with caring or not?

First—and I'll say more about this in a moment—care theory is not greatly concerned with moral credit. It is concerned with the enhancement of human life (especially moral life), and that is why it recognizes the contribution of the cared-for. The infant who responds to its parent with smiles, coos, and wriggles makes a demonstrable contribution to the caring relation, but we would not say that, by doing so, he or she should receive the sort of credit usually due to a moral agent. The same can be said for the patient's contribution to the physician–patient relation and the student to the teacher–student relation. Thus, there is a need to recognize a substantial contribution to caring that cannot itself be described as a virtue. David Hume (1983) is one of the few modern Western philosophers who recognized the contributions of pleasing personal characteristics to moral life.

Secondly, without an emphasis on the caring relation, there is no reason why we should not credit A (Case 2) with caring. She exhibits the sort of motive that might well be recognized in virtue ethics. But it is often the case that caring of this sort miscarries. It may not be received by B as caring. Indeed, parenting, doctoring, and teaching are replete with cases of this kind. A struggles to do what she thinks is right, expends much energy, and agonizes over the poor results, but B stubbornly retorts, 'You just don't care!' Sometimes, almost accidentally, A infers the need that B was trying to express, and then the relation is completed, but often we are faced with a situation in which A claims to care (or tries to care) and B, frustrated by a perceived lack of understanding on the part of A, rejects the claim. Without B's recognition, there is no caring relation.

In what does this recognition consist? Certainly it does not require an expression of gratitude. In teacher–student and parent–child relations, recognition of caring often takes the form of happy and confident pursuit by the cared-for of his or her own projects. Such indirect recognition may be enhanced by occasional smiles, shared comments, appreciative gestures, or eye contact that conveys understanding. But is the response of the cared-for *necessary* to the caring relation and, if so, must there be a caring relation in order to acknowledge the virtue of one who is trying to care?

It seems clear that the response of the cared-for is necessary to the caring relation. It would be odd indeed to say that A and B are in a caring relation but B shows no sign of recognizing it. B's response is, in fact, so important that its lack often leads to burnout in the caring professions. In talking with nurses who work regularly with comatose or severely senile patients, I have asked how they keep going without a supportive response from those for whom they provide care. Many have told me that they can detect responses that untrained people would miss; a form of response *is* there. Others have said that they need periodic rotation or transfer to work with patients who can respond. It is just too hard to serve as caregiver for long periods of time to patients who cannot respond. Thus, there is empirical evidence to support the claim that a response from the cared-for is vital to the caring relation.

A theoretical question remains: is the nurse 'caring' when there is no caring relation? It would take a cold and stubborn heart to say 'no' to this. A reasonable answer to the question reveals the strong complementarity of care theory and virtue ethics. To be recognized as a caring person, one must regularly exhibit some success in establishing caring relations. One does not become an uncaring person because one is in a situation where no response and, therefore, no relation is possible. This seems right, but we may still be uneasy. If a caregiver works only with unresponsive patients, does care theory suggest that she cannot establish the track record required to claim that she possesses the virtue of caring?

Here it helps to look at the acts performed by the caregiver. Are they to be labeled caring? If we prefer to assess acts (rather than persons) as virtuous, then we would have to say that, in the absence of relation, the caregiver's acts are properly called caring so long as (1) the carer remains receptive and continues to look for response; (2) no detectable denial of caring emerges from the cared-for; and (3) experience suggests that, if the cared-for were able to respond, the response would be positive. All of these conditions are necessary. Condition (1) is basic to the relational view of caring. If we were to depend only on (1) and (3), we might easily fall into Case 2 caring—a condition in which we feel justified in continuing our efforts at care because other patients (students, children, clients) have responded favorably and we must simply wait for this one to do so also. Thus, (2) is necessary. Similarly (3) is necessary. Without it, in the absence of a negative response (which by definition in these cases is likely to be missing), caregivers might treat unresponsive patients roughly. Caring nurses, however, handle comatose patients as gently as they would responsive patients, knowing that, if they could respond, they would regard this gentleness appreciatively.

Our description of the caring relation has a facilitative circularity. It cannot be described without attending to the consciousness of the carer, but the carer's virtue cannot be assessed without looking at the relation. From the perspective of virtue ethics, our second A may well deserve credit for caring. Care theory does not object to the credit (that is not really the point), but it advises us to analyze the situation more deeply. Is A helping to establish and maintain a caring relation, merely enhancing her own sense of goodness, or acting genuinely (but mistakenly) out of concern for the cared-for?

A fourth possibility—the most troubling of all for care theory—is that A's response really is in the best interest of B, but B does not recognize it as caring. In this case, an objective observer wants to credit A with caring but, at the same time, must admit that the relation is not (yet) one of caring, and future interactions are in jeopardy.

Often we can't tell whether we are dealing with an example of the third case (a mistake made from genuine concern) or the fourth (a move resisted by the cared-for that will prove right in the long run). I will address this case further in the discussion of teaching and learning. There are genuine dilemmas in the practical application of care theory to teaching, and they appear in every facet of teaching.

Such ambiguous cases occur frequently in personal and professional life. Parents alienate their children by insisting on projects and associations that the children hate and resist. Teachers press academic subjects on students whose passionate interests lie elsewhere. Even physicians force unwanted treatment on their patients. For example, physicians treating mental illness sometimes insist that patients continue to take certain medications even though the patients complain of disturbing side-effects, and alternatives are available (Scheff 1999). This is a classic example of the carer 'knowing best' and acting in what he or she takes to be the best interest of the patient. But it may be that the patient needs, among other things, to be considered a person whose expressed needs are heard and respected. The same is true, of course, for children in the parent–child relationship and for students in the teacher–student relationship.

There seems to be good reason, then, for preferring the phenomenological account of caring that begins with attention and motivational displacement. Starting with that description does not suggest that carers give up their values and judgments, but they do not begin with those values and judgments or allow them to obscure the message sent by the cared-for. They allow the expressed needs of the cared-for to stimulate their feeling and thinking, and they revise their responses in light of the effects their acts have on the cared-for and relation.

Caring as I have described it so far may be called *natural* caring. The word natural here means only that the characteristic attention and motivational displacement occur without recourse to principles or any special effort of will. They occur *naturally*—out of inclination or love. Obviously, this does not always happen. Sometimes attention and motivational displacement are blocked or actively resisted. The cared-for may be demanding, obnoxious, or morally wrong. A carer may be tired or lacking resources. She or he may feel that someone else should respond to B's need. When these things happen, if we value ourselves as carers, we have to draw on what I've called the ethical self—the image of ourselves at our caring best. We refer to our memories of caring and being cared for, and we then respond as carers, but our care in such cases is *ethical* caring, not natural caring. The process is very like that on which virtue ethicists depend when they describe the moral agent's reliance on character instead of abstract principles. In ethical caring, we summon our capacity to care as we would any other well established virtue.

Kant was unwilling to give moral credit for good or right acts done out of love or inclination. He insisted that, to count as moral, an act has to be done for the right reason; that is, the appropriate principle must be applied. There is a sense in which this is right. Natural caring and the contributions of the cared-for require no *ethical* effort (although those of the carer may require great physical or mental effort). Neither carer nor cared-for has to ask, Is this the morally right thing to do? What justifies my decision?

But from the perspective of care theory, natural caring is the preferred state, and ethical caring is exercised only when natural caring fails. Besides accomplishing what might have been done (under other circumstances) by natural caring, its primary purpose is to restore the conditions characteristic of natural caring. In natural caring, we respond directly to the address of the cared-for. Our response is not mediated by a principle that justifies our act. Indeed, if such mediation were sought, we might say with Bernard Williams that the carer had 'one thought too many' (1981: 17).

There is an obvious risk in ethical caring, and its recognition underscores the claim that—at least in face-to-face encounters—natural caring is the state most of us prefer. If A has to summon an image of herself as caring in order to respond as carer to B, B may detect this effort and say, in effect, 'You don't really care about me. You're just trying to look good . . .' A reaction of this sort may remind A that she really does care and help her to renew her efforts at maintaining the caring relation, or it may so alienate her that the dependence on ethical caring is increased, and the relationship becomes even more difficult. In the happiest cases, ethical caring functions to restore relations of natural caring.

In natural caring or successful ethical caring, relations are strengthened. Therefore, in most cases, when I care for another, I care also for myself. Carer, cared-for, and relation are all sustained. This mutual benefit is an important point for the caring professions, because it may help to avoid burnout. In the discussion of teaching, I will claim that teachers should choose methods that contribute to their own happiness and growth. As carers, they will, of course, be concerned with the growth and happiness of their students but, because so much depends on the health of teacher–student relations, teachers should reflect continually on the effects of their choices on themselves as well as their students and their relations.

Here we see a forward-looking or consequences-oriented concern in care theory. While natural or ethical caring may characterize the attitude and conduct of carers in direct contact with recipients of caring, a broader interest arises. Attempts to care may be blocked through no fault of either carer or cared-for by the conditions in which they find themselves. To support caring relations, carers must work toward the establishment of conditions under which caring relations can flourish. This task is closely related to the 'balanced' caring that Michael Slote (2001) has described. A cares (as I have described caring) in direct contacts, but he or she is also concerned with the well-being of those beyond the immediate circle of care. It would take us too far afield to discuss *caring about* people at a distance in time or place (but see Noddings 2002b). However, one way of acting on this concern is to work on the conditions underlying care. Caring about those beyond the immediate circle need not detract from the more personal demands for direct, person-to-person care. Indeed, such care is part of the teaching function; it shows students that caring reaches out and that care must be shared.

This work—establishing the conditions under which caring relations can flourish—is especially important for parents and teachers. Speaking of his early school years, George Orwell said, 'This was the great, abiding lesson of my boyhood: that I was in a world where it was *not possible* for me to be good . . . Life was more terrible, and I was more wicked, than I had imagined' (1981: 5). A significant moral task for every competent agent (one derived from the primacy of caring relations) is to work toward the establishment of conditions under which it is both desirable and possible to be good. In this short chapter, it is not possible to describe fully what is meant by 'good'. I mean, in the briefest terms, to act generously—without causing harm—in ways that make it possible for both the moral agent and others to attain or acquire the recognized goods of one's society.

THE VIRTUE SENSE OF CARING

The virtue use of *caring* is familiar to everyone. We say, 'He is a caring father,' 'She is a caring teacher,' 'Nurses are more caring than doctors,' and the like. When we talk this way, we usually mean that the person credited with caring exhibits an attitude of warmth, solicitude, or conscientious attention. Underlying our evaluation is the observation that the carer is one who regularly and dependably establishes or maintains caring relations. One who merely worries a lot, wrings her hands, and wrinkles her brow in sympathy does not usually earn our praise. Rather, her behavior raises doubts.

Caring, described as a virtue, is not a simple virtue. Based on the relation, it invites the question what constitutes caring, and that is answered initially by attention, motivational displacement, and response. But *attention* suggests an ability to listen, empathize or sympathize, and be moved by the plight or mood of the other. Further, a carer must do something in response, and this necessity suggests an array of other virtues: competence in the arena of need, flexibility (needs differ), cultivation of the pleasing personal qualities that make one's response acceptable, patience (one's first response may not hit the mark), open-mindedness (the needs expressed may differ from one's own), and a capacity for reflection (is my response directed to the expressed need or to a need inferred from personal or professional experience?).

We should say a bit more here on competence as a virtue related to caring. Must a carer possess 'competence in the arena of need'? Competence figures significantly in professional life, and it will be discussed more fully in the sections on teaching. But must one be competent if he or she is to be credited with caring? To insist on this invites a multitude of counter-examples and a challenge to the basic phenomenology of caring already laid out. Many parents, for example, love their children and want the best for them but lack competence as parents; they simply do not know how best to raise children in their present cultural surroundings. Immigrants, minority groups, and people who are deeply impoverished often exhibit parenting styles that may not be effective in a liberal democratic setting. But surely, we would not accuse these parents of 'not caring'. Often children of such parents acknowledge the care they have received, and caring relations have thus clearly been established. It would be better, then, to say that *striving* for competence in the area of need is the virtue characteristic of carers.

When caring as a virtue is based on the caring relation, it is complex and connotes more than an attitude. As we have seen, it involves both motives and consequences, the latter described in terms of the responses of the cared-for and the effects on the relation. It contrasts sharply with some everyday uses of the word, and it challenges attempts to operationalize it for scientific study. *Caring*, as it is used in care theory, is not simply a soft manner, and it certainly should not be identified with permissiveness in parenting or teaching. In medicine, caring implies a considerate bedside manner, but it is not synonymous with that manner.

In the past few years, researchers have created instruments to measure caring. This is a mistake unless the researcher is meticulous in probing deeply into the manifestations of each indicator on the instrument. One study, trying to identify 'caring fathers', listed such indicators as 'coaches child's Little League team'. A father who coaches his child's team may indeed be a caring father. But he may not be. An adequate evaluation asks *how* he performs as a coach. Does he form caring relations with the players? Does he help them to enter caring relations with each other or invite nasty competition? Does he establish the conditions under which caring relations are likely to be sustained or encourage unhealthy rivalry? We can study caring, but we cannot do it with a mere checklist. Virtue ethicists and care theorists agree on this and both face the task of describing caring fully enough to avoid defective cases.

Reflecting on the problem just discussed, we can probably make a general claim about all important virtues. They are rarely simple or, if they are, they appear in a complex configuration of other virtues so that we are compelled to study them, sort them out, and use contexts and histories to decide which should take priority. For this reason, virtue ethicists often draw heavily on biography and fiction. It takes a story to fill out an account of virtue (see, for example, Cunningham 2001; Nussbaum 1986). And it takes a co-authored story to fill out an account of caring.

Before turning to the discussion of teaching, it is worth pointing out that those who regularly form caring relations are often happy people (Noddings 2003b). As noted earlier, when we respond supportively to another, we contribute to the well-being of both cared-for and the relation. Hence, since we are part of the relation, we also benefit. (I am talking here about everyday, face-to-face relations, not extreme situations. There are many exceptions to the mutual benefit claim—acts that may be described as purely altruistic and even sacrificial. Their analysis is beyond the scope of this chapter.)

The caring–happiness connection is bi-directional. Caring often brings happiness, but happiness often makes us more effective carers. Parents and caring professionals are right to give attention to their own happiness because happiness becomes part of what is conveyed to the cared-for, and it also protects caregivers from burnout. Recognizing the connection between happiness and caring also underscores the need to work continually on establishing and maintaining an environment in which caring relations can flourish. When caring relations flourish, care-giving is not a grim and sacrificial duty but, rather, a way of life that enriches both carer and cared-for.

CARING IN TEACHING

The stage is now set for an exploration of caring in teaching. As carers, teachers are responsible both for the direct person-to-person caring that contributes to the growth of individual students and for the establishment of conditions under which caring can flourish.

Motivation

Part of the second responsibility of teachers is choosing a theory of motivation to guide them in making pedagogical choices. There are two general theories of motivation: Theory 1 emphasizes internal needs and wants (Dewey 1930; Maslow 1970); Theory 2, sometimes called the 'carrot and stick' theory, emphasizes external demands, rewards, and punishments. In management or teaching, advocates of the second theory ask, How can we motivate people to do what we want them to do? Under this theory, teachers are urged to 'motivate' their students to work diligently at tasks they would otherwise reject. This theory of motivation fits well with our Case 2 description of caring. Under that description, A diagnoses B's condition and decides, from her own structures of evaluation, what she should do for B. Life for these teachers is often a constant struggle to get students to do things they would prefer not to do.

Followers of Theory 1 may start by asking, Must we motivate? Recognizing that all living organisms are motivated, they ask, How should I direct this existing motivation? This theory is compatible with relational caring. It requires teachers to identify students' motivation (to listen) and to direct their interests and energies to worthwhile projects.

The difference may seem subtle to novice teachers. After all, whichever theory of motivation is accepted, teachers must teach a specified curriculum. But teachers working under Theory 1 are likely to favor a larger role for the interactive curriculum than for the pre-active curriculum; that is, much of what is learned in the classroom will come from cooperatively constructed objectives, not from preset, standard objectives. Theory 1 teachers of reading, for example, will allow students to read along lines that interest them. Not everyone in the class will read the same material. At every level, these teachers will provide a broad array of materials and topics from which students may choose. In those cases where the acquisition of particular skills is necessary and perhaps tedious, teachers will explain how the skills fit with the students' actual purposes or how acquisition of the skills will facilitate later work. This sort of work (skill building) will never dominate what is done in the classroom. Theory 1 teachers listen to their students and, when the prescribed work becomes onerous, they may turn back to the students' own motives and interests.

This is hard work. Caring teachers are not permissive; that is, they do not let students do just as they please. They recognize the truth in John Dewey's comment: 'Plato once defined a slave as the person who executes the purposes of another, and . . . a person is also a slave who is enslaved to his own blind desires' (1963: 67). Caring teachers, then, reject a system in which learning objectives are completely set beforehand and students merely execute the 'purposes of another'. But they also reject the kind of permissiveness that starts each day with, What would you like to do today? The process of constructing objectives cooperatively is one of continuous and intelligent negotiation.

There are dilemmas and uncertainties in teaching this way. Sometimes students are so used to the carrot and stick approach that they mistake a teacher's willingness to work cooperatively as permissiveness—an invitation to do as little as possible. Then it makes sense to provide incentives—because the student needs them, not because the teacher is converted to Theory 2. I once had a student who told me explicitly, 'I need to be pushed.' I responded that I'd (reluctantly) do this, and I did. However, I reminded him often about the kind of life he could anticipate if he continued to rely on others to prod him.

As carers, we face many situations in which we find it hard to judge whether we're in a type 3 episode—one in which we are pushing our own agenda too hard—or in a type 4 situation—one in which our recommendations are really in the best interests of the cared-for. In the one situation, we should back off; in the other, we should push cautiously ahead.

Some time ago, I listened to a caring art teacher struggle with this problem. She was dealing with a talented student who had a fine sense of space and color. Technically, the student was ready for detailed instruction and painstaking practice of particular skills. But the student liked to work quickly and had a host of other talents. If the teacher pushed, might the student lose interest? It was less likely that this student would get bogged down in detail and thus sacrifice her creativity (but this could be a concern with another student). This wise teacher decided to push gently and monitor the effects of her pushing. She also worked to strengthen the relationship, and she accepted the need to live with some uncertainty.

Pedagogy and Curriculum

Caring teachers (in the relational sense) must be flexible in their choice of methods, because differences in students and situations (identified through listening and responding) require differences in methods. Case 2 teachers may or may not be flexible. Out of genuine concern, they may use (or reject) a particular method that is promoted (or discouraged) by their philosophical view of teaching. Adherence to a particular method is not confined to traditional teachers. Many progressive (or 'constructivist') teachers are also inflexible with respect to the choice of methods. For example, I have encountered mathematics teachers who insist that they would *never* use rote memory or drill ("drill and kill") methods in their classes. From a relational perspective, this insistence seems mistaken. Sometimes students need to memorize and to practice routine operations. Such practice can even be restful, and it often facilitates later conceptual work. The point is to provide what students need, to remain responsive to those needs and not to an ideal model of pedagogy.

As a philosopher–teacher, I locate myself in the progressive (Deweyan) tradition, but I do not think that general agreement with Dewey's philosophy commits me to the extensive use of small groups, projects, or hands-on lessons—nor to the exclusive use of democratic processes. An emergency situation—a classroom of unruly, inattentive students—may require me to use methods more characteristic of Case 2 carers. Employing these methods with some regret, my aim would be to cultivate the conditions under which more democratic methods might be successful. As a carer, my choice of methods must depend heavily on the expressed needs and responses of my students. Even within a class for which progressive methods generally work well, I may need to use 'carrot and stick' and rote methods with some students. In these cases, my task as a carer will include helping such students to understand themselves and what their present attitudes may presage for their futures.

At the height of the behavioral objectives movement (in the 1970s) and again now with the emphasis on common standards for all, teachers are assured that they remain professionally free to choose the methods by which they will bring all students to reach the objectives or standards. Caring teachers respond to this assurance with a heavy heart, because they know that educational aims, objectives, and standards—not just methods—must all be subject to change in light of student interests and abilities. Beyond a few basic necessities such as learning to read, students must be invited to make choices on what they will learn. They must not become slaves who 'execute the purposes of another'. Without this freedom to make guided choices, students are often bored, unsuccessful, and even rebellious.

Case 2 teachers—those who have decided a priori what students need—often find the standards movement compatible with their beliefs, and they may work hard to bring students to the established standards. Their virtue in terms of conscientiousness cannot be denied. But too often, the joy in teaching and learning is lost, relationships are weakened or destroyed, and the aim of education deteriorates to passing a course, getting a good grade, graduating, and transferring the same attitudes to occupational life.

Uncertainties in the arena of curriculum abound. Much of what we now ask students to learn is material that will quickly be forgotten. Many well educated, successful adults would be unable to pass the tests we now force on children. Because caring teachers listen to their students, they know that both the coercion and the irrelevance in the current standard curriculum are deeply resented. But what should teachers do? They cannot simply ignore the material on which their students will be tested but, if they care about each student, they cannot neglect real, expressed needs. This is, perhaps, the greatest dilemma in current teaching, and it illustrates again the dual obligation of caring professionals: to care for each student *and* to work toward the establishment of conditions under which caring can flourish. Many of us believe that standardization must be rejected (Sacks 1999).

The Quest for Competence

Teacher effectiveness in the academic realm requires subject matter competence. This is generally recognized, but caring puts even more pressure on teachers to be competent. Recognizing that students come to them with very different motives and interests, caring teachers must be prepared not only with a variety of instructional methods but also with a repertoire of stories and materials that connect their subjects to ordinary purposes, to other school subjects, to the great existential questions, and to new purposes such as aesthetic appreciation and critical thinking. They must be prepared to teach something of the history, sociology, aesthetics, and epistemology of their subjects.

Competent, caring teachers want to respond to the voiced and unvoiced needs of their students. Mathematics teachers, for example, should be able to draw on history, biography, fiction, politics, religion, philosophy, and the arts in ways that enrich their daily lessons and provide many possibilities for individual students to follow their own interests and find new ones. No one topic so introduced will attract all students, but the vast multitude of direct references, allusions, stories, poems, anecdotes, and jokes will make it possible for most students to make connections with their own interests.

Subject matter preparation for teachers should become broader, not narrower, as teachers advance in their studies. Secondary school mathematics teachers, for example, need preparation that is different from that of other math majors. These days most subject matter preparation is done in Arts and Sciences, not in Schools or

Departments of Education, and too many mathematics professors believe that courses especially designed for teachers would have to be 'watered down'. I am suggesting just the opposite. Teachers, if they are to be caring teachers, need the sort of preparation discussed above, and this requires courses that are richly different, not disemboweled skeletons of "real" math courses.

From the care perspective, professors who work with pre-service teachers should be guided more by their students' needs than by the traditional curricula of their disciplines. Too many college teachers are Case 2 carers—people who are deeply concerned about their subject and about shaping their students by its standards. As a result, many teachers believe that their competence will be enhanced by more and more study of their subject. But there is a limit to the usefulness of such study for K-12, that is, primary, middle, and secondary teachers. They will not use most of this advanced material in their classroom teaching or, worse, they may force it (sometimes bungled) on unwilling students who are neither interested nor ready for it. K-12 teachers whose attitudes are shaped by subject matter specialists often become conscientious Case 2 carers themselves—teachers who fail to develop the capacity to respond to the expressed needs of their students.

Teaching is perhaps the only profession today that can, logically, welcome Renaissance thinkers. Caring teachers, widely read and conversant with material from most of the disciplines, appear to their students as models of educated persons. High school students often wonder why they are expected to learn material from four or five disciplines when their teachers know only one—and sometimes not even that one well.

Responding to the predictably wide variety of student interests, caring teachers will prepare themselves broadly, and—with a continuing commitment to caring relations—they will concentrate on developing their repertoires by adding material that contributes to their own growth and joy in learning. Care theory emphasizes the centrality of the relation, and conditions that sustain that relation include the happiness of both carer and cared-for.

Evaluation

No task is more troubling for caring teachers than grading. Grading students gets in the way of establishing and maintaining caring relations, and it often damages student–student relationships as well. Moreover, the quest for good grades may actually weaken or even destroy genuine intellectual interest (Pope 2001). In John Knowles's widely read *A Separate Peace*, the student narrator, Gene, remarks that he had a real advantage in the grade game over his nearest rival who 'was weakened by the very genuineness of his interest in learning' (1975: 46). Gene confesses that, to him, the required topics 'were all pretty much alike . . . and I worked indiscriminately on all of them' (ibid.). This is clearly a result that all good teachers would like to avoid.

There are other well-documented negative effects of grading. Students begin to confuse their achievement with their Grade Point Average and class rank. They work only as hard as the competition demands. They may also defend their own mediocre performance by pointing out that they are 'better' than some other students, and this way of establishing their own worth sometimes carries over into a lifetime of comparing themselves favorably with the very worst examples in their circle of acquaintances. Grading and ranking also lead to cheating, and teachers compound the problem when they tell students that, when they cheat, they only hurt themselves. This would be true if the system of evaluation did not involve grading and ranking. Then, indeed, students who disguise their ignorance by cheating would only hurt themselves. But they would have little incentive to do this. In the prevailing system, there is a tremendous incentive to cheat, and cheaters hurt all those whose rank they dishonestly surpass.

Case 2 teachers are as troubled by the problems of grading as are Case 1 carers. But instead of searching for a way to change the system, they often work hard to make it as fair as possible and to appeal to students' honesty and sense of fairness. These teachers can be credited with the virtues of honesty and fairness. They work hard to make the best of a bad practice. Case 2 teachers work to develop the virtue of their students in a system that itself lacks virtue; Case 1 teachers work to establish a world in which it is both desirable and possible to be good.

To establish that world, caring teachers look for another way to evaluate their students' work. Many schools refuse to grade children in primary classes (grades K-3), and quite a few use narrative evaluation (and no grades) throughout elementary and middle grades. A very few high schools and colleges also follow this practice, but they are continually under pressure to justify their refusal to give grades. Recently, faculty members from such an enlightened institution told me about their difficulties in recommending students for a teaching credential. Their state now requires that candidates for a credential maintain at least a B average. These fine educators may be forced to give grades if they want to stay in the business of preparing teachers.

What will they lose if they give way on this? The most important thing lost may be the relations of care and trust now enjoyed between faculty and students. Students should be able to ask their teachers or peers for assistance at any stage of their work, and requiring more time or assistance should not result in a lower grade. Teachers have to evaluate their students' work, but evaluation does not imply a final, summative grade. It may require asking students to rework an assignment several times in order to bring it to a satisfactory state, but it does not require giving a grade. Under this alternative practice, teacher and student work together to produce a product satisfactory to both, and often the caring relation is strengthened as a result.

All good teachers are concerned about their students' learning. Does an ethic of care provide any special guidance on the subject? We certainly cannot start with a description of caring and derive specific rules for ethical conduct as Kant did with his categorical imperative. In the preceding discussion, I've tried to make suggestions that are plausible, given a commitment to caring. I will do the same now in the discussion of learning and evaluation.

Teachers guided by an ethic of care are, I think, more likely than Case 2 teachers to change instructional objectives in light of student needs. They are more likely to ask, What has Johnny learned? rather than, Has Johnny learned X? In agreement with progressive educators, they believe that students are naturally motivated, and it is the teacher's task to connect or steer this motivation to worthwhile ends. Caring teachers are deeply concerned with learning, but they recognize that individual students need to learn, and will inevitably learn, very different things. This recognition and understanding of different needs is a direct outcome of the emphasis on caring relations. The teacher listens to students and shapes their learning experiences according to both student interests and the future demands of subject matter.

Obviously, the cooperative construction of objectives and methods makes great demands on teacher competence, and the demands are increased when teachers evaluate student work. It is far easier—although still no simple task—to evaluate all students on the basis of standard material and strict rules of fairness. Students are so accustomed to this standard mode of evaluation that they sometimes object to methods that make more generous allowances for individual students. As a mathematics teacher (and I had to give grades in that position), I once had a student object to my practice of allowing students to retake tests until they demonstrated sufficient mastery to undertake the next unit of study. He didn't object to the retaking, but he complained strenuously to my not penalizing students for several tries. 'Are you telling me,' he protested, 'that someone who makes a 95 on the second or third try is as good as someone who makes a 92 the first time?' I reminded him that the retest was always a new form (not the very same test that could be memorized) and then tried to get across the message that it is learning that matters—not how quickly it is achieved. He still insisted that my method of evaluation was 'not fair'. For this student, the object of learning was to get better grades than others, amass as many As as possible, and beat his classmates in the race for college.

Evaluation presents teachers with agonizing uncertainties. Teachers are accountable to the institutions that employ them, and they also feel a responsibility to uphold and further standards associated with their disciplines. But, even more important, caring teachers are responsible for the growth of their students as whole persons. Surely, I can't teach homemaking or pop music instead of the algebra for which I was hired. If I can include these topics in my teaching, well and good. But I must teach some algebra. Which students should be encouraged to meet the highest standards of the discipline? Which should be allowed to satisfy a merely adequate standard? Which should be encouraged to excel in other studies while they are helped to meet minimal standards in the algebra they may hate? And what are these minimal standards? Teaching is a lifelong moral quest, and evaluation is among its greatest challenges.

Moral Education

As part of that lifelong moral quest, teachers are concerned with the moral growth of their students, but views on what constitutes moral growth differ. Case 2 teachers may define moral growth in terms of students' increasing tendency to internalize the rules of their school and community. It was in part his inability to do this that led Orwell to say that, in his school days, he was in a world 'where it was not possible' for him to be good. A deeper understanding of that lament emerged later. He was in a world where it was not easy to be good in the caring sense—that is, to make it more likely that he and others would attain and acquire the real goods of democratic social life.

Carol Gilligan (1982) invigorated the field of moral education when she described an alternative to the justice orientation. Without denying the moral significance of attaining a sense of universal justice, she pointed out that a growing sense of relation with and responsibility for the well-being of others also demonstrates moral growth. An ethic of care emphasizes the value of caring relations and evaluates moral growth in terms of one's capacity to form such relations and share responsibility for the growth and happiness of others.

In earlier work (Noddings 2003a, 2002a), I have discussed four components of moral education from the care perspective. The first component is modeling. This is a component of virtually all forms of moral education. Caring teachers show what it means to care in everything they do. In acting on the choices described earlier in the discussion of motivation, pedagogy, curriculum, the quest for competence, and evaluation, teachers show students what it means to care.

Modeling of this sort is largely unselfconscious. Teachers do not say, 'I'm doing this because I care,' or 'Watch me, and you'll learn how to care.' They demonstrate caring simply because they do care. Their modeling is inescapable and usually inadvertent. The point is caring, not modeling care.

However, just as natural caring sometimes fails and moral agents must rely on ethical caring, so too caring teachers must sometimes remind themselves that—like it or not—they serve as models. Then—perhaps angry, disappointed, or tired—they must conduct themselves consciously as models. Here there is a risk similar to that incurred when we turn to ethical caring. Students may spot the effort and assess it as hypocrisy rather than virtue. A second risk is that teachers who concentrate too consciously on being models of virtue may actually fail to develop caring relations. Their attention is too narrowly focused on their own behavior. They lapse into self-righteousness.

Without making students feel overly responsible for their teachers' emotional well-being, teachers can be honest about their own feelings. One can say, for example, 'You can see that I'm angry about (what happened), but we have to give today's lesson a try. You can help me—and I'll appreciate it—by . . .' Such disclosures of genuine feeling model authenticity and help students to grow in their ability to assess feelings accurately and to respond with care.

Case 2 teachers sometimes model authenticity by displaying genuine (and justifiable) anger. Teachers must ask themselves, however, whether the display of anger is aimed at achieving closer adherence to rules or deeper concern for helping, and not hurting, others. Caring teachers help students to understand the connection between a rule and the conditions under which 'being good' is possible. If no such condition can be found, caring teachers often ignore the rule.

Exploring rules and their connection to caring relations is one function of dialogue, the second component of moral education. All teachers socialize their students, but caring teachers want their students to reflect on and understand the processes of socialization. As Diana Meyers (1989) has argued, it is through reflection that we exercise some control over our socialization.

Dialogue is fundamental not only to moral education but to caring itself. We have to engage in dialogue to learn what the other is going through. Simone Weil made the question, 'What are you going through?' basic to moral life (1977: 51), and it is certainly basic in an ethic of care. Through dialogue we learn the expressed needs of the cared-for and, through dialogue, we respond to those needs.

The alternative is to infer needs from our past experience in teaching and from our own educational philosophy. Teacher training programs usually encourage teachers to learn about the needs of young children, fifth graders, ethnic minority pupils, girls in mathematics, students with disabilities . . . Such learning can provide a useful base from which to start dialogue, but if needs-assessment ends with this general knowledge about various groups, it may work against the construction of caring relations. Genuine dialogue discloses us as individuals to one another.

The capacity to engage in dialogue calls upon some of the related virtues mentioned earlier. It requires openness, flexibility, and patience. It also requires a willingness to stay with one's partner in dialogue through difficult episodes. For example, a student may express attitudes or values that the teacher finds objectionable or even abhorrent. Should we allow the dialogue in such cases to continue?

In Gunter Grass's novel *Crabwalk*, a contemporary German adolescent becomes deeply interested in the Nazi era. His grandmother, a survivor of the Russian sinking of the German liner *Wilhelm Gustloff*, tells him about the catastrophe (in actuality, the greatest maritime disaster in history with some 9,000 lives lost, many of them children) and also about the Nazi functionary after whom the ship was named. Wilhelm Gustloff, a minor official, had been assassinated by a Jew and, as a result, had become something of a martyr. The boy, Konny, heard a distorted version of the story from his grandmother. Both of his parents were kind but aloof; he had no dialogue with them. He tried to initiate discussion by writing a thoughtful school paper on the events, but his teachers would not allow him to present or discuss it. His only recourse seemed to be a series of Internet exchanges which only heightened and further twisted his views. The tragedy that resulted might have been prevented if Konny's teachers had possessed the courage and open-mindedness to engage him in dialogue.

Grass, widely recognized as an outspoken foe of Nazism, seems to have had at least two purposes in writing *Crabwalk*: first, to creep up crab-like on stories of real and terrible German suffering during and after the Second World War (stories long repressed by German guilt) and secondly, to warn us that the repression of stories and the refusal to enter dialogue leave young people in a lost and bewildered state—searching desperately for truth and, perhaps, for a great leader who will tell it to them. As that outcome is clearly threatened at the end of Grass's novel, his narrator says, in despair, 'It doesn't end. Never will it end' (2002: 234).

Dialogue must extend beyond that between teacher and student, and a main task for caring teachers is to show young people how to engage in dialogue, and allow them to practice it (Burbules 1993). Practice is the third component in moral education, for it is from successful practice that we each build the ideal of caring that we must draw upon in ethical caring.

Guiding the practice of caring requires teachers to develop and exercise intellectual virtues, particularly those of reflection and discernment. Teacher education today is heavily loaded with what many of us regard as propaganda. It is decent propaganda, to be sure, formulated to encourage young teachers to attend to the needs of all students, to use constructivist methods, and to have high expectations for all students. But pre-service teachers are too seldom asked to challenge the claims that accompany these teachings. High expectations for all students should not mean uniform or standard expectations, and to have high expectations for a given student requires knowing that student well enough to ground one's expectations reasonably. Similarly, attending to the needs of all students requires knowing something about them as individuals. And constructivist methods are not always best. Sometimes good teachers properly use rote, drill, and lecture ('telling').

In providing opportunities for students to practice caring, new teachers might well choose to use the small, cooperative group methods so popular with constructivists today. Working together can invite caring, but it can also induce impatience, rivalry, verbal bullying, and a host of *un*caring behaviors. Teachers who reflect on the possibilities may decide, first, to remind students that the first object of working in groups is to help one another. Secondly, such teachers will design group work to support caring. This may suggest giving no group grades (a practice that often causes anger, recriminations, and a renewed round of competition) and rejecting the usual emphasis on specific roles within the group. If the object is to help one another, then it becomes less important to learn the role of leader, recorder, and so on. And without there being grades attached, students are less likely to criticize slower members of the group or to claim that they are 'doing all the work'.

Reflective teachers may also question the current practice of isolating young adolescents (ages 12–14) in middle schools (or junior highs). Students in this age group might, as part of their practice in caring, serve as models for younger children. To attend classes in the same building as younger children, to engage in cross-age tutoring, and to help in the supervision of little ones in lunchroom and playground may contribute greatly to the moral growth of young adolescents. We might do well to abandon middle schools and reorganize our schools in K-8, 9–12 or K-7, 8–12 configurations.

Modeling, dialogue, and practice are essential elements of moral education from a care perspective. A fourth component is confirmation. To confirm someone is, according to Martin Buber (1970), to bring out the best in him or her. When teachers practice confirmation, they attribute to their students' acts the best possible motive *consonant with reality*. Confirmation is not a strategy or technique. It is a way of staying with others and helping them to actualize their best selves. Teachers cannot do this unless they know their students quite well. I can't say to every student who cheats, 'I know you were trying to help your friend,' but I can say it to a student for whom I am quite sure it is true.

Case 2 teachers often use instead a model familiar in many religious communities: accusation, confession, penance, and forgiveness. This model is meant to be used with love, but frequently the effect is shame, anger, and a rupture of the caring relation. When, in contrast, a caring teacher attributes a realistically best motive to an act, a student may respond with commitment to live up to her own best as identified by this percipient person. If temptation strikes again, the hope is that the student will be stronger, remembering that 'Ms. A expects better from me.'

Supporting Caring in Schools

The choice of theories of motivation and moral education, an emphasis on interactive curriculum, the drive for broad competence, and the commitment to individual evaluation are all, in a sense, preparation for caring encounters. Such preparation does not eliminate the responsibility to respond directly to the student as cared-for when the need arises. It does, however, establish supportive conditions for caring, and it may well reduce the number of troubling cases in which students request direct personal attention. Practically, this is important for high school teachers who meet more than a hundred students every day. Such preparation is a significant attempt to care before one is directly addressed as carer, and it is clearly different from Case 2 caring in that it sets the stage for the participation of students in curriculum building, the construction of learning objectives, evaluation, and their own moral growth.

But caring teachers may still be uneasy. Their virtue as carers depends ultimately on their success in establishing caring relations. How can this be done? What conditions of schooling might support the establishment of caring relations? As suggested earlier, teachers must be free to exercise professional judgment in constructing curriculum with their students, in choosing methods, and in evaluating student work. Almost certainly, this requires the abandonment of the present standardization movement. Additionally, they must be prepared broadly so that their professional judgment can be trusted. Further, teachers should be encouraged to make choices that add to their own growth and professional happiness. In 'preparing broadly', teachers obviously can't learn everything that might interest their students; they should make choices that will increase not only their expertise but also their enthusiasm and interest as a person.

Another suggestion is to encourage teachers and students to stay together for several years (by mutual consent) instead of the usual one-year encounter (Flinders and Noddings 2001). In European elementary schools, this is a common practice. In the U.S., some schools are experimenting with a practice called 'looping'. For example, a teacher might work with the same children from first grade through to third (or from fourth to sixth) and then 'loop' back to pick up another class of first or fourth graders. The name *looping* is a poor one, however, because it concentrates attention on the teacher's experience instead of the students'—or better yet on the arrangement's effects on relations. I prefer to speak of continuity.

Continuity can be provided at the secondary level, also, and it is perhaps even more important there. We know that many children begin to lose heart and interest in school at the middle school level (another reason for abandoning that arrangement). Faced with several teachers—none of whom they get to know well—they report again and again, 'Nobody cares!' (Institute for Education in Transformation 1992). Researchers have shown, however, that teachers in the schools where this complaint is made usually *do* care, in the Case 2 sense of caring. They work hard to get their students to learn the prescribed material, but they do not listen to the students; they do not form caring relations. There is neither the time nor sufficient encouragement to form such relations. To make the formation of caring relations possible, we could encourage subject matter teachers to stay with their students throughout middle school, and the same plan could be equally effective in high school.

It is hard to overestimate the power of teacher–student continuity. At the level of graduate school, we know that the single most important factor in the success of most doctoral students is the relation between student and advisor. This relation is often continuous for the student's graduate years, and it is not unusual for it to continue over a professional lifetime. It seems reasonable to suggest that such continuity is important at every level.

CONCLUSION

Care theory is similar to virtue ethics in its rejection of fixed principles in favor of reliance on the good character of moral agents to guide moral life. It differs, however, in giving attention to the contributions of the cared-for in caring relations. In most cases, the attributes that motivate or engender these contributions would not be called virtues. They are often simply heart-warming reactions to the responses of carers. Nevertheless, I have argued that they are sustaining elements in such relations as parent–child, physician–patient, and teacher–student. They deserve inclusion in a full discussion of moral life.

Care theory is perhaps unique in making ethical caring subordinate to natural caring—relationships that require no moral effort but are sustained out of love, sympathy, compassion, generosity, good humor, and receptive attention. Ethical caring is required when, for whatever reason, natural caring fails. Then an ethical ideal composed from a lifetime of caring and being cared for is summoned to guide conduct. In this, care theory is most closely aligned with virtue ethics.

Considering the application of care theory to teaching, I have contrasted relational caring with Case 2 caring. In relational caring, teachers are more heavily guided by the expressed needs and interests of students. In Case 2 caring, teachers draw more often on their own beliefs and educational ideals. The relational perspective was applied to the choice of a theory of motivation, to pedagogy, curriculum, the quest for competence, evaluation, moral education, and the task of creating the conditions under which caring relationships can flourish. Finally, I pointed out dilemmas and uncertainties that arise in each of these areas of teaching and also the happiness that so often rewards caring teachers.

REFERENCES

Buber, M. (1970). *I and Thou*. Trans. Walter Kaufmann. New York: Charles Scribner's Sons.
Burbules, N. C. (1993). *Dialogue in Teaching*. New York: Teachers' College Press.
Cunningham, A. (2001). *The Heart of the Matter*. Berkeley: University of California Press.
Dewey, J. (1930). *Human Nature and Conduct*. New York: Modern Library.
_____ (1963). *Experience and Education*. New York: Collier Books. Original published 1938.
Flinders, D. and Noddings, N. (2001). *Multiyear Teaching: The Case for Continuity*. Bloomington, IN: Phi Delta Kappa.
Gilligan, C. J. (1982). *In a Different Voice*. Cambridge, MA: Harvard University Press.
Grass, G. (2002). *Crabwalk*. Trans. Krishna Winston. Orlando: Harcourt.
Hume, D. (1983). *An Enquiry Concerning the Principles of Morals*. Indianapolis: Hackett.
Institute for Education in Transformation. (1992). *Voices from the Inside*. Claremont, CA: Claremont Graduate School.
Knowles, J. (1960). *A Separate Peace*. New York: Macmillan.

Maslow, A. (1970). *Motivation and Personality*. New York: Harper and Row.

Meyers, D. T. (1989). *Self, Society, and Personal Choice*. New York: Columbia University Press.

Noddings, N. (2002a). *Educating Moral People: A Caring Alternative to Character Education*. New York: Teachers College Press.

—— (2002b). *Starting at Home: Caring and Social Policy*. Berkeley: University of California Press.

—— (2003a). *Caring: A Feminine Approach to Ethics and Moral Education* (2nd edn.). Berkeley: University of California Press.

—— (2003b). *Happiness and Education*. Cambridge: Cambridge University Press.

Nussbaum, M. (1986). *The Fragility of Goodness*. Cambridge: Cambridge University Press.

Orwell, G. (1981). *A Collection of Essays*. San Diego: Harcourt Brace.

Pope, D. C. (2001). *'Doing School': How we are Creating a Generation of Stressed Out, Materialistic, and Miseducated Students*. New Haven: Yale University Press.

Sacks, P. (1999). *Standardized Minds: The High Price of America's Testing Culture and what We Can Do to Change It*. New York: Perseus.

Scheff, T. J. (1999). *Being Mentally Ill*. New York: Aldine De Gruyter.

Slote, M. (2001). *Morals from Motives*. Oxford: Oxford University Press.

Weil, S. (1977). *Simone Weil Reader*. Ed. George A. Panichas. Mt. Kisco, NY: Moyer Bell.

Williams, B. (1981). *Moral Luck*. Cambridge: Cambridge University Press.

3

Professing Medicine, Virtue Based Ethics, and the Retrieval of Professionalism

Edmund D. Pellegrino

The Virtue of a Thing is relative to its proper function.

Aristotle, *NE* 1145 a 18

INTRODUCTION

In the last several decades, the traditional professions of medicine, law, and ministry have suffered a progressive erosion of their social and moral status. Concomitantly, and reciprocally, a significant degree of moral malaise has afflicted professionals themselves. There is a general loss of faith in the sustainability of the ancient links between ethics and professional practice. There is even doubt about what has been lost, why and how it was lost, and whether or not it ought to be retrieved.

The reasons for this state of affairs are many and complex, for example, the challenges to all received authority and values that accompanied the cultural revolution of the sixties of the last century; the commodification, commercialization, and industrialization of professional practice itself; the pervasive secularization of modern life; the self-regarding changes in the lifestyles of professionals; the technological bias of professional education. How one weighs, prioritizes, and interrelates these factors will shape the responses and remedies pursued or rejected.

Currently, the responses of professionals are in conflict. Some argue for a totally new ethic, shaped and changed along with contemporary mores; others deny the need for any universal set of ethical norms, preferring to leave the choices to individual patients and physicians; still others argue for a return to a putative, pristine state of professional mores, based in notions of duty, service, and altruism. Which of these pathways is chosen is of the utmost importance to all of us. At some time in our lives, we shall all need the help of one or several of these professions, usually more than once. Who, and what they take themselves to be, and what obligations we can expect them to honor are matters of the greatest personal and public importance.

This essay argues that the most significant question is the nature of the moral foundations of professionalism. This is not to deny the relevance of the socio-political, cultural, and economic milieu. Rather, it is to assert that everything depends on the moral structure of the professions. Without that being secured, the professions do indeed become simply occupations, jobs, or means of livelihood like any other. Without a moral template, the professional becomes a proletarian as happened in the last century in the totalitarian regimes.

This essay, therefore, undertakes to examine the philosophical and moral foundations of professionalism. It does so by an analysis of the act of profession, using medicine as the paradigm case. It argues that the act of profession and the specific phenomenological context within which it is performed entails certain character traits in the person making the profession. This essay thus relates being a professional to a theory of medical virtues, based in the end, or *telos*, to which the act of professing is directed, which defines medicine as a specific kind of human activity. It also argues, by analogy, that the same line of argument can apply to other 'helping' professions like law, ministry, and teaching.

Etymologically the word 'profession' derives from the Latin verb *profiteri*—to declare aloud or publicly (*The Oxford Dictionary of English Etymology* 1966). What the professions 'declare' is a claim to special knowledge and an allegiance to something beyond self-interest. They make this declaration publicly in their codes and Oaths, and privately every time they offer their services to persons in need of them. Their 'act of profession' is a solemn promise of competence, a voluntary entrance into a covenantal trust relationship. It is thus interpreted by those to whom the declaration is made.

By his act of profession, the professional is committed to the good and best interests of the person to be served, for example, the patient in the case of medicine. In this essay, I will argue that the act of profession is at the moral center of authentic professional ethics. By making this declaration, the professional binds himself to certain intellectual and moral virtues, that is, those that dispose him habitually to fulfill his promise, and the expectations his promise generates. Fidelity to these virtues makes the professional a good or virtuous professional and his act of profession becomes authentic.

The major focus for this argument is clinical medicine and the phenomena which make it a special kind of moral enterprise. A similar line of argument can be developed for social and public health medicine, and other helping professions like law, ministry, and teaching (Pellegrino 2001, 2004). Each begins with its own act of profession; each entails certain virtues that enable it best to attain its ends. These are the virtues internal to that profession required by its ends—and necessary to attainment of its ends.

My focus is professional ethics, the ethics of medicine as a profession, rather than the ethical issues that arise in the application of the techniques of medicine. These latter include end of life issues, the challenges of genetic medicine, and reproductive technology, or the dilemmas of biotechnology and a wide variety of new challenges to the ethical uses of biological knowledge for human enhancement. These issues are, of course, of extreme importance, but in this essay my concern is for the moral life of the professional. Essentially, this is a propaedeutic to a more complete moral philosophy of professionalism.

My discussion is divided into four parts. The first deals with my construal of classical virtue theory, its relationship to ends in general, and to the ends of clinical medicine in particular. The second section turns attention to the good of the patient as the specific end of clinical medicine and the specific virtues necessary to attainment of that end. The third section extends these observations to the other helping professions, and the fourth section considers some objections against the line of argument proposed here.

PART I: VIRTUE ETHICS

Virtue ethics is the most durable and complex of ethical theories. Its roots are in the classical world. It was enriched and flourished in the Middle Ages. It remained the focal point of moral philosophy until the eighteenth century when it began to be over-shadowed by theories of rights, duties, consequences, and social construction. Largely through the influence of Anscombe (1981) and MacIntyre (1984), it has enjoyed a renaissance. Many ethicists today admit the necessity of some account of virtue in any attempt to elaborate a comprehensive moral theory.

These modern and contemporary accounts are varied in their interpretations of classical virtue theory and its applicability to moral life in today's world. Some hold fast to the viability and influence of the classical account (Devettere 2002). Others emphasize modifications as well as disagreement with that account and replace it with quite different conceptions of virtue (Statman 1997; Trianosky 1997). It is impossible in this essay to take account of all these variations or the way they might affect the line of argument I present.

My argument draws heavily on classical virtue theory as I interpret it within the very specific context of professional relationships. Classical theory emphasizes the tele-ological orientation of virtue and ends and this is, I believe, particularly pertinent for the way I shall define the act of profession. Professions are distinguished by their dedication to the good of those they purport to serve and, by that fact, they commit themselves to possess the intellectual and moral virtues such a dedication requires.

Virtue theories cannot stand entirely on their own. Nor are they independent of principles and duties. They possess other limitations as well (Solomon 1997). Among these are a paucity of specific moral guidelines and disagreements about the nature of the good for humans, and a tendency to subjectivism. Despite these shortcomings, classical virtue theory has more to offer professional ethics than its more skeptical modern transmutations and substitutes.

To be sure, today's divergences about the ends and purposes of human life make it difficult to link the good with the virtues. Natural law ethicists define the good for humans in Aristotelian terms as those things needed for human flourishing (Finnis 1980; MacIntyre 1984). The Stoics identified the good with moral perfection, know-ing and doing what is right (Sandbach 1975). In any case, the good with which we are all concerned here is not the good for humans as humans in the full sense of that term, but the specific good toward which the ministrations of a given profession are oriented.

At least one deficiency of classical theory seems remediable by the teleological approach. I refer here to the difficulties of defining specific virtues and virtue in general. Too often a circular logic has been used, that is, the virtues are the character traits of virtuous person; virtuous persons are those who exhibit the virtues. Linking virtues and ends provides a way out of this circularity. If, as I argue, virtues are oriented to ends, the moral life has a vector—direction and magnitude—a starting and ending point.

Retrieving the classical notion of virtue ethics does not solve all moral questions. There is a tendency today to see virtue theory as the antidote to the ills some see in Kantianism, utilitarianism, and principlism. Virtue theory is expected to remedy the abstractness, narrowness, and neglect of the richness of the moral life some critics find in these theories. Existentialist, caring, feminist, and dialogue ethics often use virtue theory in this way as a kind of ethical panacea. Virtues, as a result, are psychologized and politicized to the detriment of their classical reasoned basis. Failing as a moral panacea, virtue ethics is then discarded.

This essay confines itself to the narrower topic of the virtues in the professions, using medicine as a paradigm case. The professions are distinct human activities in which virtues and ends can be linked. Professions have identifiable and defining ends, that is, each serves certain universal human needs. One who is ill needs to be healed; one who has been unfairly treated needs justice; one who seeks God needs religion. Other purposes may be assigned—rightly or wrongly—to medicine, law, and ministry. Without the specific end of healing, however, medicine would not exist; without the end of justice, law would not exist; without the end of linkage with God, ministry would not exist.

In each of these professions, the end or *telos* is the welfare of a human being in a particular existential state, in need of a specific kind of help. For the Hippocratic physician, the *telos* of medicine has been the good of the patient. For the lawyer, it is the good of his client. For the minister, it is the good of his parishioner. In each case, whatever the other functions they may serve, these professions have the specific good of a particular human being as their distinguishing mark. It is that distinguishing mark that determines the virtues specific to that profession.

This is the meaning of the very first sentence of Aristotle's *Nichomachean Ethics*— 'Every art and every inquiry, and similarly ever action and choice, is thought to aim at some good, and for this reason the good has rightly been declared that at which all things aim' (*NE* 1094a 1–3). This essay is, in part, a gloss on the first sentence of Aristotle's ethic using medicine as a paradigm case in which the end is the good of the patient, and in which certain virtues (excellences) 'make a person good and makes him do his own work well' (*NE* 1106a 22–4). Adapting this definition to medicine, I would define a medical virtue as a character trait which disposes the physician habitually to act well and wisely with respect to the work of medicine, its ends and purposes. A physician who exhibits these character traits is a good physician and a good person.

In the clinical encounter, the good, that is, of the patient as defined earlier is the *telos*, that is, the end toward which both the patient and the doctor are existentially oriented. To attain that end, certain virtues are required. These are both moral and intellectual. They are the virtues incumbent upon the physician if she or he is to attain the ends of medicine. These virtues are neither optional nor merely admirable. They are entailed, on the physician's part, by the nature and ends of medicine. By practicing the medical virtues, physician and person are united in the end they seek, that is, healing. By practicing the medical virtues, the physician becomes a good person, and does the work of medicine well (*NE* 1106a 21–3).

PART II: ENDS OF MEDICINE, CLINICAL AND GENERAL

a) The Ends of Clinical Medicine

I will confine this inquiry to the ends of clinical medicine rather than 'medicine' generically. By *clinical medicine*, I mean the use of medical knowledge and skill for the healing of sick persons, here and now, in the individual physician–patient encounter. Clinical medicine so defined is the activity that specifies what physicians qua physicians do. It sets them apart from other persons, like basic scientists, who may have medical knowledge but do not use it specifically in clinical encounters. Clinical medicine is the physician's ethical domain. Its definable end is a right and good healing action and decision for a particular patient (See Section IId[1]). Clinical medicine is also the instrument through which public policies ultimately affect the lives of sick persons. In this way, clinical and social medicine relate to each other (Pellegrino and Thomasma 2004). The realities of illness and disease remain universal human experiences. Their impact on individual human persons is the reason why medicine and physicians exist in the first place (Hippocrates 1972).

Using clinical medicine as a paradigm case is not to neglect the other branches of medicine, each of which has its own distinctive end. Thus, for basic scientists, the end is the acquisition of fundamental biological knowledge of health and illness. For public health officials, it is the health of the body politic. Medical knowledge becomes a part of clinical medicine and the end of the physician's act of profession when it is applied to the needs of a particular human being here and now. At this point, medical knowledge serves to advance the end of clinical medicine, that is, the good of the patient. Similarly, preventive medicine has as its defining end the cultivation of health and avoidance of illness. It centers on the use of medical knowledge to prevent illness and cultivate health in individuals. Social medicine has its end in the health of the community or the whole body politic. When the knowledge and skills of any of the other branches of medicine are used for the good of a particular person, then the ends of that branch fuse with the ends of clinical medicine. But in clinical medicine, the good of the patient is the end, the first among the other ends, the *primus inter pares*, of clinical medical activity.

Some of the difficulties in arriving at a consensus on the ends of medicine arise because these distinctions are not made clearly enough (Pellegrino 2001). Today, the tendency is to expand the definition of medicine so broadly as to absorb or 'medicalize' almost all aspects of life, like criminality, violence, juvenile delinquency, and even the 'angst' and ennui of daily life. Such an expansion confounds attempts to define ends distinctive for medicine. Ends come into conflict with each other and

---

[1] The several meanings and interrelationships of the end and the good of medicine are distinguished.

weaken any attempt to establish an order of goods among the many ends 'medicine' may serve (Nordin 1999).

b) The Idea of Ends: Re-examined

Before we go further, it is necessary to clarify my use of the term 'teleological ethics'. By this, I do not mean any form of consequentialism or its major modern expression in utilitarianism. Nor do I mean a simplistic biological or evolutionary teleologism. Rather, I refer to an ethic based in the notion of the good as the *telos* of moral acts wherein 'good' is defined in terms of the nature of the activity in question, that for which the activity exists (Veatch 1981; Cooper 1986; Hardie 1967). The medical virtues are habitual dispositions to act in such a way that the ends, the *telos* of medicine, are best achieved. The virtues thus dispose the physician to recognize and attain the ends of medicine. Such an ethic is the antithesis of an ethic of social construction in which the good is defined externally to the activity in question by what we wish or intend the activity to achieve. Elsewhere, I have spelled out the problems with a socially constructed notion of the goals, purposes, or good of medicine (Pellegrino 2001).

Today's debates about the ends of medicine arise in a long-established departure from the classical–medieval notion of ends, their relation to the good, and the relation between the idea of the good and ethics. If the end of medicine is to be redefined, the ancient concept of ends must first be retrieved from the exile imposed on it by modern and contemporary philosophy.

Aristotle (1984) began the *Nicomachean Ethics* (*NE* 1094a 1–3) with the proposition that the good is that which all men desire. The good is the end or *telos* of any human activity, and the end is that for which a thing exists, that which an act is designed to bring about what the act is good for. Ends are in the nature of things themselves. We do not impute ends to things; they are not good simply because we desire them; we desire them because they are good. We may put things like medicine to certain purposes, but whether these are good or bad uses depends upon whether they facilitate the ends for which medicine exists and which define it qua medicine.

Aristotle uses the example of medicine to illustrate his meaning of ends. Medicine, he asserts, is a *techné* whose end is health, just as a ship is the end of ship building (*NE* 1094a 7–18). These ends are also the good for each activity since they are what men seek by engaging in the activity. The activity is so structured that, by its very nature, it is ordained to the ends that define it.

Aristotle and Aquinas, in a similar fashion, were concerned chiefly with the larger conception of the good peculiar to humans as humans. Both structured their moral philosophies on the good as the end of human life. That end in its ultimate sense was, for Aristotle, a life consistent with the natural virtues, which led to happiness (*NE* 1098a 13–19). For Aquinas, it was a life lived in accord with both the natural and the spiritual virtues. Aristotle's anthropology was based in reason alone. Aquinas' ethic was based in reason plus revelation. In both the classical and medieval notion, ends and virtues were closely linked. Thus, if the ends proper to each activity are retrieved, the virtues disposing to those ends will also be retrieved. By anchoring the virtues in the ends of human life and the good, Aristotle and Aquinas linked metaphysics with ethics.

The story of the post-medieval erosion of the ancient notion of virtue and its tele-ological perspectives is long and complicated. MacIntyre (1966) and Murdoch (1993, 1999) and others have traced that story in detail. It extends through the Enlighten-ment's exaltation of autonomous, religion-free morality, to Kant's response to medi-eval metaphysics and his rooting of morality in a good will and a rational imperative. From thence it proceeds to the replacement of reason by moral sentiment in the work of Hume and the British empiricists and the discrediting of definitions of the good by G. E. Moore (1903), and most contemporary philosophers. The dismantling has been completed in the rejection by many postmodernists of any overarching found-ation for morals, together with skepticism about the possibility of ascertaining moral truth by human reason.

The upshot of all of this has been profound for moral philosophy, particularly for Anglo-American ethical theory. Emphasis on the good and on virtue has been shifted to an emphasis on rights, or to the act of valuing personal choices or social prefer-ences. For many, morality itself becomes the creation of our personal choices or of the consensus of a liberal society. The good is revealed in the choices we make. Iris Murdoch puts it this way: 'The philosopher is no longer to speak of the good as some-thing real and transcendent but to analyze the familiar activity of endowing things with value. If we want to place the definitive breach with metaphysical ethics at any point, we can place it here' (Murdoch 1999).

c) The Ends of Medicine

Aristotle and Aquinas both define the ultimate end of medicine generically as 'health' (*NE* 1094a 8). Kass defines this end a bit more specifically, as the well-functioning of the human organism (1981). These definitions are general enough to encompass clin-ical medicine as well as the basic sciences related to medicine, including social and preventive medicine. But they need to be refined for our project which is to define the ends of clinical medicine, that is, the ends of the encounter between one in need of help and one who professes to meet that need. Clinical medicine centers on the clinical encounter between someone with medical knowledge (the **professional**) and someone who needs that knowledge to restore the well-functioning disturbed by ill-ness or disease (the **patient**).

To that end, an even more proximate and immediate end must first be gained, that is, a technically correct and medically good decision made for *this* patient here and now. This decision, given the uncertainties of clinical medicine, most closely serves the good (as defined in the next section) of the patient at a particular moment and for a foreseeable future. This clinical decision must be made and safely implemented by the clinician in collaboration with the patient. It is to the extent possible a joint enterprise. This good is what the ill or sick person needs and seeks immediately, namely help, comfort, care, and cure. These are ends to which the clinician qua clinician is ordained by her medical education and experience to provide.

With respect to this end, medicine is a *techné*, but also more than a *techné*. Classic-ally, a *techné* or art is a practical knowledge of how to do, or make, a thing together with recognition of the reasons for, and principles needed, to do the task well. An art is distinguished from a science—a right way of acting with respect to truth in itself, and, from a right way of acting with respect to a human being, that is, acting well.

If medicine were solely an art, we would judge it by the degree to which its instrumental actions achieved its ends. Thus, on the classical notion of art or *techné* the physician would be like the artist. He would be judged by his mastery of the principles of diagnosis, prognosis, and therapeutics. On this view, he would not need to be a good human himself. He would need only to possess the virtues proper to his artistic activity. There is a growing inclination to see medicine this way in our time when medicine has become highly industrialized, commercialized, and bureaucratized.

However, such a partial view of the ends of medicine as only an 'art' is untenable, given the phenomena that govern the clinical encounter. Yes, the physician must master the *techné*, but he also must do so for a specific moral end as well. The necessary virtues of clinical medicine are directed to a human good, the good of a particular patient. Thus, medicine (and other true professions like law, ministry, or teaching) cannot achieve their ends unless their technical artistry serves a moral end—the good of the patient (the student, the client, or the parishioner).

The end of medicine is the act of healing, literally to 'make whole again'. Healing combines the technical and the moral ends of medicine since it is undertaken in the interests of a particular patient, that is, for the good of the patient. Healing aims whenever possible to restore health, that is, to reverse the mental and physical disruptions in the balance of a person's life. When this is not possible, healing always requires relief of pain and suffering, and restoration of function. Care for the patient is always a mandatory end of medicine and never futile. When medicine's technical powers fail to alter the progression of disease and death is inevitable, the physician must help the patient to cope with the fact of dying. The physician cannot and should not replace family, friends, and ministers. But the physician must remain a friend and helper to the end.

The good of the patient is the moral object, the intentional direction of the acts of medicine. In medicine, technical and moral good are so intimately fused that to attempt to separate them is to do violence to the practice itself. This being the case, the virtues which dispose the clinician to the end of medicine are both intellectual and moral. The virtues of medicine are entailed by both the techniques and the moral ends of medicine. Medicine is, to use the ancient terminology, *both* a right way of **doing**, and a right way of **acting**, that is, *recta ratio factibilium* and *recta ratio agibilium* (Maritain 1942).

d) The Good of the Patient: The End of Clinical Medicine

To examine these virtues and the moral foundations that necessitate them more clearly, we must delineate the good of the patient in greater detail. The good of the patient is a composite notion necessitated by the comprehensiveness of the idea of healing and the complexity of the human condition. Healing is a good of the whole person—psychosocial, biological, personal, and spiritual. Each of these dimensions of human existence may to varying degrees be compromised by illness and disease. Ideally, each must be addressed if the whole person is to be healed.

Up to this point, I have used the terms ends, good of the patient, healing, and so on. It is now important to define as precisely as possible the relations between the good of the patient and the ends of clinical medicine. The good of medicine is taken in the sense in which Aristotle uses it in the opening lines of the *Nichomachean Ethics*, 'that at which all things aim' (*NE* 1094a 3). The good aimed at varies with each art and activity, and, in the case of medicine, that good is 'health' (*NE* 1094a 7). This is the ultimate end of medicine as medicine. This *ultimate end*, again following Aristotle, is served by subordinate ends, which I shall call *proximate* and *immediate*—those more immediately related to the concrete and specific phenomena of clinical medicine.

Within this schema, the *proximate end* of the clinical encounter has several possible dimensions depending on the clinical context, that is, curing disease when possible, relief of suffering, always providing comfort, care, and counseling, and so on. The *immediate end* is the first step toward both the proximate and ultimate end. The immediate end is making the right and good decision which shapes the action to be taken to answer the patient's need, that is, to know what is wrong, what can be done about it, how and at what cost in suffering, and so on. These are the three elements of the medical good, that is, the aim and purview of the clinician qua clinician. Each in its way serves the ultimate end of health, and, taken together, these ends serve *healing*, that is, to make whole to the extent possible.

What I have just described are components of the medical good. But the medical good is not the whole of human good. It exists within a larger frame of the good for humans, which of course goes beyond the medical good. In this sense, the good of medicine serves the good of the patient as a human person. The physician is primarily responsible for the medical good of his patient. However, he also has responsibility for assessing the other levels of the patient's good—that is, the patient's own opinion of what is good for him, the good of the patient as human being with rights and intrinsic dignity, and his spiritual good. The physician often plays a secondary role in addressing goods beyond the strictly medical. Yet it is his responsibility to detect needs beyond the medical, to refer the patient to the proper professional, and to work cooperatively with that professional.

Within the classical concept of virtue as a character trait that habitually disposes an agent to the good, the medical virtues are those character traits that dispose habitually to the medical good as defined above.

The Hippocratic Oath addresses the end of medicine as beneficence: 'I will follow that system or regimen which, according to my ability and judgment, I consider for the benefit of my patient and abstain from whatever is deleterious and mischievous' (Hippocrates 1972b: 299). Thomasma and I have suggested that the good of medicine is a composite of four elements or ends in general (Pellegrino and Thomasma 1987). The first has as its end the medical or physiological good, that for which the patient immediately presents herself. The second level is the personal good, that is, the good as perceived by the patient, that which the patient expects medical good to serve; third is the good of the patient as a human being, that is, the good for humans as humans, those goods common to all humans by virtue of their common humanity. The fourth is the spiritual good, the patient's perception of her good in relationship to some transcendent reality, to a source of good beyond man. Each patient is unique in the way she defines and orders these goods.

For some, this quadripartite hierarchy of good is an ascending order of good. For others, it is not. As a result, the moral relationship between, and among, these levels of good is peculiar to the patient in question. It distorts the integrity of the good of a patient to exaggerate or neglect one good to the exclusion of another. Each should be served to the extent the contingencies of the clinical situation allow.

(1) The Medical Good

The medical good is that which relates most directly to the art of medicine, that part which is uniquely medical. The medical good aims at the return of physiological function of mind and body, the relief of pain and suffering, by medication, surgical interventions, psychotherapy, and so on. At this level, the patient's good depends on the right use of the physician's knowledge and skill, those that are intrinsically part of the medical *techné*.

But the medical good must be brought into proper relationship with the other levels of the patient's good. Otherwise, it may become harmful. What is medically 'good' simply on grounds of physiological effectiveness may not be 'good', if it violates the patient's good as he perceives that good. For the Jehovah's Witness, medically indicated blood transfusion may be a medical good, but certainly not a spiritual good. For a Christian Scientist, antibiotics might cure pneumonia, but it would not be a 'good' for the patient. For a secular humanist, the medical good is the fulfillment of what he values as the good, or simply the relief of suffering by any means.

(2) The Patient's Perception of the Good

To be morally valid, the medical good should serve the many complex facets of what the patient perceives as his own good. Here, we are concerned with the patient's personal preferences, choices, and values, the kind of life he wants to live, and the balance he strikes between the benefit and burdens of the proposed intervention. These qualities and values are unique for each patient and cannot be defined by the physician, the family, or anyone else. They are determined by the interrelationships between and among age, gender, station in life, occupation, and so on, in the narrative of a particular patient's life. To serve the patient's perception of the good, the medical good must be placed within the context of *this* patient's life-plans. The strictly medical or physiological good may not coincide with the patient's conception of his own good or with his conception of the good for humans as humans. In that case, the medical good may be technically correct but morally wrong.

(3) The Good for Humans

Medical good and the patient's perception of the good life are related to the good for humans as humans. This is the good Aristotle and Aquinas sought to define as the *telos* of human life. At this level, we are concerned with the good peculiar to humans, self-preservation, preservation of dignity of the human person, respect for his rationality as a creature, someone who is an end in himself and not a mere means, whose value is inherent and not determined by wealth, education, position in life, and so on. The patient is a fellow human with the physician. The physician is bound to the patient by solidarity and mutual respect.

It is at this level that some of the more familiar principles of medical ethics are philosophically rooted, like autonomy, beneficence, non-maleficence, and justice. In American bioethics, these principles are taken to be prima facie principles grounded in a 'common morality' (Beauchamp and Childress 2001). This suggests that they could be changed if the 'common morality' were to change. For natural law ethicists this is not the case. The good for humans is not merely subject to social or cultural construction. It is inherent of human nature and a requirement of the natural law. At this level, the good for humans is the good peculiar to humans as beings of a specific kind.

In the clinical encounter, the medical good and the personal good must, in their turn, be consistent with, and protect, the good for human beings. Physicians who ignore the patient's notion of what is good violate the good of the patient as a self-determining rational being. Denial of care to the poor violates their dignity and value as human beings. Devaluing the lives of the handicapped does the same. Putting patients at experimental risks that outweigh potential benefits, even with informed patient consent, violates the precept of doing good and avoiding evil. These are all instances of violations of human rights, that is, those based in the dignity of the human person (see the United Nations Declaration of Human Rights).

(4) Spiritual Good

For many patients, the highest level of good which must be served in the clinical encounter is the patient's good as a spiritual being, that is, as one who, in his own way, acknowledges some end to life beyond mere material existence. This may, or may not, be expressed in religious terms. Most patients acknowledge some realm of 'spirit', however differently they may define it. Many may consider this good the most important one for themselves or others. Not all do, of course. This realm of spirit gives ultimate meaning to many human lives. It is that for which some humans will often make the greatest sacrifices. For many, the realm of the spirit coincides with a specific religion. This is expressed in a set of specific beliefs or doctrines that carry ultimate weight in many decisions. They are particularly important in end-of-life decisions.

Spiritual good, however, refers not necessarily to religious belief, but rather to the answers a patient has arrived at about the ultimate questions—that is, What is it to be human? What meanings should be attached to life?, and so on. In brief, it is the patient's own 'philosophy of life'. Having such a philosophy is part of being a rational, reflective, inquiring, and responsible human person. Whether one shares the patient's philosophy or religion, the physician must take it into account so that treatment of the body will not injure the patient's perception of the good.

How to attain this good, how to deal with differences between what a patient may wish in this respect, and what is attainable is beyond the scope of this essay. My intent is to signal this realm as part of the context of a human's life experience. Recognizing this dimension does not imply that the good and virtuous physician must comply with all patients' wishes, even if they violate his or her moral integrity. Physician and patient owe each other mutual respect. Their differences must be managed in an ethically sensitive way.

e) Some Complexities

In many clinical encounters it may not be possible to assess each of the four levels of patient good and establish a clear order of moral priorities among them. This is the case with infants, children below the age for responsible decision-making, the intellectually disabled, the elderly, or those in permanent vegetative states. In these circumstances knowledge about the patient's personal preferences or spiritual beliefs may be lacking. Yet, clinical ethics imposes the duty to come as close as circumstances permit to an estimate of the patient's good as a whole and the levels within it of special concern to that patient.

In such cases, two levels of the good are still accessible—that is, the medical good, and the good of the patient as a human being. In the case of infants it is impossible to know about preferences, and so on. Surrogates and others must be relied upon to represent the particularities from prior knowledge of the patient's personal or spiritual preferences. How these are best balanced with medical good is a matter for more extended analysis than possible here. Surrogates, to be morally valid proxies, must be without significant conflicts of interest. In the end the physician is still responsible for what is done for the patient and must therefore remain a guardian of the patient's interests, good, or welfare especially for the most vulnerable patients.

In a pluralist society, a particular patient's preferences, world-views, and religious practices may conflict with the physicians own beliefs about what is good for the patient. I have emphasized the primacy of the good of the patient. However, the good, as perceived by the physician, must also be respected as well. The dictum of the primacy of the good of the patient does not override the physician's conscience or his judgment of what is good medicine, what he thinks of the human life issues, and the spiritual destiny of himself and his patient. Resolutions of conflicts in these areas of interest are frequent occasions for ethics consultation.

Whatever the patient's spiritual or religious beliefs, the physician must decide whether accommodation to them is consistent with his or her own perceptions of medical good. Physicians cannot be expected to sacrifice personal and scientific integrity to satisfy every patient's preferences. Patients who expect healing to mean satisfaction of their personal preferences distort the healing purposes of medicine. What is required is a sensitivity to those preferences, that is to say, a recognition of their existence, importance, and kind. The physician must take them into consideration consciously to understand if he can concur and still maintain personal and professional integrity.

As our society becomes ever more pluralistic ethnically, culturally, and spiritually, it becomes even more obligatory that physicians be aware of the broad outline of the beliefs and values they may encounter. To this end, the John Templeton Foundation has funded programs in 'spirituality' in medicine in nearly a dozen American medical schools. These programs alert medical students to cross-cultural attitudes in their patients so that they can be more sensitively confronted in the clinical encounter.

'Spiritual' and 'religious' are not synonymous terms. Spirituality, as I am using it above and elsewhere, refers to the recognition of some entity, force, power, source, outside of, and beyond, the material aspects of human constitution and the visible structures of the world around us. Religion, on the other hand, is a specific form of spirituality; one's religion resides in the existence of some divine power to whom worship is due in some prescribed manner.

Many people today characterize themselves, in surveys, for example, as 'spiritual' but not 'religious'. Many who label themselves as 'religious' do not attend church or worship regularly. Clearly, in today's world, a wide variety of beliefs fit under both rubrics, that is, 'spiritual' or 'religious'. They are important in people's lives and often have a role in how they wish to be treated medically. To understand these, to respect them, without capitulating to them is a delicate, but genuine, element in professional ethics.

Similar difficulties are encountered in the interpretation of clinical futility. This is a central criterion in deciding the medical good especially in decisions to withhold or withdraw life-sustaining measures. Clinical futility can be defined as the balancing of a relationship between the effectiveness, benefits, and burdens of intervention. Effectiveness is an objective assessment of whether a treatment will change the natural history of the disease; benefit is the patient's or surrogate's estimate that the treatment will serve some value of the patient's; burdens are the physical, emotional, and fiscal costs of the treatment. To be worthwhile, there must be some acceptable proportionality in the ratio of effectiveness, benefit, and burdens. But this calculus may result in different or opposing conclusions about whether it is morally permissible to discontinue treatment (Pellegrino 2000). The physician, the patient, or the patient's proxy may differ seriously on what is 'good' for the patient in these circumstances.

From the moral point of view, there is no obligation for the physician to provide futile or disproportionately burdensome treatments. This would be to do harm, not good. Yet, some patients' families want 'everything' done, including cardiopulmonary resuscitation even when the data show it would be unsuccessful. These and many other conflicts in the interpretation of the 'good' of the patient are frequent in the clinical encounter today. They promise to become even more widespread in our morally polyglot society.

These complexities emphasize the need for greater clarity in the ethics of the process of clinical ethical decision-making. They do not vitiate or trivialize the importance of a definition of the ends of medicine. Indeed without some clarity on those ends, the process of ethical decision-making would become even more difficult. Making choices does not equate with the right choices (Taylor 1980). Unscrambling wrong choices and conflicts of choices is a recurrent problem in clinical ethics.

f) Virtues in Role Related Ethics: Medicine as a 'Practice'

Most discussion of virtues concentrates on general ethics, that is, the relation of virtue to the good of human life, that is, the good for humans. Virtue within a specific activity like medicine (special ethics in the terminology used here) has a narrower meaning, existentially if not essentially. In this respect, MacIntyre's work on virtues defined within the concept of practices is helpful.

MacIntyre offers a very 'tentative' definition of virtue: 'A virtue is an acquired human quality the possession and exercise of which tends to enable us to achieve those goods internal to practices and the lack of which effectively prevents us from achieving any such goods' (1984: 191). By 'practices' MacIntyre means:

> any coherent and complex form of socially established cooperative human activity through which goods internal to that form of activity are realized in the course of trying to achieve those standards of excellence which are appropriate to, and partially definitive of, that form of the activity, with the result that human powers to achieve excellence and human conceptions of the ends and good involved are systematically extended. (1984: 187)

Medicine is cited by MacIntyre as a practice in this sense (1984: 194). It possesses an internal good, a set of rules and obligations related to that good, and a set of virtues requisite for achieving the internal good and without which that good is unattainable. The virtues of medicine are the standards of excellence needed to actualize its internal good, which is the good of the patient as I have described it earlier in this essay.

The health professions in general fit MacIntyre's definition of 'practices'. Thus, for a health profession, there is a specific end (good) which defines it as a 'practice' and which, if executed with excellence, enables the end to be achieved excellently, and which makes the professional a good professional. The good internal to health professions, as defined above, is multi-faceted, for example, healing: helping, caring, curing, and comforting sick persons. These are actions for the good of the patient, and they are subsumed under the broad heading of healing, that is, to make whole again, to restore function, cure disease, relieve pain and suffering, to the extent possible. The professional who heals well does his or her work well and becomes, by that fact, a good professional. Healing is the internal good of the practice of medicine which must be pursued for itself and not for the external goods which may accompany it, that is, profit, pleasure, prestige, or power.

Thus, the physician or nurse who performs well, with respect to the internal good of the clinical encounter, is a virtuous, a 'good', nurse or physician. Exercise of the right virtues for the right reasons makes the nurse or physician a good person and makes him do his (her) work well (*NE* 1106a 22–4).

g) Professional Ethics and the Act of Profession

If we are not to see the professional virtues as merely admirable traits, we need some grounding for them beyond subjective opinion. Such grounding can be derived for the medical virtues from three existential phenomena of the healing relationship—the human relationship between one who is ill and one who 'professes' to heal. Three phenomena are central: the *fact* of illness, the *act* of profession, and the *art* of medicine (Pellegrino 1976, 1979; Pellegrino and Thomasma 1981). From the ethical point of view, the act of 'profession' is the moral impetus, which entails the virtues required of the good physician.

The *fact of illness* is the inescapable reality that the sick person is in a state of vulnerability, in need of help, dependent upon others for help and technical knowledge. The sick person is exploitable, anxious, often in pain or suffering. The humanity of the patient, that is, her capacity to pursue her life goals in her own terms, is compromised to a significant degree.

With the patient in that vulnerable state, the physician or other health professional makes a private act of profession—that is, she declares aloud and voluntarily that she is a healer, one who can help and offers to help. This act of profession is made the moment the professional offers to help. This is what being a 'professional' means etymologically. The act of profession is made every day with every encounter with a sick person. It is then a private act of profession—a promise made to an identifiable person. It is made in a more public and general way at the beginning of medical school when the medical student first dons a white coat. It is repeated at graduation when some variant of the Hippocratic Oath is recited. These public acts make the graduate a 'professional', much more than the fact that she has expert knowledge, has a degree in medicine, belongs to a professional body, or is licensed to practice medicine (Freidson 2001: 12). These are the sociological definitions of a 'professional', but the grounding for its moral meaning for each physician is its promise to help an identifiable human person in need of help.

This act of profession elicits an expectation on the patient's part that one who so professes has the requisite knowledge and will use it in the interests of the one seeking help. The act of profession signals the initiation of a covenant of trust on the part of the professional. That covenant promises fulfillment of the patient's expectations of expertise and the use of that expertise for the benefit of the patient. The patient who agrees to be treated by the doctor or nurse accepts the promise and expects it to be fulfilled with fidelity. The patient's part of the covenant is to facilitate, or at least not frustrate, the physician's ability to meet his covenantal obligations.

The 'art' of medicine incorporates the healing acts the patient expects to be undertaken to attain the good he seeks (help, care, cure, and so on). This is what is promised by the physician's act of profession. This art encompasses the many actions available in modern therapeutics—diagnostic procedures, medications, surgery, psychotherapy, and so on. Whatever form it takes, the art of healing must be carried out safely, competently, and with respect for the person of the patient. Thus, competence is an essential component of any realization of the internal good of the clinical relationship. In the end, then, the art of medicine requires a fusion of a morally right and a technically correct decision and action. This is the promise held out in the act of profession and it entails both the moral and the intellectual virtues.

Individual and private acts of medicine, acts of promise, are made daily in the encounter with each patient. These private acts are, however, embedded in a more public act of promise or profession when the physician takes an Oath at graduation. Today these Oaths vary in content considerably, but their symbolic and existential meaning remains unchanged (Orr, Pang, Pellegrino, and Siegler 1997). Graduation Oaths are public declarations of commitment to the use of acquired medical knowledge for something other than selfish self-interest. With the Oath, those who have received a medical degree enter the profession. However, the medical degree per se does not make the physician a true 'professional'. It is a certificate of qualifications only.

Having participated in the public declaration, however, the graduate elicits expectations in the public and social realm. Even if the graduate engages in mental reservations about what he is willing to promise, he is committed unless he publicly disowns the oath he has taken. He must make his dissent clear so that he will not be identified as one who is committed to the use of his knowledge for the good of others.

h) Moral Virtues Entailed by the Act of Profession

Given the existential status of the sick person, he or she must finally trust the physician's character. One may search out the physician's credentials, reputation, or other attributes, but in the end, the patient must trust the physician to act well with reaction to the patient's good. This fact does not grant the physician the privileges of authoritarian paternalism. Rather, it imposes obligations to exhibit the virtue of fidelity to trust. Indeed, fidelity to trust is entailed by the act of profession and the circumstances in which it is made. It is a central and indispensable medical virtue.

'Entailment' is used here in its sense of a conclusion that follows from the premises. Certain virtues can be inferred from the existential reality of the act of profession. Without them, the act of profession is meaningless. This sense of virtue entailment extends to other virtues requisite to the attainment of the internal goods of the medical encounter. Some of the most important of those virtues are benevolence, some degree of effacement of self-interest, intellectual honesty, compassion, courage, and humility. Each virtue disposes the physician to act in such a way that the good of the patient is sought to the degree possible given the particular exigencies of the patient's physical, physiological, and emotional state.

On this view, benevolence goes beyond preventing harm, which is the bare minimum of moral responsibility, equivalent only to what is required by law. Benevolence must also mean seeking the good of the patient even when it means some effacement of the physician's self-interest, that is, when doing the good requires some loss of time, convenience, or money on the physician's part. This is not to demand absolute or heroic activism more than is expected of non-professionals.

In a similar vein, intellectual honesty requires disclosure of the limits of one's knowledge and skill. This enables patients to make free choices and give informed consent. The virtue of compassion is necessary if care is to be personalized. Compassion allows for those changes in approach that come from putting oneself in the patient's place, that is, feeling something of the uniqueness of the patient's predicament. Courage is needed to assure that care is not compromised by fear of contagion, or censure for being the patient's advocate in relations with institutional policies or administrative policies deemed injurious to the patient. Humility assures that the enormous powers of medicine to heal and harm are used not to advance the physician's own self image, interests, or pride. It acknowledges the limitations of the art. It is the antidote to the vice of physician arrogance that demeans the person of the patient.

Another, essential virtue in today's environment of self-interest is suppression of self-interest, at least to some degree. Physicians hold medical knowledge in trust. They were given a social mandate that allowed them to dissect human bodies, to participate in the care of patients, and to perform procedures before they were qualified to do so. Even though, under supervision, participation by medical students and residents slows down patient care and can increase its discomfort, as well as morbidity. Therefore, responsibility for care of the sick is an obligation owed to society in return for the social contract implied in society's sanction for the idea of clinical training.

These are some of the most important moral virtues required to attain the internal good of the clinical encounter in almost any case of significant illness (Pellegrino and Thomasma 1993). Others may be required and they will be identified if the clinician possesses the virtue of practical wisdom or *phronesis*. Here we enter the realm of the intellectual virtues, those essential for medical decisions and acts to be technically sound, safe, and competent. These are the virtues that dispose to truth, what some today call the 'epistemological' virtues (Zagzebski 1996; Hockaway 1994).

i) The Intellectual Virtues, the Act and the Art of Profession

Aristotle, and Thomas Aquinas after him, both recognized that truth and good are intimately related. For Aristotle, 'a good action and its opposite cannot exist without a combination of intellect and character' (*NE* 1139a 33–4). Aristotle lists the intellectual virtues—those ordered to truth—as five: 'art, knowledge, practical wisdom, philosophic wisdom and comprehension' (*NE* 1139b 4–5). These virtues are understood differently in Aristotle's time from what their names might suggest in ours (Ross 1959). Thus, knowledge is 'the state of capacity to demonstrate' (*NE* 1139b 31) the starting of reasoning by induction and syllogism. Art, which is right reason with respect to doing things (*NE* 1140a 1–23), is an art of making, not acting. Practical wisdom, or *phronesis*, deals with a true disposition toward action, a power of deliberation about the things good for oneself (*NE* 1140a 24–30; 1140b 1–30). Intuitive reason is the power to grasp a universal truth as self-evident. Theoretical wisdom is, for Aristotle, the highest science and it deals with the 'highest' things. It is distinguished from practical wisdom however, which is concerned with deliberation about action (*NE* 1141a 1–15).

Thomas Aquinas, following Aristotle, lists the intellectual virtues as: wisdom, science, art, understanding, and prudence. These are virtues of the speculative intellect suited to the consideration of truth. They are not moral virtues. Persons may possess intellectual virtues yet not use them to pursue good ends (*ST* I-II Q 57 art. 1,2). Aquinas carefully distinguishes the intellectual and moral virtues (*ST* I-II Q 58). Thomas, like Aristotle, however, puts special emphasis on the intellectual virtue of prudence (*phronesis* in Aristotle), that is, practical wisdom.

For clinicians, the intellectual virtues as a whole are essential to the technical correctness of necessary medical acts for good. Prudence, however, is the most crucial for the clinician. It is the virtue which is 'right reason about things to be done (and this not merely in general but also in particular)' (*ST* I-II Q 58 art. 5). Prudence links the intellectual and the moral virtues, thus: 'Consequently an intellectual virtue is needed in the reason, to perfect the reason and make it suitably affected toward things ordained to the end, and this virtue is prudence' (*ST* I-II Q 57 art. 5).

In the clinical realm, prudence is the central intellectual virtue. Aristotle defines it as 'a true and seasoned capacity to act with regard to the things that are good or bad for man' (*NE* 1140a 24–1140b 21; 1140b 4–5). Within the narrower confines of a role-related, or professional, ethics like medicine, prudence would refer to the reasoned capacity to act with regard to the things good for the patient—both technical and moral. Prudence enables the clinician to evaluate clinical facts, to relate the particulars of a case to the moral implications of each, to put the other virtues into proper relationships to each other, and to choose the right means to a morally right end in complex and previously unencumbered situations. Prudence is the analogue of clinical judgment in the moral sphere.

Thus, the individual virtues (intellectual and moral) are 'entailed' by the act of medicine, that is, by the promise of professional competence. They orient us to the medical good of the patient and enable us to take the right steps, in proper order, and put into practice the right orientation of values for this particular person if his good is to be achieved. Prudence links the intellectual and moral virtues with the end of the medical act of profession. Prudence provides reasoned guidance to the other virtues, and it is essential to the fusion of the technically correct, and morally good of the moral and intellectual virtues. '[T]he choice will not be right without particular wisdom; any more than without virtue; for the one determines the end and the other makes us do the things that lead to the end' (*NE* 1145a 4–6).

PART III: IMPLICATIONS FOR THE OTHER HELPING PROFESSIONS

The conceptual schema proposed in this essay to redefine the virtues of medicine in terms of the good of the patient and the act of profession has applicability beyond medicine. With proper definition of the ends peculiar to each profession, this schema also defines the good of the lawyer's client, the teacher's student, and the minister's penitent or parishioner. As with medicine, the ends of these other helping professions are linked to a particular activity specific to each profession. Each profession has its own 'act' of promise which invites trust and entails certain virtue as a result. Each has a morality internal to its end and the kind of activity it is.

Law, ministry, teaching, and medicine share a common phenomenological ground. They all deal with human beings in compromised existential states. The persons they serve are dependent, anxious, in distress, and lacking something essential to human flourishing. That lack in medicine is health; in law it is justice; in education, knowledge; and in ministry, union with God. Humans in these compromised existential states are eminently vulnerable and exploitable. Persons in that state are invited by the promissory act of each profession to trust the professional. Each, indeed, *must* trust that professional in order to be helped or healed. In each instance, the untrustworthy professional could exploit the patient's vulnerability for personal power, profit, or prestige. In each case, the character of the professional is the final safeguard of the subject's bodily and psychological integrity. In each case, the end of professional activity is the good of the person in need of help.

As with the medical relationship, the 'good' in each of the other three helping professions has four components: (1) a level of technical good, (2) the good perceived by the person served, (3) the good needed for the person to flourish as a human being, and (4) the spiritual good. Each profession operates primarily on one or other of the four levels. But, regardless of its specific focus, each profession also attends to the totality of the good of the person served by that profession.

For example, the lawyer focuses on obtaining justice for his client. Justice is a good of the client as a human being necessary to fulfillment of his human nature. But the lawyer cannot attain that end unless he is also concerned with the first level of the good—the legal good—that is, he must be competent in legal practice. He must be fully competent in legal procedures and in those techniques necessary to press his case in court, negotiations, or depositions. These are necessary for a right verdict but not entirely sufficient for a good verdict, for the lawyer must also be aware of the other levels of the client's values.

Thus, at the second level: What does the client deem justice to be in his case? To what degree does he wish to risk gain or loss, to settle out of court, to demand retribution? At the third level, the lawyer's success or failure is attendant on the degree to which he can gain for his client the human right of justice, freedom, vindication, or, if his client is guilty, a fair sentence. Finally, at the fourth level, to the extent that his client's religious or spiritual beliefs shape his plea for justice, they must be taken into account. For example, the client may be willing to forgo certain of his claims in the name of charity for his opponent. Thus, as in medicine, all four levels of the good must be factored into the outcome or ends of the morally valid lawyer–client relationship.

Teaching may be similarly treated. As he is the possessor of knowledge and skill, the teacher's major emphasis will be at level three. Knowledge and truth are goods essential to human flourishing and fulfillment. To help others to achieve those goods, the teacher must, at the first level, possess the knowledge and skill specific to the art he purports to teach. He must have mastery of the teaching methods, sources, and technical apparatus without which the end of knowledge transmission cannot be attained. At the second level, teachers must also adapt, to some significant degree, to the interests, learning modes, work habits, and career aspirations of the student. In the interests of the good of the student, teachers also may have to modify, restrain, or replace their own interest to some degree if they interfere with the end of learning. At the third level, that of the good for humans, teachers are required to treat their students with the dignity owed to persons, to treat them fairly, honestly, and so on. Finally, at the fourth level, spiritual beliefs must be respected, allowed to flourish, and integrated with the more technical or academic dimensions of the student's education.

The priest–parishioner or minister–parishioner relationship has its moral dimension most specifically at level four, the *level of the spiritual good*. This is what the parishioner and penitent seeks from the minister, that is, counsel on his relationship with God; how to be reconciled with God after sin; how to grow in the spiritual life; how to decide moral questions in light of revelation or church teaching; how to adapt to death, hardship, and so on in accordance with Divine Will. For religious persons, the spiritual good takes precedence over the other levels of good. But the other levels cannot, by that fact, be ignored since they are part of the integral good of the person served. Physician, minister, lawyer may need to work closely together to effect the necessary synthesis.

At the first level, therefore, priests must be skilled in the ends of the activities specific to the priestly vocation, that is, mastery of the theological or pastoral skills required to make their counsel serve the good of the penitent. At the second level, they must take into account the parishioner's unique values, the uniqueness of his spiritual predicament, his station in life, preferences for spiritual charisma, styles of prayer, life situation, and so on. At the third level, the priest must protect the good of the parishioner as a human being, that is, maintain the seal of the confessional, help the penitent to integrate his spiritual and his temporal good, appreciate his dignity as a child of God, and so on.

In each profession, the four components of the client's good are arranged in some hierarchical order. For many, the spiritual good (as defined above) takes precedence over all, followed, in descending order, by the good for humans, the personal evaluation of the good, and, at the lowest level, the technical good specific to each profession. Moral decisions in the course of professional activities are 'right' if they conform to the *techné* of each profession at the first level. But to be morally 'good', they must also conform at the other levels as well. For each person, the order of priority between and among levels will be unique.

In sum, the four 'helping' professions share a common end, a common devotion as it were, to the good of vulnerable persons who need their expertise. Each profession 'professes' to act for the good of the person served. This act of profession makes it a true profession. Each profession by this act invites the trust of the person that the promise to act for his or her interest will be fulfilled. Fidelity to trust and other virtues required to achieve the good of the person are entailed by the *initial act of profession*. Each act of profession entails both the moral and the intellectual virtues which are necessary to assure that what is done and advised is technically right and morally good.

On the view I have been presenting, virtue theory, at least for the professions, is not locked in an iron circle of logical redundancy. In each case, the beginning of professional virtue theory is the private or public act of profession, the act that promises fidelity to an end, that is, the good of the patient (client, student, or parishioner). This is the beginning point, the *terminus a quo*. From the outset, the end is the good peculiar to a profession, that is, the *terminus ad quem*, the end specific to the profession in question. There is therefore a linear direction, a purposeful, teleological moral trajectory that energizes professional ethics.

Another aspect of a virtue-based moral philosophy for the professions is the existential distinction it implies between *being* a professional and *having* a profession. Gabriel Marcel (1965) made this point in a brilliant essay in which he distinguished possessing something and being something.

It is one thing to *have* the qualifications of a profession—a formal education, a degree, a title commensurate with both, as well as a position, a set of responsibilities, and mastery of certain skills and knowledge sufficient to be accepted socially as a physician. It is quite another to *be* a physician, to be transformed as a person, to be the kind of person healing others requires. Such a person would exhibit character traits or virtues that dispose him or her predictably to act in such a way that the healing purposes of medicine are fulfilled. To *be* a physician or other true professional is to have assimilated the medical virtues into one's person in such a way that one's perspectives on illness, suffering, death are permanently altered.

Today there are many more physicians who 'have' a profession than persons who 'are' physicians. Some part of the moral malaise afflicting medical ethics and professionalism today is the failure to understand the reality of Marcel's distinction. Clearly, 'having' a profession might well include having completed a course in medical ethics. But having does not automatically translate into being. It is more than the sociological fact of membership in a group labeled 'professional' by certain external standards. Rather, being a professional is to live in a certain way, in so far as the sick person is concerned.

PART IV: SOME OBJECTIONS

The line of argument developed here with respect to the virtues in medical practice derives from a philosophy of medicine I suggested in 1976 (Pellegrino) and subsequently developed in a series of books and articles co-authored with David Thomasma (1981, 1987, 1993).

To ground an ethic of medicine in a philosophy of medicine does not entail commitment to an idiosyncratic ethic or philosophy limited to medicine. Nor does it mean that every profession or art must possess its own peculiar ethic. Instead, this account begins with the realities and phenomena of the medical or healing relationship. These phenomena define medicine as the specific kind of human activity it is. This sets it apart from other activities. It brackets specific ethical theories. Once having arrived phenomenologically at the nature or *eidos* of the medical encounter, existing ethical theories can account for the specific virtues, duties, obligations required of both physician and patient if the defined end (the good) of the patient is best to be achieved. Central place is given to the principle of promise-keeping as it is specified in the phenomenology of the act of profession.

Admittedly, I employ a combination of a classical theory of virtue and ends with some elements of modern phenomenological realism. I do not, however, begin with a specific normative content, as would be the case with well-established ethical theories. Thus, Kantian deontology would commit us to the categorical imperative, utilitarianism to the utilitarian calculus, consequentialism to the results of acts, social construction and dialogue ethics to consensus, and so on. Methodologically, my approach does not per se rule out any of these theories, which one may use from time to time in resolving ethical dilemmas. Rather, I ask which existing theory fits most closely the existential realities of the medical encounter, that is, which one enables the moral agent most closely to attain the end of the encounter?

This methodology differs from the usual, in which a well-established theory of norms or principles is applied to the dilemmas of medical practices. The method pursued here starts instead with the phenomena of clinical medicine and, from them, it adduces an 'internal' morality of medicine, one rooted in the kind of activity medicine is. But, as such, it is not *sui generis*, an independent system of morals.

An example is the act of profession as described earlier in this essay. The act of profession is a promise made by the physician to act in the interests of the patient, that is, to act for the patient's good in its several dimensions. As a promise made voluntarily, it must be kept in accordance with the norms of the ethics of promise making and fidelity to trust relationships. This method is not an instance of the naturalist fallacy. It develops no new norm, an ought is not derived from an 'is'. Rather, the actualities of the 'is' require application of the ethics of promise keeping. They do not establish that ethic. An internal morality of medicine, then, is not a morality independent of established theories. Rather, it defines which of those theories are entailed by the phenomena of medicine. It leaves open the debate about the validity of one ethical theory over another. It does argue in this essay for a realist epistemology and metaphysics as possessing greater coherence than other theories.

In this essay, the theory entailed is virtue theory. But virtue theory does not stand alone. It is related to other theories, with the determinative factor again being the kind of activity medicine is essentially and existentially. The *telos* of the clinical encounter defines the virtues, as well as the norms, an ethically sound physician–patient relationship requires.

I accept the existence of certain moral principles, virtues, duties, and so on derived from pre-existing theories. I do not invent them to fit the phenomena of clinical medicine. I attempt, rather, by a reflection on the phenomena, and by bracketing ethical theories to discover which principles, duties, or virtues are specifically required to reach the *telos* of medical acts. The moral content of professional medical ethics derives from the phenomenon of the act of promise. The act of promise generates the obligation to be faithful to the promise.

In 1994, Daryl Koehn based professional ethics in a public commitment and promise which entailed obligations. Koehn rejected the usual sociological descriptive signs of a profession as the source of its moral status. Koehn put emphasis on the act of profession as I do, but there are significant differences. Koehn's account does not derive specifically from a philosophy of medicine. It makes no connection with virtue theory, ancient or modern, or with ends in any teleological sense. Koehn's analysis is more consistent with a social contract foundation for professional ethics. This work is a valuable contribution to a better understanding of the meaning of profession and professionalism, but, in my opinion, it is insufficiently fundamental as a basis for profession in ethics.

Some contemporary ethicists would object to the implications that Koehn as well as Thomasma and I believe follow from the nature of the act of profession. They take the virtues to be supererogatory, that is, beyond what virtue or duty require. McKay (2002) argues that entering medicine presupposes 'unqualified' supererogation because of the risks the physician incurs when he enters medical practice. O'Neill argues for supererogation of another kind—not in the categories of duties physicians assume, but in the degree to which the performance of these duties should exceed ordinary measures of duty (1996).

Downie, on the other hand, sees no virtue, or altruism, in the physician's work. Therefore, there is no supererogation possible. Acting for the patient's best interests is simply part of the doctor's job description (2002). In a similar vein, Veatch, maintaining his customary skepticism about virtues and the capacity of physicians to know anything about a patient's good, also doubts that physicians' Oaths have any genuine meaning (2002).

Many physicians will agree in principle with the argument presented in this essay, but object that it is too 'idealistic' or impossible to observe in the commercialized managed care milieu of medical practice today. They paraphrase Machiavelli's advice to his Prince that one cannot be virtuous and survive when everyone else pragmatically ignores virtue (2003). Many physicians today follow Machiavelli's advice in the name of survival. They argue not without reason that managed care, the market ethos, and malpractice suits 'force' them to be practical. In a way, they confirm the suspicions of medicine's harshest criticism, that physician self-interest is so ubiquitous as to make virtuous ethics a fantasy.

Unfortunately, there is enough truth in the assertions of these self-styled realists that some physicians take refuge in a Hobbesian defense of self-interest. These criticisms notwithstanding, they cannot erase the ineradicable fact that the physician's character traits are the locus on which trust pivots in any serious bedside decision. Fortunately, there are still enough physicians who recognize that the medical virtues are not supererogatory, but intrinsic to the moral status of the clinical relationship.

Making and keeping promises is, after all, the most rudimentary of moral obligations. Any human relationship not based in confidence that a promise will be kept is morally bankrupt at the outset. The act of profession which initiates the physician–patient relationship entails certain virtues as this essay argues. Fidelity to the trust invoked by the physician's act of profession is a sure measure of the degree to which a clinician is a physician in his being, as opposed to simply having a profession.

REFERENCES

Anscombe, G. E. M. (1981). *Ethics, Religion and Politics*. Minneapolis: University of Minnesota Press, 3.

Aquinas, S. T. (1981). *Summa Theologica*. Complete English Edition in Five Volumes, Translated by Fathers of the English Dominican Province. Allen, TX: Christian Classics, 2: 827–37.

Aristotle (1984). *The Complete Works*. Revised Oxford Translation, edited by Jonathan Barnes. Princeton, NJ: Princeton University Press, I: 1729, 1735, 1747, 1798–802.

Beauchamp, T. L. and Childress, J. F. (2001). *Principles of Biomedical Ethics* (5th Edition). New York: Oxford University Press.

Becker, L. C. (ed.) and Becker, C. B. (associate ed.) (1992). *A History of Western Ethics*. New York: Garland.

Cooper, J. M. (1986). *Reason and Human Good in Aristotle*. Indianapolis: Hackett, 88.

Devettere, R. J. (2002). *Introduction to Virtue Ethics*. Washington, DC: Georgetown University Press.

Downie, R. S. (2002). 'Supererogation and Altruism: A Comment'. *J. Med. Ethics*, 28: 75–6.

Finnis, J. [1982], c1980 (1986 printing). *Natural Law and Natural Rights*. Oxford: Clarendon Press; New York: Oxford University Press.

Friedson, Eliot. (2001). *Professionalism, the Third Logic: On the Practice of Knowledge*. Chicago: University of Chicago Press.

Hardie, W. F. R. (1967). 'The Final Good of Aristotle's Ethics', in *Aristotle: A Collection of Critical Essays*, J. M. E. Moravcsik (ed.). Garden City, NY: Doubleday, Anchor Books, 296–322.

Hariman, R. (ed.) (2003). *Prudence: Classical Virtue, Postmodern Practice*. College Station: Pennsylvania State University Press.

Hippocrates (1972). *Ancient Medicine*, with English translation by W. H. S. Jones. Cambridge, MA: Harvard University Press, I/iii: 17.

_____ (1972). *The Oath*, with English translation by W. H. S. Jones. Cambridge, MA: Harvard University Press, I/III: 299.

Hockaway, C. (1994). 'Cognitive Virtues and Epistemic Evaluation'. *International Journal of Philosophical Studies*, 2: 211–27.

Kant, I. (1964). *The Theory of Virtue*. University of Pennsylvania Press.

Kass, L. (1981). *Regarding the End of Medicine and the Pursuit of Health, Interdisciplinary Perspectives*. J. McCartney (ed.). Reading, MA: Addison Wesley, 4: 18.

Koehn, D. (1994). *The Ground of Professional Ethics*. New York: Routledge, 4: 54–68; 5: 69–88.

Machiavelli, N. (2003), *The Prince*, translated with notes by George Bull; introduction by Anthony Grafton. New York: Penguin Books.

MacIntyre, A. (1966). *A Short History of Ethics: A History of Moral Philosophy from the Homeric Age to the Twentieth Century*, Reprint edition. New York: Macmillan Press.

_____ (1984). *After Virtue: A Study in Moral Theory* (2nd edn.). Notre Dame, IN: University of Notre Dame Press, 187.

_____ (1990). *Three Rival Versions of Moral Enquiry: Encyclopedia, Genealogy, and Tradition: being Gifford lectures delivered in the University of Edinburgh in 1988*. Notre Dame, IN: University of Notre Dame Press, 137–9.

McKay, A.C. (2002). 'Supererogation and the Profession of Medicine'. *J. Med. Ethics*, 28: 70–3.

Marcel, G. (1965) *Being and Having*; a translation by Katharine Farrer of *Être et avoir*. New York: Harper and Row.

Maritain, J. (1942). *Art and Scholasticism, with Other Essays*, translated by J. F. Scanlan. New York: C. Scribner's Sons, 5–7.

Moore, G. E. (1903). *Principia Ethics*. Cambridge: Cambridge University Press.

Murdoch, I. (1993). *Metaphysics as a Guide to Morals*. New York: Penguin.

_____ (1999). *Existentialists and Mystics: Writings on Philosophy and Literature*, Peter Conradi (ed.), foreword by George Steiner. New York: Penguin, 60.

Nordin, I. (1999). 'The Limits of Medical Practice'. *Theoretical Medicine*, 20: 105–23.

O'Neill, O. (1996). *Towards Justice and Virtue: A Constructive Account of Practical Reasoning*. Cambridge: Cambridge University Press, 207.

The Oxford Dictionary of English Etymology (1966). C.T. Onions (ed.) with the assistance of G. W. S. Friedrichsen and R. W. Burchfield. Oxford: Oxford University Press, 713.

Orr, R. D., Pang, N., Pellegrino, E. D., and Siegler, M. (1997). 'Use of the Hippocratic Oath: A Review of Twentieth Century Practice and a Content Analysis of Oaths Administered in Medical Schools in the U.S. and Canada in 1993'. *Journal of Clinical Ethics*, Winter: 377–88.

Pellegrino, M.D., Edmund D. (1976). *The Fact of Illness and the Act of Pro-Fession*, Some notes on *Source of Professional Obligation*, in McCullough, Laurence B. and James Polk Morris (eds.), *Implications of History and Ethics to Medicine—Veterinary and Human*. Texas: Texas A and M College.

_____ (1979). 'Toward a Reconstruction of Medical Morality: The Primacy Act of Profession and the Fact of Illness'. *J. Medicine and Philosophy*, 1: 32–56.

_____ (1997). 'Profession, Patient, Compassion, Consent: Meditations on Medical Philology'. *Connecticut Medicine*, 42: 175–8.

_____ (1998). 'What the Philosophy Of Medicine Is'. *Theoretical Medicine and Bioethics,* Dave Thomasma, Gerrit Kimsma, and Evert Van Leeuwen (eds.), 19/6: 315–36.

_____ (1999). 'The Goals and Ends of Medicine: How Are They to be Defined?'. *The Goals of Medicine: The Forgotten Issues in Health Care Reform*, Mark J. Hanson and Daniel Callahan (eds.). Washington, DC: Georgetown University Press, 55–68.

_____ (2000). 'The Use and Abuse of the Concept of Futility Proceedings'. *Fifth Assembly of the Pontifical Academy for Life.* Vaticano: Libreria Editrice, 219–41.

_____ (2001). 'The Internal Morality of Clinical Medicine: A Paradigm for the Ethics of the Helping and Healing Professions'. *Journal of Medicine and Philosophy*, 26/6: 559–79.

_____ (2001). 'Philosophy of Medicine: Should it be Teleologically or Socially Construed?'. *Kennedy Institute of Ethics Journal*, 11/2: 169–80.

_____ and Pellegrino, A. A. (1988). *Humanism and Ethics in Roman Medicine*, Translation and Text Commentary on a text of: Largus, Scribonius, *Literature and Medicine: Literature and Bioethics.* 7: 22–38.

_____ and Thomasma, D. C. (1981). *The Philosophical Basis for Medical Practice.* New York: Oxford University Press.

_____ (1987). *For the Patient's Good.* New York: Oxford University Press.

_____ (1993). *The Virtues in Medical Practice.* New York: Oxford University Press.

_____ (2004). 'The Good of Patients and the Good of Society: Striking a Moral Balance', in M. Boylan (ed.), *Public Health Policy and Ethics.* The Netherlands: Kluwer Academic, 17–37.

Ross, W. D. (1959). *Aristotle: A Complete Exposition of His Works & Thought.* New York: Meridian Books, 184.

_____ (1988). *The Right and the Good.* Indianapolis: Hackett, 75–133.

Sandbach, F.H. (1975). *The Stoics* (2nd edn.). Indianapolis: Hackett, 28.

Sidgwick, H. (1988). *Outlines of the History of Ethics.* Indianapolis: Hackett.

Solomon, D. (1997). 'Internal Objections to Virtue Ethics'. *Virtue Ethics: A Critical Reader*, Daniel Statman (ed.). Washington, DC: Georgetown University Press, 165–79.

Statman, D. (1997). 'Introduction to Virtue Ethics'. *Virtue Ethics: A Critical Reader*, Daniel Statman (ed.). Washington, DC: Georgetown University Press, 1–41.

Taylor, C. (1980). *Sources of the Self.* Cambridge, MA: Harvard University Press, 84.

Trianosky, G. V. (1997). 'What is Virtue Theory About?'. *Virtue Ethics: A Critical Reader.* Washington, DC: Georgetown University Press, 42–55.

Veatch, H. B. (1981). 'Telos and Teleology'. *Studies in Aristotle*, Dominic J. O'Meara (eds.). Washington, DC: Catholic University of America Press, 279–96.

Veatch, R. M. (2002). 'White Coat Ceremonies: A Second Opinion'. *J. Med. Ethics*, 28: 5–6.

Zagzebski, L. (1996). *Virtues of the Mind: an Inquiry into the Nature of Virtue and the Ethical Foundations of Knowledge.* New York: Cambridge University Press.

4

Doctoring and Self-Forgiveness

Jeffrey Blustein

1. SELF-FORGIVENESS: A PROBLEM FOR PHYSICIANS

In the vast philosophical literature in moral psychology on the subject of forgiveness, most attention by far has been directed to its interpersonal version, that is, to forgiveness of others rather than forgiveness of self. There is a relatively small number of philosophical papers that explicitly takes up self-forgiveness in a sustained way (Snow 1993; Hughes 1994; Holmgren 1998, 2002; Dillon 2001). Most discussions of forgiveness do not mention self-forgiveness or mention it only in passing, perhaps because it is thought that the concept of self-forgiveness is problematic or that the analysis of other-forgiveness can be transposed without significant alteration to cases of self-forgiveness or for some other reason (Downie 1965; Haber 1991). There is indeed much that we can learn from accounts of other-forgiveness that can help illuminate self-forgiveness as well, and the following discussion will reflect this. But it would be a mistake, a kind of essentialist fallacy, to suppose that there is some single thing, namely forgiveness, that can indifferently take as its object either another person or oneself. With respect to concerns about conceptual coherence, it may be doubted that what is called 'self-forgiveness' can be seriously seen as a species of forgiveness at all. Since standard forgiveness involves an innocent party (the one who forgives) and a guilty party (the one who is forgiven), how can one person be both forgiver and forgiven? Clearly, if forgiveness is to be applied reflexively, some of its usual implications will be lost. But it is worth noting that we are familiar enough with other cases where this happens and we do not question the legitimacy of the reflexive application ('self-taught', for instance).

Assuming, as I shall, that someone can, more or less literally, forgive him- or herself, the theoretical core of this chapter—sections 2 through 4—explores the constitutive elements of self-forgiveness and the conditions under which it is morally warranted, referring, where appropriate, to accounts of interpersonal forgiveness. Developing an account of the nature and ethics of self-forgiveness, however, is really only my secondary aim here. My primary aim is to use this account to illuminate an aspect of the role of physician that has not been dealt with in the philosophical literature of medical ethics. One would expect self-forgiveness to be discussed, if it were discussed at all, by those who have turned to virtue ethics as a corrective to principle-based approaches that have not been sufficiently attentive to the importance of character in defining the role responsibilities of physicians. But this has not been the case. Edmund Pellegrino and David Thomasma, for example, have written at length on the virtues of the good physician (1993; Pellegrino 1995), pointing out that what we prize in a good physician is not just her outward conformity to moral prescriptions but her characteristic motivational structures. The good physician, they claim, is one who puts the good of the patient before her own and practices such virtues as compassion, benevolence, honesty, fidelity to promises, and at times, courage. But there is no mention of the role of self-forgiveness in the physician–patient relationship or discussion of its place within a conception of the good physician.

I find this somewhat surprising, since self-forgiveness (or the lack thereof) would seem to be of particular relevance to the practice of doctoring, given the culture of the medical profession as it currently exists. Physicians, by virtue of the sort of training and socialization they receive and in some instances also by temperament, expect themselves to live up to the highest standards of professional excellence. This is certainly commendable—but it has a downside. Beginning in medical school and continuing in residency training and beyond, a consistent and clear if largely implicit message is conveyed: physicians are not permitted to make mistakes since mistakes can have grave consequences; physicians should not acknowledge uncertainty to patients since an admission of medical fallibility will alarm them; physicians who cannot cure have failed their patients. Physicians are taught to maintain an aura of infallibility in their dealings with their patients (Katz 1984: 42), and the impact of this training goes deeper than the management of appearances: they also come to expect the same of themselves. They are taught to view themselves as healers who are engaged in an aggressive war against death and disease, where anything less than victory is second best, a proof of failure. But of course infallibility, perfection, and mastery of nature inevitably elude them, and if they are unequipped with adaptive means for coping with this reality, they respond by adopting defensive strategies of one sort or another (Hilfiker 1984; Newman 1996; Wu 2000). This process is reinforced by concerns about professional reputation and malpractice litigation.

Cultivating a norm of high standards among physicians is highly desirable. It is the counterpart of a fundamental goal of medical education, namely, developing the physician's sense of responsibility for his or her patient. A commitment to high standards of professional practice expresses and underscores the seriousness of the physician's vocation, its ethic of serving the sick by aiming at cure, prevention, or amelioration of disease. However, traditionally the processes that motivate physicians to maintain standards of excellence in practice have not fostered development of the skills, attitudes, and traits physicians need to deal constructively—non-evasively and non-self-punitively—with their perceived limitations, shortcomings, and lapses.[1]

---

[1] This is a claim that is often made in the literature on medical professionalism. For example, Novack et al. note that while writers stress the 'importance of activities that promote personal awareness in medical education', including acceptance of one's limitations and the limitations of one's craft, 'medical school and residency curricula often do not include these activities' (Novack et al. 1997: 502). Similar observations are also found in Quill (1990); Longhurst (1988); and McCue (1982). For a discussion of the emotional, developmental issues that arise for students in medical school and their implications for medical pedagogy, see Marcus (1999, 2003).

Failures to meet one's own or others' expectations of perfection and control over death and disease always occur and may cause the physician enormous emotional distress, but the opportunities to discuss them among colleagues in a supportive environment are limited. The one forum where physicians can talk candidly about their mistakes, the Mortality and Morbidity Conference, is designed more to promote group solidarity and reinforce medical hierarchy than to encourage participants to discuss their mistakes and their emotional responses to them openly (Bosk 1979; Orlander and Barber 2002). In some cases, because of the lack of social supports to mitigate stress, the physician may be plagued by recurring self-doubt or lapse into neurotic behavior to deal with her anxiety and guilt (Hilfiker 1984).

Self-forgiveness has not been on the agenda of medical education and training; it is rare to find it included in the lexicon of the medical profession. Though there is growing recognition of the need to emphasize personal awareness in medical education and training, as the burgeoning literature on medical professionalism attests, change is slow in coming. Not enough has been done in a serious and sustained way to help physicians in training distinguish between those situations when self-reproach is reasonable and those when it is not, or to teach them how to respond properly and constructively to the former. They may therefore blame themselves for untoward medical outcomes even though guilt and remorse are out of place, since they did not do anything wrong or anything that they should not have done. When self-reproach makes sense and is justified, as it sometimes is, they might attempt to shirk responsibility by blaming adverse events on deficiencies in the organization of the care delivery system (Lo 2000: 263) or, if this proves unsuccessful, they might be left with feelings of worthlessness that they must cope with on their own and for which their training has not adequately prepared them. The burden of dealing with mistakes and personal failings commonly falls on the physician alone without other significant social processes being available to assist her in the task of self-forgiveness (Baylis 1997). Clearly the emotional impact on the physician of some perceived wrongdoing or deficiency on her part can seriously disrupt her professional and personal life (Novack et al. 1997; Christensen 1992). Self-forgiveness does not insulate her from all such bad feelings, nor should it. But it enables the physician to cope better with those feelings by regulating and modulating them.

To understand why self-forgiveness should be included among the virtues of the physician, however, we have to look beyond the effects on the physician him- or herself. Alasdair MacIntyre's account of the virtues (1981) provides one way of approaching this question. According to MacIntyre, virtues have both inherent and instrumental worth, the latter deriving from their relationship to what he calls 'practices'. Practices are complex and demanding activities with standards of excellence and goods or ends 'internal' to them, and a profession like medicine can be viewed as a practice in this sense. In order to realize the goods internal to a practice, practitioners must submit to the rules of the practice and align themselves with the traditions that have given rise to its canons of excellence. A virtue on this account is a learned human quality without which one cannot attain these goods. From this perspective, the virtues of the physician are those acquired traits of character that are necessary to realize the goods internal to medicine and that should be cultivated for this reason. To establish that self-forgiveness is among the virtues necessary to practice medicine, then, we need to identify what these goods or ends are and to show why the set of dispositions associated with proper self-forgiveness is indispensable to their realization.

It may be argued that since it is so difficult to determine what the ends of medicine are, this is not the best or most helpful way to account for the status of self-forgiveness as a virtue of physicians (Arras 2001). I believe a strong case can be made, however—and I will say more about this in Section 5—that physicians need this virtue if they are to do well as physicians, according to widely shared conceptions of excellence in the practice of doctoring. The good physician does not hold herself to standards of professional practice that demand a degree of control or flawless performance that exceeds in magnitude what most people would find reasonable. If she possesses this virtue, her feelings of self-reproach are responsive to reasonable beliefs about her fault and the faultiness of her conduct. She does not persist in blaming herself when it is inappropriate to do so and, as we shall see later, this has important implications for her continuing to care for patients who are beyond her ability to cure. In other situations, when it is appropriate to blame herself she does, but she knows how to manage these feelings so that she is not dominated by them. She also takes responsibility for her lapses and mistakes, which includes owning up to or acknowledging them, expressing regret and remorse, and making apologies. As Pellegrino notes, 'the vulnerability and dependence of the sick person forces him to trust not just in his rights but in the kind of person the physician is' (1995: 78), and this trust is not well-placed if the physician's difficulties with self-forgiveness, as manifested in inappropriate or excessive self-reproach, interfere with the care that she ought to provide and that her patients, in their vulnerable state, depend upon.

Self-forgiveness has been ignored as a practical matter in the education and socialization of physicians, where little has been done to encourage appreciation of its value and much has been done to discourage it. The problem to which I am drawing attention is not only or mainly a matter of individual psychology, and I am certainly not claiming that every physician has difficulties with self-forgiveness. Rather, difficulties enacting self-forgiveness are widespread if not universal, and to a large extent they are rooted in the culture of medicine and professional training that shapes the self-conceptions of physicians in ways that are potentially harmful to themselves, their patients, and the relationship between them. This neglect of self-forgiveness provides the context and much of the impetus for the investigation that follows. Specific recommendations for how to change the practices of mainstream medicine are beyond the scope of this essay. My aim is rather to contribute to the literature on a virtue-based ethic of medicine by reflecting on the meaning and importance of self-forgiveness in the physician–patient relationship. But first I want to examine self-forgiveness from a broader perspective as an interesting and important topic in its own right.

2. THE CONCEPT OF SELF-FORGIVENESS

In this section, I discuss conceptual relations among self-forgiveness, emotions of self-reproach, and the sense of self-worth. Self-forgiveness, I claim, is a matter of overcoming the self-reproach that accompanies a diminished sense of self-worth.

What We Forgive Ourselves For

Concerns about self-forgiveness are often occasioned by wrongdoing that actually caused or nearly caused harm to others. There is no good reason, however, to restrict the notion of self-forgiveness in this way. We may reproach ourselves for not developing our talents, for personal shortcomings, failures of character, evil thoughts, malicious desires, and more, and it makes sense to reproach ourselves for these flaws and failings, as well as for our wrongdoings, as long as they implicate our agency and responsibility can be taken for them (Calhoun 1992; Murphy 1998; Dillon 2001: 59). This expanded notion of self-forgiveness, I believe, conforms to common usage. For example, one may say things like, 'I cannot forgive myself for having let myself be talked into going for surgery' or 'I cannot forgive myself for wishing that my patient would just die.' Such remarks import notions of responsibility and self-reproach or self-blame and raise philosophical questions about their appropriate application.

Distinguishing Self-Forgiveness from Condonation

We need to be clear at the outset about what self-forgiveness is not. It does not involve canceling the judgment that I did something wrong or that it was mean-spirited of me to wish someone ill, for example. Forgiveness, of others as well as of oneself, takes place in the face of ongoing acknowledgment of these facts. Nor is forgiving oneself, as R. S. Downie (1965) argues, really a matter of condoning, that is, excusing or overlooking or treating indulgently something about oneself or one's actions. Admittedly, we sometimes say we forgive ourselves when what we have done is trivial, harmless, or of no importance, or when we admit that what we did was wrong but excuse ourselves for it. However, use of the term in such cases is, strictly speaking, idiosyncratic (Hampton 1988: 40). For if we collapse self-forgiveness into condonation and deny the former a conceptual space of its own, we would have no basis for claiming that sometimes it is condoning rather than forgiving, and sometimes the converse, that is the correct response to what we have done. Nor could we sensibly make the observation that condoning is frequently used as a morally inferior substitute for self-forgiveness, since it is often psychologically easier to play down the extent of the injury one is responsible for by condoning it than to face up to it honestly and engage in the process of self-forgiveness. For these reasons a distinction between self-forgiveness and condonation in terms of the gravity of what we have done and our responsibility for it needs to be retained.

Self-Forgiveness as Overcoming Self-Reproach

Self-reproach is the general term I will use to characterize the range of negative emotions of self-assessment that the achievement of self-forgiveness overcomes, emotions which include guilt, shame, self-loathing, and self-contempt, to name some. Forgiveness is essentially a matter of changing how one feels about or sees a person who has done wrong or is in some way deficient, and that person may be oneself or another. I do not forgive another if I continue to harbor hostile feelings towards him but just do not outwardly display them. Similarly, I do not forgive myself if I do not let go of self-hatred and other painful emotions engendered by my past behavior or personal shortcomings. Of course, one can come to feel differently about a person by just no longer experiencing the same emotions toward him. Self-forgiveness, however, involves the overcoming of self-reproach not necessarily its elimination, so self-forgiveness is possible even if self-reproach endures. What is required to overcome self-reproach is a change in the way one experiences the emotion so that, as Robin Dillon puts it, 'one is no longer in bondage' to self-reproach, 'no longer controlled or crippled by a negative conception of oneself and the debilitating pain of it' (Dillon 2001: 83). In this sense, one 'lets go' of the painful feelings that accompany the negative self-assessments.

Painful feelings about oneself motivate the work of self-forgiveness, but self-forgiveness is not to be treated as merely one way among others of lessening the power of self-reproach, such as going to a psychotherapist to have the bad feelings taken away, or talking yourself into a better frame of mind by telling yourself that what you did wasn't so terrible after all, or even forgetting what you have done. Being freed from the grip of these bad feelings is the upshot of the achievement of self-forgiveness; but self-forgiveness has a complex moral structure that remains hidden so long as it is viewed as just another form of psychological therapy.

The Centrality of Shame in Self-Forgiveness

Though self-reproach covers a range of emotions, shame occupies a central place in the analysis of self-forgiveness. The question asked by those who struggle with self-forgiveness is not whether they can or should forgive their misdeeds, but whether they can or should forgive themselves for their misdeeds. In other words, self-forgiveness is ultimately concerned with one's self and not with what one has done or, rather, only with what one has done insofar as it reveals something about an aspect of oneself or about the kind of person one is. Moreover, one's sense of self-worth is normally called into question when one is revealed to oneself in this light, and it is this that makes it appropriate to talk about self-forgiveness in these cases. If a person committed harmful acts in the past for which he holds himself responsible and he is a morally conscientious person who recognizes that he stands in certain normative relations to other people, his sense of worth is bound to be diminished, and concerns about self-forgiveness, about whether and how he can forgive himself and whether he should do so, would gain a foothold. We can also speak of self-forgiveness, as H. J. N. Horsbrugh observes, when no other person has suffered harm because 'one's moral image can sustain a severe fracture' (1974: 276) as a result of actions for which one reproaches oneself even in these cases. In neither type of situation, of course, is the injury to one's sense of worth what one forgives oneself for.

Someone who is struggling with self-forgiveness, with whether he can and should forgive himself, may feel shame or guilt acutely or chronically. Shame, as commonly understood, is felt upon the discovery of shortcomings in oneself that call into question the worth one thought one had, and in the light of what I have said about the relationship between self-forgiveness and the sense of self-worth, we can understand why shame is particularly closely associated with self-forgiveness. According to Gabriele Taylor, shame also has an especially close connection with self-respect: loss of self-respect is generally registered emotionally as shame, and the prospect of experiencing shame inhibits one from doing things that would injure one's self-respect: 'To respect the self . . . is to do that which protects the self from injury or destruction . . . And shame is the emotion of self-protection: It may prevent the person concerned from putting himself into a certain position, or make him aware that he ought not to be in the position in which he finds himself' (1985: 81).

Of course, a serious violation of a rule can both engender guilt and damage one's self-respect, if adherence to that code of conduct is among one's core commitments, so both shame and guilt can be aroused by the very same act. Nonetheless, it is shame, not guilt, that, as Dillon notes, 'is at the core of the negative stance' (2001: 63) that self-forgiveness addresses and would overcome.

Self-Forgiveness as Requiring Injury to One's Sense of Worth

One way in which the sense of one's worth may be diminished is by an injury to one's self-respect, and an injury of this sort has a number of different explanations, depending on the kind of self-respect at issue. There is, first, a kind of self-respect that involves the belief that one has equal status in a system of moral rights and that one is entitled to recognition of this status by others. Thomas Hill's examples of the overly deferential wife and the extremely self-deprecating person illustrate how one might fail to have this type of self-respect (1991). When an individual acquiesces in disrespectful or degrading treatment that denies her her basic rights as one person among other persons, and she acknowledges and holds herself at least partly responsible for this, she likely suffers an injury to her self-respect. Secondly, among morally concerned and decent persons, self-respect is grounded in part in taking one's moral responsibilities seriously and caring about the rights and interests of others. Awareness of one's wrongdoing, and even of one's involvement in causing harm to others (as, for example, when a system sets up a physician to make a mistake that causes significant harm to the patient) may damage this type of self-respect. A third type of self-respect, of which the second may be viewed as a particular instance, involves developing and living by commitments and attachments that ground a set of personal (or in the case of the physician, professional) standards by which the individual is prepared to judge his self-worth. These standards may or may not be ethical ones, and the individual may or may not criticize others or all others for not having the same ones. As he sees it, they may be standards that apply only to himself, or only to others in the same profession. The standards implicate his sense of self-worth because the commitments and attachments are constitutive of his self and because it is impossible to have constitutive commitments and attachments without having some view of what is expected or required to sustain them. The view need not be very articulate and may only become so under special circumstances, but if he fails to live up to these self-imposed expectations, he fails to be himself. On this account, to have a conception of self-respect is to have a sense of one's constitutive commitments and attachments, and one has self-respect to the extent that one is disposed to act in accordance with them.

A distinction is sometimes drawn between self-respect and self-esteem and it is important to say something about how this distinction figures in the analysis of self-forgiveness. Gabriele Taylor distinguishes them in the following way:

> The person who has self-esteem takes a favorable view of himself, while he who lacks it will think of himself in unfavorable terms . . . . There is a connection between self-esteem and emotional pride: the person who is proud of this or that enjoys, at the time of feeling proud, an increase in his self-esteem; he can now take a more favorable view of himself (in some respect) . . . . For a person to have self-respect does not mean that he has a favorable attitude toward himself, or that he has any particular attitude toward himself at all. Nor is self-respect connected with emotional pride. (1985: 77–8)

Pauline Chazan also argues that self-respect and self-esteem are distinguishable from one another: self-respect involves 'aspects of a person which are experienced by her as essential parts of what she is', whereas self-esteem, like pride, involves 'evaluations of some aspect or aspects of the self' that may belong to one merely contingently (Chazan 1998: 147, 149). To be sure, as both writers point out, self-respect and self-esteem are not unconnected: a lack or loss of self-respect will adversely affect how good one feels about oneself and retaining one's self-respect is always a ground for self-esteem. But a lowering of one's self-esteem does not necessarily undermine one's self-respect.

Given the distinction between self-respect and self-esteem, we may now ask whether self-forgiveness is only a matter of addressing damaged self-respect or whether diminished self-esteem can also be a proper occasion for self-forgiveness. As I understand it, it is conceptual of self-forgiveness that one's sense of worth has been called into question. Sometimes the blow to one's self-esteem will be of such a nature that one's sense of worth will also be diminished, but this is not always the case. Someone who suffers a loss of self-esteem, for example, may be deeply disappointed with himself, may be dispirited, but these emotions are not the same as, nor need they involve, a diminished sense of worth. So it is appropriate to speak of self-forgiveness when there has been a loss of self-esteem only when this loss is serious enough to upset one's sense of worth. Injury to self-respect, by contrast, always strikes at one's sense of worth, and it is the grounds for a diminished sense of worth which is just what self-forgiveness addresses.

I close this section with a few words comparing self-respect in other-forgiveness and self-forgiveness. In the case of other-forgiveness, we forgive someone for what he has done or the sort of person he has been, and this is similar to self-forgiveness. But being mistreated by another only sometimes damages our self-respect, since we may not share the offender's belief that we do not deserve to be treated well, whereas a central case of self-forgiveness is addressing damaged self-respect. Further, sometimes forgiving another can indicate a lack of self-respect, if, for example, it is motivated by the belief that we don't deserve any better treatment than we have received and so have no grounds for resentment. Self-forgiveness can also sometimes show a lack of self-respect—although not in quite the same way—if one forgives oneself prematurely or without having done the necessary preparatory work.

3. THE ETHICS OF SELF-FORGIVENESS

In this section, I explore a number of ethical issues pertaining to self-forgiveness. I discuss two sorts of cases: in one, self-forgiveness is ethically improper, because one is being too easy on oneself; in the other, self-forgiveness is improperly withheld, because one is being unduly hard on oneself. To possess the virtue of self-forgiveness is to be characteristically disposed to regard one's flaws or failings neither too leniently nor too sternly. Finally, in accord with Aristotle's claim that virtues benefit their possessors, I suggest various ways in which the virtue of self-forgiveness does so.

Being Too Easy on Oneself

Self-forgiveness for actions or attitudes that have shown disrespect for another may seem morally suspect because it deflects attention from the one who has been wronged and what the offender must do to make it up to him. Surely, if I have committed a wrong against you or harmed you, I cannot simply eliminate justifiable guilt at will. To suppose otherwise, Richard Swinburne argues, is to fail to 'take seriously the fact that the act is an act by which you are wronged, and in the wiping out of which you ought therefore to have a say. One consequence of my harming you is just it is in part up to you whether my guilt is remitted' (1989: 87). Often the victim will require at least some minimal attempt at atonement on the part of the offender such as an apology and an effort to do what she can to repair the injury, even if this is not very much. Alternatively, the victim may in a spirit of generosity or out of compassion forgive the one who has wronged him even if repentance is not forthcoming, and perhaps it is good that he should sometimes be willing to do so. Whatever the victim chooses to do, the remission of guilt depends in part on his willingness to forgive the offender, and self-forgiveness may be morally troubling because it seems to be something entirely internal, a matter of the self's relation to itself only. And if it is entirely internal, self-forgiveness is incompatible with respect for the one who has been wronged.

These remarks express a legitimate concern that self-forgiveness will substitute for or bypass the often painful task of seeking forgiveness from those one has wronged, and indeed self-forgiveness without consideration of the person one has wronged and his willingness to forgive may be a kind of moral self-indulgence or moral arrogance. Or as the theologian Paul Tillich succinctly observes, self-forgiveness in a vacuum 'is simply a self-confirmation in a state of estrangement', and this is 'just the opposite of what forgiveness means' (Gartner 1992: 25). In the absence of forgiveness by the one wronged, a morally conscientious person would carefully consider whether he is deceiving himself about having met the conditions for justified self-forgiveness. Perhaps he is making matters too easy for himself by assuming that he has done all he needs to do to earn the other's forgiveness and that the other is being unreasonable not to grant it. Seeking forgiveness from someone we have wronged, after all, is a humbling undertaking that in serious cases we usually approach with some trepidation and anxiety, in part because of the possibility that the other will reject our apologies and offers of atonement. Because of this we may be tempted to take the path of least resistance and grant ourselves the forgiveness we have not received from the person we have wronged but that we are convinced we deserve.

This is not to say that forgiveness by the one we have wronged is necessary for justified self-forgiveness. Though arguably there is no duty to forgive another, the one who has been wronged may be intransigent without an adequate justification. If the offending party has repented and atoned in such a way that a reasonable person would grant forgiveness, but his efforts are rebuffed or disregarded by the wronged party, the offending party may nevertheless be justified in forgiving himself. After all, he may reason, I have done everything that I can reasonably be expected to do to make up for what I have done or the sort of person I have been, and this is not so terrible as to be unforgivable. Again, there is a danger of self-deception here, and depending on how likely this is thought to be, the morally conscientious person may want to give the wronged party the benefit of the doubt. In a loose sort of way, then, forgiveness by the one who has been wronged functions as a moral constraint on forgiveness of self. We can put the connection between self-forgiveness and forgiveness negatively: when the wronged party is justified in not forgiving the wronging party, the latter is not justified in forgiving himself.

The criticism we level against the person who attains self-forgiveness without making himself available to the one he has wronged is that his self-forgiveness has not been earned. This is an instance of the more general point that self-forgiveness is not warranted unless one has worked through various tasks, tasks that may be daunting for the offender, especially if he has seriously wronged another. The importance of fulfilling these tasks can be explained in different ways. They may be regarded as signs of a change of heart on the offender's part brought about by reflection on the wrong he has committed or the kind of person he has been (Calhoun 1992); they may also be taken to constitute his taking responsibility for what he has done or been. Thus, a person who manages to overcome self-reproach without exposing himself to the justified anger and resentment of the one he has wronged, or without seeking to make amends to the other, or without resolving through moral self-improvement to become a better person, and so forth, has clearly done nothing to evince a change of heart of the requisite sort or to take responsibility for what he has done or been. He may therefore be said to be too ready to forgive himself, or to forgive himself prematurely, or to be too easy on himself. In other related cases, there may be individuals who deny that they did anything wrong, or who do not regard their failings as failings, or who dismiss wrong acts and failings from their mind because they simply do not care that they are wrongs or failings. Strictly speaking, these individuals do not forgive themselves too easily, for self-forgiveness just does not arise as an issue for them. But they can be criticized for being too easy on themselves nonetheless.

Can Self-Forgiveness Be a Virtue?

A lingering suspicion that the self-forgiver is making matters too easy for herself may lead us to question whether self-forgiveness can have the status of a virtue at all. For virtues, according to Aristotle, are about what is difficult and self-forgiveness, it seems, is all too easy, since the offender is the judge of the adequacy of her own reparative efforts: she is like the criminal pardoning herself. But the persuasiveness of this objection depends on how self-forgiveness is understood, that is, on whether self-forgiveness is thought of as: (a) just a psychological state characterized by an absence or diminishment of self-reproach; or (b) an achievement with a particular history, a history, roughly speaking, that includes working through a process of honestly addressing one's wrongs and shortcomings and learning from them and the emotions they arouse. (See the point in Section 2 about self-forgiveness as just another form of psychological therapy.) The latter is what Margaret Holmgren calls 'genuine self-forgiveness' (2002: 113) and the offender is not the sole judge of how well this process has gone and of the 'genuineness' of his self-forgiveness. Moreover, there is a virtue of self-forgiveness in part because self-indulgent generosity toward oneself is a common temptation. (Genuine) self-forgiveness is a virtue for the same reason that Philippa Foot claims courage and temperance are virtues: it is a 'corrective disposition' 'standing at a point at which there is some temptation to be resisted' (1978: 8).

Being Too Hard on Oneself

I have discussed cases in which self-forgiveness comes too easily, and self-forgiveness under these circumstances is not the manifestation of a virtue of self-forgiveness. Consider now a different sort of case in which the wronged party forgives the offender and is in fact justified in doing so. The latter, however, does not forgive himself. Of course, he may have good reason for not doing so. He may, as Norman Care suggests (2002: 217), suspect that the victim's reasons for forgiving him do not properly address the substance of what he did, or that the wronged party is only forgiving him because he (the one who was wronged) does not believe that he deserves to be treated well. But we may suppose that he has properly satisfied himself that these suspicions are without merit. Nevertheless, he refuses to accept the wronged party's forgiveness of himself as sufficient for self-forgiveness and continues to castigate himself for his wrongs or deficiencies. He does not just continue to reproach himself: he is controlled and debilitated by self-reproach.

Such a person, we might say, is being unduly hard on himself, the counterpart, at the other end of the continuum of self-forgiveness, of being too easy on oneself. It is an interesting and difficult question whether there are some acts for which one should not forgive oneself, no matter how remorseful one feels or how much one atones for them or works to repair the damage one has caused or resolves to become a better person. Given that forgiveness by the wronged party has a moral bearing on self-forgiveness, we can also ask whether there are some acts whose forgiveness would be incompatible with the wronged party's self-respect. If there are acts for which one should not forgive oneself—either because of what was done or whom it was done to—then one is not being unduly hard on oneself by not doing so.

I am inclined to think that there are some acts for which, because of the enormity of the wrong one has committed, one ought not to forgive oneself, but I will not attempt to argue for this here (Lang 1994; Govier 2002: 100–18). If there are such acts, then a person who possesses the virtue of self-forgiveness will be sufficiently attuned to differences in the moral quality of his actions that he will not regard all of them as equally forgivable if they are not. In any case, concerns about one's openness to self-forgiveness do not usually arise in connection with acts that are as extreme as this, assuming that such acts exist at all, so I set them aside in what follows. I am mainly interested in persons who cannot let go of self-reproach, who are unwilling or unable to forgive themselves, even though what they reproach themselves for does not fall in the category of the unforgivable. They may, however, erroneously consider it to be unforgivable.

The Middle Ground between Being Too Easy and Too Hard on Oneself

A person who is too easy on himself is improperly self-forgiving (if he thinks about self-forgiveness at all) and one who is too hard on himself is improperly unself-forgiving. The former overcomes self-reproach without going through or completing the tasks that are preliminary to self-forgiveness, or he does not reproach himself when there is reason for him to do so. The latter does not or cannot overcome self-reproach even if he takes responsibility for what he has done or been—indeed, his taking responsibility may only deepen his self-reproach—or he reproaches himself for something that a reasonable person would not reproach himself for. And insofar as these extremes of being too easy and too hard on oneself are characteristic of a person, he lacks the virtue of self-forgiveness.

Virtues, as Aristotle famously argued, are dispositions not only to act but to feel emotions, and in the person who possesses the specific virtue of self-forgiveness, the emotion of self-reproach will be felt and manifested at such times, on such matters, for such reasons, and in such ways as are proper. Putting this in terms of Aristotle's doctrine of the mean (Urmson 1980), we can say that he has a mean or intermediate disposition regarding the emotion of self-reproach and the actions that manifest it, and this is one excellence of character. One diverges from the mean in the direction of deficiency when one does not experience and exhibit self-reproach at all when one should, or when one experiences it but not to the degree that one should, or when one overcomes self-reproach for reasons that do not address the substance of what one reproaches oneself for. And one diverges from the mean in the direction of excess when one reproaches oneself too often, about trivial as well as important matters, or for too many reasons, or when self-reproach is resistant to modification by rational means.

We might also explain deviations from the mean in terms of a continuum of self-regard. Narcissistic self-love (Fiscalini 1995: 334)[2] and self-hate are the extremes on this continuum and proper self-criticism the mean, and these, it might be said, under-lie respectively excessive, deficient, and proper self-forgiveness. (Thus, excessive self-forgiveness corresponds to deficiency with respect to self-reproach, and so forth.) In both cases of excessive and deficient self-forgiveness, there is something wrong with the person who is so disposed, a lack of proper self-regard, and this lack can be exhib-ited in one's life generally or only in some specific sphere or role. Whether because of temperament or upbringing or training or a combination of these, some individuals may find it exceedingly difficult to let go of negative moral emotions such as guilt and

---

[2] I use the term 'narcissism' here in something closer to its ordinary rather than its technical sense to refer to a pejorative self-love.

shame. They see themselves as having done things that the person they took themselves to be would not do, and while almost anyone would feel that she has been a failure in a particular instance and suspect that she is not much good under these circumstances, their self-deprecation is deep and long-lasting. There are also those who, as we might say, love themselves too much or in the wrong way, and are seldom bothered by pangs of self-reproach.

How Self-Forgiveness Benefits the Individual

Aristotle also claimed that virtues benefit their possessors, that human beings need the virtues in order to live well, and the benefits of self-forgiveness can be demonstrated in a number of ways. First, it provides psychological benefits of relief from loneliness, anxiety, and other debilitating emotions. Chronic feelings of dejection and unworthiness may sap one's interest in people, things, or activities, and engender desperate and futile appeals for reassurance of one's goodness to counteract self-hate. In psychoanalytic theory, the inability to forgive oneself is explained in terms of a failure to attain an integrated, realistic view of oneself that contains both good and bad aspects (Gartner 1992). Those who are capable of self-forgiveness and who work to attain it draw upon their resources of self-love and attempt to come to terms with disabling feelings that interfere with their enjoyment of life. It might be argued that one can be freed from debilitating emotions simply by denying or repressing or downgrading the seriousness of what one has done, and therefore that one can achieve healthy psychological functioning without satisfying the conditions of proper or warranted self-forgiveness. This will of course depend on how the normative notion of 'healthy' psychological functioning is understood, but generally there is significant overlap with those conditions.

Secondly, self-forgiveness benefits the individual by contributing toward the regaining of effective agency, including moral agency. Care clarifies this notion as follows: 'What this recovery is of [namely "agency"] is then lots of things, including a sense of oneself as intact in a way that allows responsible forward-looking action, plus a measure of self-worth, and perhaps even the capacity to find in oneself interests and enthusiasms with enough strength to give meaningfulness to certain of one's activities' (1996: 131). Self-reproach, when dominating and unremitting, undermines self-confidence, the sense that one is, within realistic limits, in control of what happens in one's life and has the personal resources effectively to meet challenges and difficulties that life may throw in one's way. Moreover, while one can be an agent without being a moral agent, there are no cases in which the converse is true. The psychological capacities required for the possession and exercise of agency are presupposed by moral agency, so when the former suffer the corrosive effects of despair and persistent self-reproach, moral agency is undermined as well.

Thirdly, and closely related to the recovery of agency, self-forgiveness helps restore self-respect. As I noted earlier, the issue of self-forgiveness arises when reflection on one's actions or features of one's self leads to a diminished sense of self-worth, although, as also noted, it is not the diminishment in the sense of self-worth for which one needs to forgive oneself. The proper objects of concern are one's actions, traits, and the like, and the persons whom one has wronged by them, but the person whose self-respect has been damaged can through self-forgiveness 'recover enough self-respect to recognize that she is a valuable human being in spite of what she has done' (Holmgren 1998: 76). She recovers self-respect by working through the process of self-forgiveness and taking responsibility for what she has done or been, thereby demonstrating to herself and others that she is a decent person, despite her discreditable past. In this way, self-forgiveness allows her to absorb the full impact of the wrong without losing sight of her basic humanity. Admittedly, one may need some degree or kind of self-respect to begin the process, and it may be out of respect for oneself that one takes on the process of restoring self-worth through self-forgiveness. But what is restored if self-forgiveness is attained is different from the abiding self-acceptance, what Dillon calls the 'basal self-respect' (2001: 73), that grounds the work of self-forgiveness and makes it possible. In addition, in repairing the damage to self-respect, the individual gains an important good, since without self-respect, or with a diminished sense of self-worth, enjoyment of other goods diminishes. No matter how much wealth and power, or how many opportunities, one has, enjoyment of these goods is likely to be transitory if one lacks self-respect. One is also unlikely to see much point in striving to rectify character flaws or habits that have caused injury to self or others in the past.

It is a fairly common view that the aim or the result of forgiveness of others is reconciliation, and it is worth reflecting on whether this view, if correct, tells us something true and important about self-forgiveness as well. Thus, according to Robert Roberts, the practice of forgiveness is 'at home in an ethic of community or friendship—one underlain by a sense of belonging to one another'. Forgiveness is characteristically motivated by a desire for 'reconciliation—restoration or maintenance of a relationship of acceptance, benevolent attitude, and harmonious interaction' (1995: 294, 299). The forgiving person seeks reconciliation because she tends to feel uncomfortable with the anger she feels toward the offender and with the alienation from him that her anger brings. Reconciliation is not all that matters to the virtuously forgiving person, of course: she may be open to seeing the offender in a different light, as one with whom she can (re)establish a harmonious relationship, but she will not seek reconciliation in ways that betray her self-respect, for example.

A notion of reconciliation is also central to some understandings of self-forgiveness. Thus, Beverly Flanigan, for example, characterizes the psychological state of those who have not achieved self-forgiveness as one of conflict with the 'enemy within', conflict which is 'ended, at least where peace is the result, through self-forgiveness . . . .When we forgive ourselves, we make peace with ourselves. We restore trust in ourselves' (1996: 57–8).

Now if by reconciliation we mean the maintenance or restoration of harmonious and cooperative relations, as in Roberts, then it is doubtful that forgiveness of others always achieves reconciliation. It is doubtful too that reconciliation in this sense is the point or goal of forgiveness. It seems quite possible for A to forgive B (truly to forgive B and not just pretend to do so) and, despite this, not to want to have or be able to have a relationship of acceptance, benevolent attitude, and harmonious interaction with B. Such a relationship may sometimes be achieved, but it is a sort of idealistic fantasy to suppose that this is always the case. Rather than jettison the notion of reconciliation altogether, however, we may do better to reinterpret it. If we mean by reconciliation something like the establishment or re-establishment of relations of mutual respect and trust that ought to exist between people, this seems to capture much better what forgiveness accomplishes (Thompson 2002: 50–1). This, and not necessarily maintaining or restoring a harmonious relationship with one another, is how those who forgive and those who are forgiven put the past behind them.

I would say something similar about self-forgiveness. The notion of being at peace with oneself is misleading insofar as it suggests that one is free of inner conflict regarding one's past behavior or that one has 'got over' or 'got beyond' what one has done in such a way that one no longer reproaches oneself for it. Self-forgiveness, as I noted before, is compatible with self-reproach, even persistent self-reproach, so long as this is not disabling. Here, as with forgiveness of others, it is better to think of reconciliation in terms of establishing or re-establishing relations of respect, not exactly in the same way as with forgiveness of others, of course, but something analogous. Specifically, we can understand self-forgiveness as a process of self-reconciliation that restores damaged self-respect and self-trust, rather than one that eliminates self-reproach in any form or to any degree.

To sum up, the virtue of self-forgiveness benefits the one who possesses it in various ways. It enables persons who feel guilt for having wronged another or shame for having been a certain sort of person to recover and live well, not merely at peace with themselves. The way in which these benefits are attained is critical for the virtue of self-forgiveness, since some ways of possibly attaining these benefits are precluded by it. In particular, the benefits must be secured as a result of examining oneself realistically and honestly, taking responsibility for what one has done and been, confessing and seeking forgiveness for one's wrongdoings and flaws, and resolving to prevent repetition and to improve. The person who does not take responsibility, or who takes responsibility only half-heartedly—not just on particular occasions but so repeatedly that we can say it is characteristic of her not to do so—does not show respect for the victims of her wrongdoing and does not have the virtue of self-forgiveness. Even if she manages to achieve some measure of contentment and self-confidence, she will not be living well in doing so, and in any case, such contentment and self-confidence are likely to be tenuous at best.

The virtue of self-forgiveness benefits its possessor, but its value cannot be understood in self-regarding terms alone. For one thing, a person who has unreasonably high expectations of himself and so cannot forgive himself when he errs might also be unforgiving of others even for minor missteps. The offending party might beg for forgiveness and be deeply repentant, but the offended, expecting nothing less than perfection of himself and others, is unmoved, thereby denying the offender the reconciliation he seeks. Even if the unself-forgiving person does not hold others to the same impossibly high standard to which he holds himself, he might withdraw from those he has wronged because their presence is a painful reminder of his misdeeds, and this withdrawal might compound the initial injury. In addition, there are certain role relationships in which the virtue of self-forgiveness has special other-regarding significance because of the particular demands of the relationship. I spoke about one of these, the physician–patient relationship, at the beginning of this essay and I will return to it in the concluding section.

4. RESPONSIBILITY, BLAME, AND SELF-FORGIVENESS

The assumption of responsibility is central to the self-reproach that self-forgiveness enables us to overcome. It makes no sense, or is at least irrational, to speak about self-forgiveness in relation to something for which one bears no responsibility. But there are different views concerning when an agent is and can be held responsible for wrongdoing. (As I noted earlier, self-forgiveness also arises in connection with certain mental states and traits, but I do not address here the issue of responsibility for them.) According to one, an agent is responsible for wrongdoing if and only if she is culpable: when and only when she deliberately commits wrongs, for example, or negligently allows unjustified harm to occur, or fails to prevent wrongs when she has a responsibility to do so and no legitimate excuse for not doing so. According to the other, it is not necessary that an agent be culpable in order to be responsible for wrongdoing. It is sufficient that she has violated the rights of another or failed to fulfill a reasonable expectation, even though her action or failure to act might be excusable (Thompson 2002: 44–5). Those who subscribe to the first view think that ascription of responsibility is appropriate only insofar as the person in question is blameworthy; in other words, both could have and should have acted differently. Those who subscribe to the second believe that it may be appropriate even if no blame may be attached. They may also believe in the existence of what are called 'moral remainders'.

There is a well-known case discussed by Joel Feinberg that illustrates this phenomenon (Feinberg 1978: 102). It involves a backpacker high in the mountains who encounters an unanticipated blizzard that threatens his life. Fortunately he stumbles upon an unoccupied cabin, and though it is clearly someone's private property, he breaks in, helps himself to the food supply, and warms himself by burning some of the cabin furniture. Feinberg claims that the backpacker's actions were, all things considered, justifiable. At the same time, however, he believes that the backpacker owes compensation to the owner of the cabin for the damage he has done. After all, he has violated the owner's property rights, so done wrong, even though this can be justified as necessary to save his life. The backpacker himself, if he is a morally decent person, is likely to be pained by what he did and wish that he had not had to act as he did. As Michael Walzer says, expressing a common intuition, 'when [moral] rules are overriden, we do not talk or act as if they had been set aside, canceled, or annulled . . . . They still stand and . . . we know we have done something wrong even if what we have done was also the best thing to do on the whole in the circumstances' (1973: 171). We have done wrong and are responsible for it, and though, having acted justifiably, we cannot rightly be blamed for it, we ought to do something to repair the damage we have done.

I use the case of moral remainders in order to make the following point: the sense of responsibility that is operative in discussions of self-forgiveness should not be tied too closely to blameworthiness. One can be and feel responsible for having wronged another even though it was a justified wrong, and one can be distressed that one has done this, that is, distressed not just at what happened but at its having been done by oneself. If we allow that self-reproach can cover a range of painful feelings of negative self-assessment, self-reproach in cases of the moral remainder type is not necessarily irrational and may very well be reasonable. And if the self-reproach is occasioned by one's having done something that strikes at one's sense of worth, then the conditions have been met for being able to speak sensibly about self-forgiveness.

Moral remainder cases are not the only ones that could be used to make the point about the relationship between self-forgiveness, responsibility, and self-blame, but I will not pursue this here. (We might also mention cases illustrating what Bernard Williams calls 'agent-regret', such as that of a lorry driver who, through no fault of his own, accidentally runs over a child (Williams 1982).) In general, the grounds for attributing responsibility and the grounds for assigning blame may come apart. There may be a stronger case for the former than the latter, and it is responsibility rather than blame that is required for self-forgiveness. Of course, self-blame for wrongdoing is sometimes appropriate, and these are perhaps the standard cases in which the issue of self-forgiveness arises. But even if self-blame is warranted, this does not imply that it will always be best from the point of view of securing reparation for damage done to encourage wrongdoers to blame themselves for their misdeeds.

5. THE PHYSICIAN–PATIENT RELATIONSHIP REVISITED

I argued in the opening section that the characteristic normative self-conception that has long been shaped and sustained by medical training and practice does not leave much room for the virtue of self-forgiveness. This would not be a serious criticism if self-forgiveness turned out not to be a virtue after all, or at least it would not be a serious criticism of the *physician* if there were no reason to include it among the virtues particularly needed in this role. Neither view is correct, however. With respect to the latter, I have claimed that self-forgiveness is a virtue that physicians need to possess because of the nature of their role, since without it they are less likely to perform well as physicians. It is now time for me to try to make good on this claim. I propose to do this by focusing on two problem areas in clinical medicine—caring for the incurable and disclosing medical mistakes—and by considering what light the previous discussion of self-forgiveness can shed on why physicians often do not respond well in these types of situation and what it would take for them to respond well. If the importance of self-forgiveness in these situations is established, this will go some way toward showing that physicians need the virtue of self-forgiveness if they are to do well in the demanding job of looking after the sick.

Caring for the Incurable

'There is a specific form of abandonment that is particularly common among patients near death from cancer,' writes Sherwin Nuland, 'abandonment by doctors' (1995: 257). The point, I believe, has considerably wider application than to terminal oncology patients alone. Emotionally, and sometimes physically as well, many physicians tend to disappear when their efforts to cure, or if not cure, significantly to prolong life, fail. Many reasons have been given for this disturbing and lamentable tendency of physicians to turn away from their patients in their time of great need. Nuland mentions two. One is a heightened degree of personal anxiety about dying: 'We become doctors because our ability to cure gives us power over the death of which we are so afraid, and loss of that power poses such a significant threat that we must turn away from it, and therefore from the patient who personifies our weakness' (1995: 258). The feeling of invulnerability that is reinforced by working among the sick while being healthy is, on this account, a defense against the physician's fear of illness and death, and the illusion of invulnerability is maintained by staying at a distance from the patient whose condition she cannot reverse or whose death she cannot prevent.

Another reason given by Nuland is the intense need to exert control over nature: 'When control is lost, he who requires it is also a bit lost and so deals badly with the consequences of his impotence' (1995: 258). Physicians are trained to try to control disease processes and naturally are frustrated when that can't be achieved. Many physicians, however, regard their failure to prevent death or to cure disease not just as a failure of medicine but as personal defeat. Rather than accept that the powers of even the most competent physician to extend life and cure disease are severely limited, they persist in viewing death and disease as enemies that must be vanquished, and they are likely to deal with their sense of defeat by putting emotional distance between themselves and the painful reminders of their impotence (Brusstar 2001; Gunderman 2000; Novack et al. 1997).

In addition to patient abandonment, the physician's defensive need to shun acknowledgment of his limited powers as a physician, most acutely experienced in relation to patients who are near death, may have other consequences that do a disservice to patients and their families. Nuland notes that 'having lost the major battle, the doctor may maintain a bit of authority by exerting his influence over the dying process' (1995: 259), by unilaterally determining the manner and timing of the patient's death. The physician, unable to prevent death, can continue to maintain the illusion of his power by controlling how and when the patient dies. In this way, 'he deprives the patient and the family of the control that is rightfully theirs' (1995: 259). This disempowerment of patients and families is facilitated by the physician's lack of candor about the efficacy of her treatments and the patient's prognosis, a lack of candor that itself often results from the physician's sense of therapeutic impotence. When her efforts to prolong life are frustrated, the need to maintain control may get displaced from treatment decisions on to the medical decision-making process.

The physician's limited powers to extend life and eliminate disease are to a large extent, of course, attributable to the current state of medical science, not necessarily to any incomplete or imperfect mastery of available knowledge or personal shortcoming on the part of the individual physician. Physicians have a theoretical awareness of the limitations of medical knowledge, of the humbling truth that even with medical and technological advancement, disease and death will not be eradicated, but this often gets suppressed when they turn their attention to the care of patients. As a consequence, undesired outcomes get attributed to some individual failing rather than to deficiencies in collective professional knowledge and physicians blame themselves for outcomes for which they are not at fault. The tendency to personalize, to take personal responsibility (in the sense of culpability) for adverse medical outcomes that do not in fact indicate substandard care on the part of the individual physician, is widespread and fostered and reinforced by professional medical training. It is also facilitated by a long-standing and deeply entrenched feature of clinical practice, namely, that physicians, generally speaking, do not see themselves as part of a system and resist collaborative approaches to patient care.

It should be clear from this description what role the virtue of self-forgiveness can play in such situations. A person who has the virtue of self-forgiveness steers a middle course between being unduly hard on himself and being too easy on himself, and there are several ways in which the former can occur. Self-reproach can become all-consuming, so that one is constantly absorbed in trying to atone for what one has done or been; it can be out of proportion to the seriousness of that for which one reproaches oneself, that is, although one did wrong or was in some respect deficient, one greatly exaggerates how bad one is; and, what is of particular relevance here, one's self-reproach can be misplaced, in other words, one reproaches oneself for something that does not warrant self-reproach or at least this kind of self-reproach. Physicians who blame themselves for ignorance or ineptitude when an adverse event is instead due to limitations of present medical knowledge are being unduly hard on themselves in this latter sense. If part of the virtue of self-forgiveness is the ability to discern whether there is any need to forgive oneself for what one has done or failed to do, physicians who are prone to this sort of self-blame are deficient with respect to that virtue. Admittedly, there may be situations in which, with good reason, it is difficult to distinguish between the respective contributions of personal and collective deficiencies to an adverse event. Self-blame may or may not be warranted in these cases, but the virtue of self-forgiveness will protect the physician from reaching hasty conclusions in this matter.

An analogy might help explain why I include this sort of case in a discussion of the virtue of self-forgiveness. Someone who possesses the virtue of courage not only knows how to act when confronted with danger, and so acts, but also has true or at least reasonable beliefs about what is dangerous. A paranoid person may run from danger, but it is not chiefly for this reason that we would say he lacks the virtue of courage. He lacks this because his perceptions of danger are regularly distorted by his paranoid delusions. Similarly, the physician who is prone to blame himself for doing things that were not wrong or faulty because he has exaggerated expectations of his competence is to this extent lacking in the virtue of self-forgiveness. This is not because he does not let go of feelings of self-reproach. Arguably, people might properly continue to reproach themselves for their wrongdoing even if they possess the virtue. It is rather because his self-conception or self-ideal distorts his assessment of his blameworthiness, and he does not (consciously) recognize that it operates in this way. Among other things, the virtue of self-forgiveness functions as a corrective to erroneous or unreasonable beliefs about one's fault and hence to unreasonable self-blame. Moreover, since unreasonable self-blame can in various ways, as I have indicated, interfere with good and respectful patient care, it is an important virtue that needs to be cultivated in medical training for the sake of patients and their families.

Disclosing Medical Errors

Failures to cure or prolong life are not necessarily wrongs nor do they necessarily involve wrongs. No rights of the patient may have been violated or reasonable expectations gone unfulfilled. The commission of a medical mistake, however, is clearly different, since patients are entitled to expect that they will receive care that meets existing professional standards. Since serious mistakes as well as various kinds of moral wrongdoing can be objects of self-forgiveness, I examine next what role the virtue of self-forgiveness can play with respect to how the physician responds to her awareness that she has made or been involved in a mistake.

First some distinctions. Adverse outcomes or events in medicine are of various types. The undesired outcomes may be neither preventable nor predictable; they may be unpreventable but foreseeable, in the sense that they occur with predictable frequency even when the standard of care is practiced; or they may be preventable, either because they result in large measure from remediable deficiencies in the delivery system (i.e. system errors) or from carelessness or ignorance or ineptitude on the part of individual health providers (i.e. human errors). Human errors are more idiosyncratic and less predictable than system errors, and they include both errors of commission, for example, prescription errors, and errors of omission, 'failure or delay in making a diagnosis or instituting treatment, and failure to use indicated tests or take precautions to prevent injury' (Leape et al. 1991: 381). Sometimes a human error is caught in time so that serious injury does not result; sometimes the error is not detected or corrected until it is too late to prevent harm.

Even when treatment does not fall below the standard of care and the physician has done everything that could reasonably be expected of her, there is no guarantee of a positive outcome. The science and practice of medicine are such that adverse outcomes are always possible and not uncommon. Adverse events are never welcome, of course, but it is especially difficult for physicians to acknowledge to themselves and admit to others that an adverse event was caused by an error they were involved in or committed, perhaps a result of some deficiency in their own knowledge, skill, or attentiveness (Banja 2001; Novack et al. 1997). Christensen et al. account for this by noting that the 'processes that motivate the physicians to maintain excellent standards of practice do not incorporate the notion of fallibility' (1992: 430).[3] Echoing this explanation, a recent report from the Veterans Health Administration states, 'No one likes to admit responsibility for an error or to face a person they may have harmed. Perhaps no group of professionals likes this less than physicians, whose profession "values perfection" and whose prime directive is to "do no harm"'(2003: 4). The connection between difficulties with disclosure of mistakes and the ideal of infallibility is noted by many authors (Levinson and Dunn 1989; Newman 1996). There are other factors as well that help explain the reluctance of physicians to reveal medical

---

[3] The authors go on to suggest that 'the absence of fallibility as a category in physicians' concepts of their profession may be a product of the lack of serious discussion of mistakes in medical training, in the medical literature, and in the conferences, grand rounds, and symposia through which physicians are continuously socialized into the way that medicine works.'

mistakes, including concerns about legal and financial risks and fear of damage to reputation and loss of respect or status among colleagues (Lo 2000; Finkelstein et al. 1997).

Recent reports by the Institute of Medicine (2000) and the Quality Interagency Coordination Task Force (2000) have stressed the need for a systems approach to reducing the incidence of medical errors. Unfortunately, this emphasis on faults in the health care delivery system as the leading cause of medical errors may make it easier for physicians to deny their responsibility for the commission of medical errors by placing blame on some other part of the health care system. There is a morally significant distinction to be drawn between errors caused by flaws in the health care delivery system and those caused by individual ignorance or ineptitude, but individual physicians are not necessarily exempt from responsibility in the former situation. Responsibility for the commission of an error is sometimes shared between the physician and other elements of the system and sometimes primarily the physician's, but in either case the physician (alone or with others) owes the patient or family some acknowledgment of the harm that was done, some expression of remorse or at least regret, and an apology for the mistake (Wu et al. 1997; Gallagher et al. 2003).

The moral arguments for at least informing patients that a mistake was made are compelling (Vogel and Delgado 1980; Wu et al. 1997; Veterans Health Administration 2003). According to one line of argument, a consequentialist one, the benefits of disclosure for patients, physicians, and other involved parties outweigh the harms, at least when the benefits and harms to the patient are weighted more heavily than the others, as they should be. Some but not all of these benefits can only be secured if the physician himself discloses. For patients who have been harmed by an error, failure to disclose can deny them the opportunity to seek further treatment to restore health or mitigate harm and to obtain financial compensation. Disclosure can also benefit physicians by relieving them of some of the emotional burden of guilt. A second line of argument is duty-based and looks to the fiduciary character of the physician–patient relationship. The ethical principles upon which this relationship is grounded, including those that require the physician to further the health of his patient and to respect his patient's autonomy, argue in favor of disclosure. Since the relationship of trust is between a particular patient and a particular physician, disclosure of an error by someone other than the responsible physician will not be morally sufficient. Compatible with this line of argument is a third, which I have pursued in this essay: it argues for disclosure from the standpoint of virtue ethics. On this view, the moral reason for disclosing, and no doubt for doing more than just this, is that this is what a physician, who has and exercises certain virtues, would characteristically do in circumstances in which he has made or been involved in a medical error. Among these virtues is that of self-forgiveness.

Ethical arguments notwithstanding, physicians often do not disclose mistakes they have made, and it is the obstacles to disclosure relating to personal ideals that are most pertinent in the context of a discussion of self-forgiveness. I offer the following hypothesis: a physician who expects herself to be infallible will tend to repress evidence of her fallibility, and since few things bring home her fallibility as effectively as confronting those she has mistakenly harmed, she will tend to avoid them or at least to act around them as if nothing untoward has taken place. From one point of view, such a physician is taking the easy way out by not facing those she has harmed. But from another, such a physician is being unduly hard on herself: not because she has not done anything wrong (after all, she has made a mistake, in contrast to the cases discussed earlier under the heading of caring for the incurable), but because she has inflated and unrealistic expectations of herself, and she engages in defensive man-euvers to avoid self-acknowledgment of her failure to live up to them. She does not therefore properly take responsibility for whatever errors she commits, which consists in part in stepping forward and disclosing her mistakes, especially to those she has harmed, and exposing herself to their judgment and anger. Among other things, she may chalk up the error to "the system" and refuse to take any personal responsibility for it.

Once again we see the importance of cultivating the virtue of self-forgiveness in the training of physicians and its value in the physician–patient relationship.[4] Pos-sessing the virtue of self-forgiveness, the physician would have a proper appreciation of the nature and extent of her involvement in medical error, and would neither evade responsibility that she ought to accept nor take on more responsibility than is warran-ted. The discussion of disclosure of medical errors, like that of caring for the incur-able, bears out the adage that 'the perfect is the enemy of the good,' where 'good' here refers to qualities of the virtuous physician.

I will not comment on the training methods to be used (Goldberg et al. 2002), other than to say that it is important to devise approaches that avoid the traditional reliance on blame: blame is of limited usefulness in fostering the virtue of self-forgiveness, since it discourages candor and encourages defensiveness. Moreover, the individual physician is not always responsible (in the sense of culpable) for the mistakes he makes. Of course, even with much greater attention to the virtue of self-forgiveness, problems might remain. The legal and institutional context within which physicians practice medicine may continue to make it difficult and costly for physicians to disclose error to the patient or the patient's family, even if they are so disposed.

Finally, it may be said that few physicians make mistakes, or many mistakes, or at any rate serious mistakes, so the preceding discussion is not a very persuasive way of making the case for the virtue of self-forgiveness. Against this, Atul Gawande claims that 'virtually everyone who cares for hospital patients will make serious mistakes, and even commit acts of negligence, every year' (Gawande 1999). Moreover, with the

---

[4] As Nancy Berlinger notes in a recent article about medical harm:

in conversations I have had with clinicians and hospital chaplains on the topic of forgiveness after medical error, *self*-forgiveness has emerged as a constant theme. All stressed that some form of self-forgiveness (their phrase) was essential in restoring confidence and morale after incidents of medical harm, even as one physician acknowledged that while self-forgiveness is 'something we all have to face when we make an error that harms someone'. . . . It is hard to get physicians to think in these terms. (Berlinger 2003: 33–4)

Berlinger's report is particularly significant because of what it reveals about the perceptions and concerns of practicing health professionals, a group that includes more than physicians in training.

advent of managed care, arguably the incidence of errors, especially errors of omission, is likely to increase, since physicians are under intense pressure to increase their productivity and control costs. Gawande's statement may be an exaggeration. But even if most physicians seldom makes serious mistakes, the argument I have presented for why the good physician has the virtue of self-forgiveness is not predicated on the assumption that the individual physician will in fact frequently make serious mistakes. The virtue of self-forgiveness is one of the virtues of the good physician because it involves disclosure of mistakes when they are made, because there are compelling ethical reasons to disclose, and because the nature of medical practice is such that serious mistakes are always possible. What we expect of the virtuous physician is that she will be neither unreasonably hard nor unreasonably easy on herself when mistakes are made and, further, that she has the trait of character that justifies patients in trusting her to own up to her mistakes and disclose them when they occur.

REFERENCES

Arras, J. (2001). 'A Method in Search of a Purpose: The Internal Morality of Medicine'. *Journal of Medicine and Philosophy*, 26/2: 643–62

Banja, J. (2001). 'Moral Courage in Medicine: Disclosing Medical Error'. *Bioethics Forum*, 17: 7–11.

Baylis, F. (1997). 'Errors in Medicine: Nurturing Truthfulness'. *Journal of Clinical Ethics*, 8/4: 336–40.

Berlinger, N. (2003). 'Avoiding Cheap Grace: Medical Harm, Patient Safety, and the Culture(s) of Forgiveness'. *Hastings Center Report*, 33/6: 28–36.

Bosk, C. (1979). *Forgive and Remember: Managing Medical Failure*. Chicago: University of Chicago Press.

Brusstar, G. (2001). 'Recovering the Heart to Heal: New Programs, Perspective Revitalizes Physicians'. *Michigan Medicine*, 100: 20–6.

Calhoun, C. (1992). 'Changing One's Heart'. *Ethics*, 103: 76–96.

Care, N. (1996). *Living With One's Past*. Lanham, MD: Rowman and Littlefield.

_____ (2002). 'Forgiveness and Effective Agency', in S. Lamb and J. Murphy (eds.), *Before Forgiving: Cautionary Views of Forgiveness in Psychotherapy*. Oxford: University Press, 215–31.

Chazan, P. (1998). *The Moral Self*. London: Routledge.

Christensen, J., Levinson, W., and Dunn, P. (1992). 'The Heart of Darkness: The Impact of Perceived Mistakes on Physicians'. *Journal of General Internal Medicine*, 7: 424–31.

Dillon, R. (2001). 'Self-Forgiveness and Self-Respect'. *Ethics*, 112/1: 53–83.

Downie, R. S. (1965). 'Forgiveness'. *Philosophical Quarterly*, 15: 128–34.

Feinberg, Joel (1978). 'Voluntary Euthanasia and the Inalienable Right to Life'. *Philosophy and Public Affairs*, 7: 93–123.

Finkelstein, D., Wu, A., Holtzman, N., and Smith, M. (1997). 'When a Physician Harms a Patient by a Medical Error: Ethical, Legal, and Risk-Management Considerations'. *Journal of Clinical Ethics*, 8/4: 330–5.

Fiscalini, J. (1995). 'Narcissism and Self-Disorder', in M. Lionells et al. (eds.), *Handbook of Interpersonal Psychoanalysis*. Hillsdale, NJ: Analytic Press, 333–75.

Flanigan, Beverly (1996). *Forgiving Yourself*. New York: Macmillan.

Foot, P. (1978). 'Virtues and Vices', in *Virtues and Vices and Other Essays in Moral Philosophy*. Berkeley: University of California Press, 1–18.

Gallagher. T., Waterman, A., Ebers, A., Fraser, V., and Levinson, W. (2003). 'Patients' and Physicians' Attitudes Regarding the Disclosure of Medical Errors'. *Journal of the American Medical Association,* 289/8: 1001–7.

Gartner, J. (1992). 'The Capacity to Forgive: An Object Relations Perspective', in M. Finn and J. Gartner (eds.), *Object Relations Theory and Religion: Clinical Applications.* Westport, CT: Praeger, 21–33.

Gawande, A. (1999). 'When Doctors Make Mistakes'. *New Yorker,* 1 Feb.

Goldberg, R., Kuhn, G., Andrew, L. B., and Thomas, H. A. (2002). 'Coping with Medical Mistakes and Errors in Judgment'. *Annals of Emergency Medicine,* 39/3: 287–92.

Govier, T. (2002). *Forgiveness and Revenge.* London: Routledge.

Gunderman, R. (2000). 'Illness as Failure: Blaming Patients'. *Hastings Center Report,* 30/4: 7–11.

Haber, J. (1991). *Forgiveness.* Savage, MD: Rowman and Littlefield.

Hampton, J. (1988). 'Forgiveness, Resentment, and Hatred', in J. Murphy and J. Hampton (eds.), *Forgiveness and Mercy.* New York: Cambridge University Press.

Hilfiker, D. (1984). 'Facing Our Mistakes'. *New England Journal of Medicine,* 310: 118–22.

Hill, T. (1991). 'Servility and Self-Respect', in *Autonomy and Self-Respect.* Cambridge: Cambridge University Press, 4–18.

Holmgren, M. (1998). 'Self-Forgiveness and Responsible Moral Agency'. *Journal of Value Inquiry,* 32: 75–91.

—— (2002). 'Forgiveness and Self-Forgiveness in Psychotherapy', in S. Lamb and J. Murphy (eds.), *Before Forgiving: Cautionary Views of Forgiveness in Psychotherapy.* Oxford: Oxford University Press, 112–35.

Horsbrugh, H. J. N. (1974). 'Forgiveness'. *Canadian Journal of Philosophy,* 4: 269–82.

Hughes, P. (1994). 'On Forgiving Oneself: A Reply to Snow'. *Journal of Value Inquiry,* 28: 557–60.

Institute of Medicine, Committee on Quality of Health Care in America (2000). L. T. Kohn, J. M. Corrigan, and M. S. Donaldson (eds.), *To Err is Human: Building a Safer Health System.* Washington, DC: National Academy Press.

Katz, J. (1984). 'Why Doctors Don't Disclose Uncertainty'. *Hastings Center Report,* 14/1: 35–44.

Lang, B. (1994). 'Forgiveness'. *American Philosophical Quarterly,* 31: 105–17.

Leape, L. L., et al. (1991). 'The Nature of Adverse Events in Hospitalized Patients'. *New England Journal of Medicine,* 324/6: 377–84.

Levinson, W., and Dunn, P. M. (1989). 'Coping with Fallibility'. *Journal of the American Medical Association,* 261: 2252.

Lo, B. (2000). 'Disclosing Mistakes', in *Resolving Ethical Dilemmas* (2nd edn.). Philadelphia: Lippincott, 263–70.

Longhurst, M. (1988). 'Physician Self-awareness: the Neglected Insight'. *Canadian Medical Association Journal,* 139: 121–4.

McCue, J. D. (1982). 'The Effects of Stress on Physicians and Their Medical Practice'. *New England Journal of Medicine,* 306: 458–63.

MacIntyre, A. (1981). *After Virtue.* Notre Dame, IN: University Press.

Marcus, E. R. (1999). 'Empathy, Humanism, and the Professionalization Process of Medical Education'. *Academic Medicine,* 74/11: 1211–15.

—— (2003). 'Medical Student Dreams About Medical School: The Unconscious Developmental Process of Becoming a Physician'. *International Journal of Psychoanalysis,* 84: 367–86.

Murphy, J. (1998). 'Jean Hampton on Immorality, Self-Hatred, and Self-Forgiveness'. *Philosophical Studies,* 89: 215–36.

Newman, M. C. (1996). 'The Emotional Impact of Mistakes on Family Physicians'. *Archives of Family Medicine*, 5: 71–5.

Novack, D. H., Suchman, A. L., Clark, W., Epstein, R. M., Najberg, E., and Kaplan, C. (1997). 'Calibrating the Physician: Personal Awareness and Effective Patient Care'. *Journal of the American Medical Association*, 278/6: 502–9.

Nuland, S. (1995). *How We Die*. New York: Vintage.

Orlander, J. D., and Barber, T. W. (2002). 'The Morbidity and Morality Conference: The Delicate Virtue of Learning from Error'. *Academic Medicine*, 77: 1001–6.

Pellegrino, E. (1995). 'The Virtuous Physician and the Ethics of Medicine', in J. Arras and B. Steinbock (eds.), *Ethical Issues in Modern Medicine*. Mountain View, CA: Mayfield, 77–85.

⸺ and Thomasma, D. (1993). *The Virtues in Medical Practice*. New York: Oxford University Press.

Quality Interagency Coordination Task Force (2000). 'Doing What Counts for Patient Safety: Federal Actions to Reduce Medical Errors and Their Impact.' Washington, DC.

Quill, T. E., and Williamson, P. R. (1990). 'Healthy Approaches to Physician Stress'. *Archives of Internal Medicine*, 150: 1857–61.

Roberts, R. (1995). 'Forgiveness'. *American Philosophical Quarterly*, 32: 289–306.

Snow, N. (1993). 'Self-Forgiveness'. *Journal of Value Inquiry*, 27: 75–80.

Swinburne, R. (1989). *Responsibility and Atonement*. Oxford: Clarendon Press.

Taylor, G. (1985). *Pride, Shame, and Guilt*. Oxford: Clarendon Press.

Thompson, J. (2002). *Taking Responsibility for the Past*. Oxford: Blackwell.

Urmson, J. O. (1980). 'Aristotle's Doctrine of the Mean', in A. Rorty (ed.), *Essays on Aristotle's Ethics*. Berkeley: University of California Press, 157–70.

Veterans Health Administration, National Ethics Committee (2003). Disclosing Adverse Events to Patients. Washington, DC: Department of Veterans Affairs.

Vogel, J., and Delgado, R. (1980). 'To Tell the Truth: Physicians' Duty to Disclose Medical Mistakes'. *UCLA Law Review*, 28: 52–94.

Walzer, M. (1973). 'Political Action: The Problem of Dirty Hands'. *Philosophy and Public Affairs*, 2: 160–80.

Williams, B. (1982). 'Moral Luck', in *Moral Luck*. Cambridge: Cambridge University Press, 20–39.

Wu, A., (2000). 'Medical Error: The Second Victim: The Doctor Who Makes the Mistake Needs Help Too'. *British Medical Journal*, 320: 726–7.

⸺ Cavanaugh, T., McPhee, S., Lo, B., and Micco, G. (1997). 'To Tell the Truth: Ethical and Practical Issues in Disclosing Medical Mistakes to Patients'. *Journal of General Internal Medicine*, 12: 770–5.

5

Virtue Ethics as Professional Ethics: The Case of Psychiatry

Jennifer Radden

In the following discussion I explore the applicability of a virtue ethics framework to professional ethics using the case of psychiatry.[1] This inquiry is motivated in several ways. Possession of a virtuous character, over and above an exhibition of exemplary deeds, has long been seen as requisite for ethical medical practice, and medicine most generally understood has been judged a place where the virtues have special relevance (Drane 1988; Dyer 1988, 1999; Churchill 1989; May 1994; Pellegrino and Thomasma 1993). In addition, recent philosophical writing has urged that a virtue ethical framework should be applied to all professional practices owing to features shared by such practices (Kronman 1993; Oakley and Cocking 2001).[2] Psychiatry requires special attention because of its apparent uniqueness as social and medical practice. The particular vulnerabilities of psychiatric patients, combined with the nature of mental health treatment, call for special virtues and an especially virtuous character in psychiatric practice (Dyer 1988, 1999; Christianson 1995; Radden 2002; Crowden 2003; Bloch and Green 2006).[3] At the same time, psychiatric practice introduces extra challenges for the application of virtue ethics that do not arise in the same way, or at least with the same force, in other professional practices. For example, I explore how aspects of the psychiatric patient and of psychiatric treatment combine to permit and even invite the feigning of certain virtues in a way not possible in other settings. Arguably, then, psychiatry represents one of the

---

[1] The term 'psychiatry' here indicates treatment offered mentally disordered patients by medically trained practitioners, although much of what is asserted will have application to others providing mental health care.

[2] As Oakley and Cocking have argued, the teleological approach to right action in terms of good functioning relative to appropriate ends makes virtue ethics especially applicable here; this is because good functioning can be understood in terms of the good performance of a role, and virtue ethics can then evaluate the good performance of the role and the appropriateness of certain dispositions to a particular profession according to how well those roles and dispositions serve the proper ends of that profession (2001). For a useful discussion of role morality without the presuppositions of a virtue ethics framework, see Applbaum (1999).

[3] In claiming that psychiatry stands alone as a social and healing practice, I am not suggesting that these characteristics are entirely unique to psychiatry; most are found in other practices. Psychiatry's uniqueness derives from the combination and concentration of these features.

most urgent but at the same time one of the most complex and difficult cases for the application of virtue ethics to professional practice.

If a certain character in the practitioner is required for ethical psychiatric practice, what kind of character would that be? The ethical psychiatrist needs many traditional moral virtues such as integrity, justice, benevolence, and fidelity. However, I shall argue that in addition to these traditional moral virtues an ethical psychiatrist must also possess character traits which, outside the context of professional practice, are morally neutral—neither virtues nor vices—or are at most prudential and intellectual virtues, rather than moral ones. Some of these role-specific traits required in psychiatric practice are traits whose sole value lies in furthering the good of professional practice (the quality of 'unselfing' is provided as an example of this kind); others, while valuable in other contexts, acquire the status of moral virtues here because they either further the good of professional practice (realism is an example), or are preconditions for certain other, more traditional virtues also called for by the practice (self-unity and self-knowledge, because they can lead to the moral integrity, illustrate this kind of role-specific virtue).

Rather than undertaking a complete analysis of the character of the ethical psychiatrist, I develop my discussion around examples of four traits which appear to be role-constituted virtues the psychiatrist must posses—self-unity, self-knowledge, 'unselfing', and realism.

In the second part of the chapter some of the implications of the relationship between professional role morality and character are explored. I introduce the problem of feigned virtues as one complication raised by the suggestion that psychiatric practice invites or even requires the possession of a certain character in its practitioners, and explore the moral psychology of feigning virtues with particular emphasis on the context of psychiatric practice.

PART 1: WHICH VIRTUES?

The so-called health care virtues prescribed for those working in medical settings have been said to include benevolence, truthfulness, respect, friendliness, and justice (Drane 1988), as well as compassion, *phronesis*, fortitude, temperance, integrity, and self-effacement (Pellegrino and Thomasma 1993). Virtues required for caregivers within the mental health setting include trustworthiness and respect for confidentiality (Dyer 1988); compassion, humility, and fidelity (Christianson 1995); warmth and sensitivity (Beauchamp 1999); perseverance and humility (Dickenson and Fulford 2000); *phronesis* (Fraser 2000; Crowden 2003); and caring (Bloch and Green 2006).

In addition to these, many virtues have been seen as required across all professional practices. Dentists, accountants, teachers, and lawyers, as much as doctors, are governed by professional codes of conduct presupposing that they are honorable, just, and respectful of the basic contractual relationship between provider and recipient of professional services. Traits such as trustworthiness, fidelity, honesty, and integrity have even been identified with professional status: to have a profession, as distinct from having mere technique, it has been said, implies 'the possession of certain character-defining traits or qualities' (Kronman 1986: 841). Among the traits or qualities called for by every professional—and, indeed, every practical—setting, the most obvious one may be the Aristotelian virtue of *phronesis*, a quality as necessary for the ethical practice of law, or business, as medicine. Any professional practice will require the grasp of particulars, cleverness, perception, and understanding which combine in *phronesis* to direct us toward right action. That said, some have argued that *phronesis* has its own special application in psychiatric practice. For instance, Allan Fraser argues that only *phronesis* bridges intellectual knowledge about the properties and appropriate use of remedies such as medication and the needs of the patient understood not as a biological system but as a person (Fraser 2000).

There are quite significant differences between the traits enumerated above. Some are not moral virtues in the sense that their absence generally invites or entails a corresponding vice. Others may be found in the service of vices, as sensitivity seems to be implicated in the vice of cruelty, for instance. Moreover, the *phronesis* emphasized in some analyses is a kind of meta-virtue, a judgment ensuring the appropriate application of other virtues to particular situations. Each of these virtues and each of these kinds of virtue (professionals' virtues most generally understood, health care virtues, and mental health virtues) are arguably found in the ethical practitioner. (Many of them are also general and traditional virtues as well, of course: required for anyone to be virtuous in any setting.)

A complete account of all the mental health care virtues and of the setting and professional practice demanding their cultivation is beyond the scope of this discussion. But a few examples allow us to see how features of the mental health setting might call for not only (a) certain distinctive virtues (such as unselfing) but (b) greater virtue in its practitioners (more integrity, greater self control, outstanding trustworthiness, and so on), than is required by other roles and settings: (i) a group as seemingly vulnerable to exploitation as psychiatric patients will require exceptional compassion, justice, trustworthiness, and fidelity on the part of the psychiatrist; (ii) disorders so frequently affecting their sufferers' communicative and reasoning capabilities will likely call for special perseverance, compassion, and humility; (iii) in a cultural context where mental disorder is still controversial and subject to misunderstanding and stigma, the intimate, personal and private details regularly explored in healing practice will require extra discretion and trustworthiness on the part of the psychiatrist; (iv) attempts to change the patient may be unsuccessful, partial, temporary, or in some other way incomplete, but potentially the healing project in psychiatry is often sweeping: nothing less than replacing deficiency and disorder with the cherished traits of sanity, rationality, and autonomy. The profundity of this project seems to demand unusual integrity and benevolence. Finally, and perhaps most important, (v) the psychiatrist is vested by society with the unique power of restraining and treating innocent adults against their wishes—a power calling for a special degree of moral integrity in those who exercise it.

The above vulnerabilities in patients and features of psychiatric practice in no way imply that practitioners of psychiatry are more exploitative than other people (any more than child protection laws cast aspersions on the character of parents taken as a group). Because these features of practice accord such power to the practitioner however, they permit and sometimes invite exploitative responses, or even ingrained vices, against which any practitioner requires special protection in the form of character virtues such as benevolence, trustworthiness, restraint, and self-control. Consider, for example, that psychiatrists must sometimes repel openly seductive behavior from patients without conveying personal rejection, losing the patient's trust, or otherwise damaging or jeopardizing the therapeutic relationship. That practitioners do not always succeed in this endeavor does not detract from the point made here: the challenge such an endeavor presents to, and the demands it imposes on, the ethical practitioner's character.

Most of the dangers of the power accorded the practitioner are less obvious and less apparently tied to the appetites as traditionally understood. Moreover the corrupting influence and temptations associated with imbalances of power between persons are not well acknowledged in traditional virtue ethics. But the aspect of human nature which is exploitative and predatory nonetheless allows us to recognize the many non-sensual temptations to which the practitioner in psychiatry is exposed: the desire to feel superior at the expense of the other, to 'play God' with another's life, to take a prurient interest in the other's personal story, to indulge bias and prejudice, to strive to preserve self-esteem, and so on. Occasions to act on non-appetitive desires like these occur as frequently in psychiatric practice as do occasions to act from the more commonly acknowledged vices. And because such occasions are part of psychiatric practice, the practitioner's character must be strong enough to endure their temptations as well.

Useful Virtues

In the case of psychiatry, we can identify two distinct rationales supporting the importance of the virtues. The first is that ethical psychiatrists must cultivate certain character traits because such traits are called for by the particular demands of the mental health care setting, as in examples (i)–(v) above. The second is that the cultivation of certain traits will be useful to therapeutic effectiveness.

Consider the psychiatrist who refuses extravagant gifts from his patient. There will likely be two reasons to refuse the gifts, and each reason may be construed as deriving from different virtues. The first is that the patient is rendered vulnerable by her impulsive generosity. She must be protected from her yearning for acceptance and love, her failure of judicious concern over her own interests, or her incautious nature. These attributes leave the patient at risk of exploitation and, recognizing them, a virtuous practitioner will not take advantage of her by accepting the gifts. Here, the mental health care setting demands the refusal of gifts: it is a compassionate response to the patient's evident vulnerability. Hence we might think of these kinds of reasons as 'traditional' role-constituted reasons, since they are required of the virtuous professional in the role context and are commonly recognized as moral reasons for virtuous behavior.

Instead, the refusal of gifts might derive from a different sort of disposition. In fostering the therapeutic relationship, the psychiatrist may wish to model honesty, appropriateness, or good judgment; to express that his caring is not dependent on receiving 'rewards' of this kind; to point out the message or strategy behind the proffered gift, or to open up some discursive possibilities around the patient's attitudes toward her self and her values. The practitioner's more general ethical stance vis-à-vis the features of the mental health care setting motivates the first sort of response; his commitment to a successful therapeutic alliance stimulates the second.

Each reason for refusing the gifts is a moral reason, broadly understood. The psychiatrist's professional—and personal—moral code requires he avoid exploiting his patient's vulnerabilities, so his first reason is obviously a moral reason for him. But his professional code also requires him to achieve therapeutic effectiveness, which will in turn require that he possess the dispositions grounding the second kind of rationale for refusing the gifts. So the ethical psychiatrist has two types of reason to cultivate a good character, each discovered in a different way. He will possess and should cultivate any virtues which, based on his professional (and personal) *ethos*, appear to be called for by the mental health care setting, and we can find out what these particular virtues are by examining that setting. In addition, if certain dispositions and responses are required for and/or markedly enhance the effectiveness of treatment in psychiatry, he will also possess and should cultivate those traits because of his professional duty to maximize therapeutic effectiveness, and we can ascertain which those are by examining the ingredients of therapeutic effectiveness.[4]

The significance of the therapeutic reasons for being virtuous is pronounced in the case of psychiatry, where the personal conduct and character of the practitioner are represented as a sine qua non of healing and the psychiatrist uses her persona in forming, maintaining, and fostering the relationship or alliance with the patient out of which healing derives. The importance of these therapeutic reasons for being virtuous is thus heightened because of the nature of psychiatric practice, although some non-psychiatric practice may also be enhanced by the practitioner's persona (even whether the patient doubts or has faith in his surgeon may affect healing to some degree). To the extent that a virtue ethics framework is applicable to other professional practices requiring particular personal traits for effective ethical practice, the same layered moral description will be required. Those role-specific virtues demanded of the ethical practitioner regardless of that practice's outcome, will be distinguishable from those whose possession will enhance that outcome.

---

[4] Although the difference noted above between virtues called for by the setting and virtues that are effective in practice is rarely encountered in writing about virtues in practice, we do find it acknowledged in a brief discussion of the importance of compassion for medical ethics. Charland and Dick separate clinical from ethical aspects of empathic compassion: the principle of respect for persons imposes the ethical requirement that physicians be compassionate towards patients, they argue (1995: 417), while the clinical advantages are several. Compassion contributes, they assert, to 'professional objectivity and overall clinical state, while addressing the special needs of patients to be understood, and maintaining a level of communication needed for therapeutic diagnosis and benefit'. (1995: 418). It is difficult to deny, they insist, that ' "feeling understood" is a positive clinical therapeutic phenomenon for patients' (1995: 416). In some respects this separation between the clinical and ethical reasons for compassion in the character of the practitioner is useful, but it is misleading in its suggestion that these two sorts of reasons represent moral (ethical) and non-moral (clinical) reasons to cultivate compassion. It is argued in the present chapter, that the ethical practitioner devoted to the good of healing is motivated morally in responding with compassion to her patient.

One of the purposes of introducing the distinction between outcome-indifferent and outcome-sensitive role-constituted reasons for being virtuous is to begin to sort out what the character of the ethical psychiatrist might be like. To do so, I want to situate this discussion within claims that have been made about professional roles and role morality. Each of the professions imposes special duties on its practitioners, it is generally agreed, requiring dispositions and conduct conducive to furthering the particular good of that profession (Churchill 1989; Veatch 1991; May 1992; Pellegrino and Thomasma 1993; Applbaum 1999; Oakley and Cocking 2001). Medicine most generally understood demands the promotion of health and healing, and for the practitioner in psychiatry, this becomes the promotion of mental health and healing.[5] Within a virtue ethics framework, then, this demand is for the possession and cultivation of certain traits that promote health and healing. Although they are role-constituted moral virtues within the practice setting, outside that practice setting, these are not necessarily moral virtues whose absence is a vice, and sometimes are not virtues in any sense. This point has been explained by Justin Oakley and Dean Cocking:

> a virtue ethics criterion of right action in the context of a professional role ... would be directed towards the proper goal of the profession in question ... For example, in a medical context ... the character of the virtuous doctor would be constituted by dispositions which serve the goal of health in appropriate ways. Thus, on a virtue ethics approach to professional roles, something can be a virtue in professional life—such as a doctor's acute clinical judgment in making a correct diagnosis from a multitude of symptoms—*which might be neutral in ordinary life*. (Oakley and Cocking 2001: 129, my emphasis)

Our virtuous psychiatrist refuses gifts out of a kind of compassionate recognition of the patient's vulnerability, but equally out of an acute sensitivity to the implications for therapy of the patient's motivation, needs, and understandings, a sensitivity which marks an effective practitioner. The refusal of gifts, we might say, derives from these two, equally important virtues of compassion and sensitivity. A kind of practical wisdom allows the therapist to know how to respond here, so we can add *phronesis* to the virtues demonstrated in this example. Sensitivity may be a virtue of some kind in everyday morality, though it appears to be an intellectual rather than a moral virtue. It nonetheless is made up of traits which, as Oakley and Cocking point out, may be neutral in everyday morality but have become role-constituted moral virtues in this context: a good memory, an ability to pick out and understand emotional saliencies, a skill at reading the patient's extra-verbal expressions and paying close attention to small cues, the gentleness to refuse the gift without hurting the patient's feelings, skills of timing and phrasing, and so on. A much quoted, partial definition by Alisdair MacIntyre has proposed that a virtue is 'an acquired human quality the possession and exercise of which tends to enable us to achieve those goods which are internal to practices and the lack of which effectively prevents us from achieving any such

---

[5] Conceptions of mental health vary, even within our culture. Nonetheless, in their broadest outlines, there is considerable agreement over the traits marking mature social and psychological adjustment, and practitioners are more likely to disagree over the methods of achieving those goals than over the goals themselves.

goods' (MacIntyre 1981: 178). Because of its instrumentalist emphasis, this definition has been criticized (Pincoffs 1986: 96; Crisp and Slote 1997: 11–13). Yet what makes it insufficient as a complete definition for all virtues fits it as a definition for role-constituted virtues, such as sensitivity was shown to be. They are qualities whose possession and exercise tend to enable us to achieve those goods which are internal to a professional practice.

The previous reasoning requires a clarification of the notions of character and virtue. Character sometimes refers to the set of a person's moral virtues and perhaps even their vices, those traits Aristotle saw as acquired through early habituation and, in the case of moral virtues at least, the correct rational deliberation. More broadly understood, a person's character is made up of a range of characteristic traits, positive, negative, and morally neutral. Thus, for example, Kupperman defines character as a normal pattern of thought and action (for any given X who possesses that character) 'especially with respect to concerns and commitments in matters affecting the happiness of others or of X, and most especially in relation to moral choices' (Kupperman 1991: 17). Interestingly, on a common interpretation even Aristotle's *arête* is rendered with the broader 'excellence', to indicate that it spans both moral virtues and additional non-moral traits (Irwin 1985; Kupperman 1991) although this broader interpretation of *arête* has been contested (Beresford 2005).

Relying on the narrow notion of character which excludes morally neutral traits, we might have said that the *ethical* practitioner possesses moral virtues, while the *effective* practitioner possesses useful traits. After all, we can envision an ethical though ineffective practitioner, or an effective but otherwise unethical one. Whether or not we allow character to comprise useful traits as well as moral virtues, and whatever way we understand the Aristotelian term *arête*, this set of distinctions proves insufficient when we turn to the useful traits that are part of the role morality of the ethical practitioner. The tenets of role morality require us to understand the designations 'moral virtue' and 'useful trait' to be relational, so that *within the professional context,* useful traits *acquire the status* of moral virtues.

Role morality seems to come in weaker and stronger forms. Weak role morality acknowledges the more stringent obligations imposed by roles. The demands of weak role morality never override, but they add to, the dictates of 'broad based' morality applicable to the rest of society. Thus, for example, weak role morality may forbid consenting sexual relations between unmarried, adult doctors and their unmarried, adult patients, even though broad based morality permits consenting sexual relations between unmarried adults. More controversial, strong role morality, allows that what is morally permissible or even morally required by a role is not necessarily required and may not even be permitted on the broad based morality. Arguably, for instance, adherence to adversarial principles underlying the lawyer's professional role may permit forms of manipulation and communication unacceptable according to broader based standards of civility and honesty. It does not seem that the psychiatric role imposes any similarly controversial features, however. What is defended here is weak role morality.

Many virtues are required in psychiatry merely because its practitioners are professionals and doctors. But some role-constituted virtues are more practice-specific.

I want to focus attention on a handful of these that seem to function in different ways within the character of the virtuous psychiatrist: self-knowledge, self-unity, 'unself-ing', and realism. Though not moral virtues on traditional definitions (self-knowledge and self-unity are intellectual virtues, perhaps, on the Aristotelian schema, 'unself-ing' is not a virtue at all, and realism is at best a prudential virtue), each of these are role-constituted virtues, in the sense that they are called for by the psychiatric setting, or appear to be useful for effective psychiatric practice. Moreover, the traits of self-knowledge, self-unity, and realism are implicated in the psychiatric project in a third way: they are cultural ideals that find expression in conceptions of mental health.

Self-Knowledge, Self-Unity, and Moral Integrity

Understood as ends consciously sought, self-knowledge and self-unity are not easily separated. Self-knowledge can be characterized as understanding of one's own sub-jectivity, psychic states and traits, life, and character. Self-unity or integration is a condition of psychological coherence and consistency. At the very least, these two qual-ities will likely be sought, although perhaps not always found, together. Insight and the exercise of reflective self-examination characterizing self-knowledge is usually con-strued as the means to achieving the psychological integration involved in self-unity. We can envision self-unity occurring in an unreflective psyche, however, and there may be alternative paths to integrity other than the self-conscious and rationalistic efforts associated with acquiring self-knowledge, as thinkers such as Martha Nussbaum and Nomy Arpaly stress (Nussbaum 1996; Arpaly 2003). Moreover we can envision a degree of self-knowledge not motivated, or accompanied, by a unified psyche. So while related as personal ideals, self-knowledge and self-unity are separate qualities.

The trait of self-unity, at least, if not self-knowledge, seems close to the trans-parently moral virtue of integrity.[6] Schauber (1996) has distinguished 'moralizing integrity' from 'self-unifying integrity' where moralizing integrity refers to coherence and consistency in moral judgment and righteous action, and 'self-unifying integrity' indicates a more coherent subjectivity and memory. I will continue to speak of moral integrity and self-unity to emphasize, along with Schauber, that these two sorts of integration are distinct. Nevertheless, there seems to be an interrelationship between them. Just as self-unity is often sought through self-knowledge, so the coherence and consistency of moral integrity seem to derive from a psychological coherence and con-sistency. Such an integrated psychological subjectivity seems to auger, and may be a precondition for, the moral virtue of integrity.

That the mental health care setting calls for moral integrity in its practitioners has long been emphasized. This much seems incontrovertible. The particular vulnerab-ilities of their patients each demand that psychiatrists be persons of moral integrity, whether these vulnerabilities involve a risk of exploitation, the nature of the mental health care setting, or the psychiatric undertaking with its potentially profound effects on and appraisal of the patient's life and experience. The link with self-unity and

---

[6] The complex virtue of integrity requires a fuller discussion than these brief references provide, and readers are directed to the valuable literature on integrity (Taylor 1985; McFall 1992; Diamond 1992; Sutherland 1996; McKinnon 1999; Cox, Lacaze, and Levine 2003).

the importance of moral integrity are nicely conveyed by William May. Integrity, he insists, '*makes possible* the fiduciary bond between the professional and the client' (my emphasis) because it signifies 'wholeness or completeness of character; it does not permit a split between the inner and the outer, between word and deed' (May 1994: 87). If May is right, any professional practice depends on the integrating aspect of moral integrity in the practitioner, which in turn depends on self-unity and self-knowledge.

While called for by the mental health care setting because of their relationship to moral integrity, self-knowledge and self-unity are also dispositions likely required for therapeutic effectiveness. Descriptions sometimes portray the psychiatrist's function as an exemplar in the therapeutic relationship, representing a person or character whom the patient can emulate. It has been claimed, for example, that the patient tends to 'identify with', and 'model herself on', the psychiatrist (APA 1998: 2). In addition, the encounter and task of psychiatry can be a dialectical exchange, in which the psychiatrist and patient together actively interrogate the patient's experience, sharing an exploration into the meaning of the patient's life understood in the most holistic terms (Havens 1987; Frank and Frank 1991; Lomas 1999; Jackson 1999; Luhrmann 2000).[7]

Self-knowledge and self-unity, then, become traits of professional character, which the practitioner will not only exemplify, but also explore with the patient in the dialectical therapeutic setting. Almost certainly there are other traits as well whose cultivation will be valuable within psychiatric practice. But on the assumption that effective treatment outcomes depend on certain dispositions in the practitioner, the practitioner will at the least need to acquire and cultivate self-knowledge and self-unity.

Over and above their status as role-constituted virtues, self-knowledge and self-unity are each strongly associated with the goal and good of psychiatric practice: mental health. Whatever other personal changes they seek, patients' conceptions of the ideal they strive to achieve will almost certainly include self-knowledge and self-unity, if only because of the perceived instrumentality of these traits in bringing other ends, such as autonomy. In the patient's normative project—what sort of changes he hopes to make in himself—these dispositions and habits of mind will likely be central. The patient wishes to understand himself more fully and to become a more unified and coherent person. Indeed, and not incompatibly, a striving for integrity of a more ambitious and moral kind has also been attributed to patients and to the psychotherapeutic project (Lomas 1999; Glover 2003).

We can attribute the goals of self-knowledge and self-unity to psychiatric patients with some confidence in part because within the present Western, twenty-first-century culture self-knowledge and self-unity are values which, though often implicit,

---

[7] Acknowledgement of the psychotherapeutic treatment model presupposed here is not as common as it once was and managed care delivery systems and psychopharmacology seem together to be fast reducing access to the kind of in-depth, long-term, psychotherapy through which this model of therapy can be most fully and easily realized (Emanuel and Emanuel 1992). But regardless of the truncated approach employed to bring about the goal, the therapeutic project remains a normative one of profound significance, in which, as some more thoughtful proponents of the new approaches have recognized, nothing less than a transformation of self or character is envisioned (Kramer 1993; Dickenson and Fulford 2000).

are widely shared. The unitary and integrated self of Western individualism and modernism is cherished as a cultural ideal; so too is the insightful and introspective modern self. And as a normative project, psychiatry will inevitably be situated this way, embracing the prevailing values of the context within which it is practiced. The cultural embeddedness of mental health norms has most commonly been acknowledged with respect to another of our cultural ideals: autonomy. Although autonomy has received more attention and recognition within discussions of the values underlying psychiatric practice, however, self-unity and self-knowledge have a comparable claim as mental health norms.

Unselfing

For want of a better term, 'unselfing' will be used to identify the personally effaced yet acutely attentive attitude adopted by the effective practitioner toward the patient in an effort to uphold the boundaries circumscribing the therapeutic relationship. Maintaining this attitude of unselfing toward the patient is a central aspect of the ethical and effective psychiatrist's professional role.

This trait has some parallels in the attitudes required of all professionals toward their clients. Any recipient of an expert's paid services is entitled to that professional's undivided attention; moreover, to greater and lesser degrees boundaries are maintained in most professional relationships, where conflicts of interest are regularly codified and proscribed. Within psychiatric practice though, concern to maintain the formal frame around the relationship is intense (Plaut 1997; Gabbard and Gutheil 1998; Gabbard 1989, 1999; Kroll 2001; Radden 2001; Gutheil, Norris, and Strasburger 2003). This is in part because of the extra vulnerability of many psychiatric patients, and in part because of the belief that more casual or everyday elements in the relationship will likely interfere with the effectiveness of the alliance, and hence the treatment. The concept of unethical boundary violations has given rise to an elaborate codification of every nuance of gesture, conduct, and communication in the therapeutic relationship, to a set of metaphors, and to the vocabulary which is the lingua franca of much psychiatric ethics today.

Unselfing plays a different part in the character of the ethical psychiatrist from that of self-knowledge and self-unity. Though not moral virtues outside the setting in which they are role-constituted virtues (within which, we saw, they are even emblematic of mental health), self-knowledge and self-unity are widely valued as intellectual virtues. Unselfing, in contrast, seems to have little currency in everyday life. In ordinary relationships, the attentiveness associated with being a good listener *is* valued, it is true, and unselfing involves that kind of attentiveness. But in everyday settings we also value mutuality and equality of exchange. Indeed, like emotional detachment, reserve is sometimes judged a hindrance to intimacy and mutuality, and thus undesirable.[8]

---

[8] Although the value of unselfing is widely accepted within professional psychiatry, there is disagreement over its *extent*, expressing itself in challenges to the enumeration of boundary violations in codes of ethics (Plaut 1997; Kroll 2001). Moreover, outside professional psychiatry certain approaches such as feminist therapy have challenged the inequality and lack of mutuality implied in this model (Brown 1994).

Perhaps closest to, but nonetheless different from, the trait of unselfing is professional detachment, which has been the subject of some philosophical attention and analysis (Fried 1976; Postema 1980; Applbaum 1999; Curzer 1993; De Raeve 1996; Oakley and Cocking 2001; Halpern 2001). Professional detachment involves an emotional distancing from the states or plight of the client: a denial or submersion of one's own feelings (typically, of compassionate distress), in favor of a controlled, unemotional 'professionalism'.

Professional detachment is similar to unselfing in two ways: it requires vigilant self-control and because it seems to represent a departure from everyday, more reciprocal attitudes toward others, it may be taken to require some justification.[9] But here the parallels end. Detachment is an attitude, an inner state of almost Stoic reserve. In unselfing, the practitioner adopts the appearance of reserve, and closely controls the expression of feeling toward the patient, but at the same time experiences and unflaggingly monitors her inner feelings and attitudes. Moreover, the practitioner who maintains boundaries around the therapeutic relationship is concerned to control more than her feelings and their expression. Unselfing requires her to control many less obviously private and personal aspects of her identity—her reactions and responses, her social and cultural background, her ideas, every facet of her non-professional life. Finally, unlike professional detachment, which is morally controversial because of disagreement over its supposed contribution to practice, the unselfing required to maintain boundaries is widely believed essential to effective psychiatric practice.

The latter difference, in itself, illustrates the apparent uniqueness of psychiatric practice. Because the relationship between practitioner and patient is so important and because that relationship so depends on the self-presentation of, and boundary conservation by, the psychiatrist, maintaining and supporting the relationship through the exercise of the virtue of unselfing becomes a critical ingredient in therapeutic success.

Realism

A final example of a role-constituted virtue is realism. Realism is not always a trait valued in everyday life, although it is more valued in some settings than others—we want our air traffic controllers to be realists though not, perhaps, our artists or lovers—but when honored, it is customarily as a prudential rather than a moral virtue, useful in promoting one's own good. Realism implies that one's thoughts, beliefs, and responses are kept in line with the facts, at least as the facts are understood by those around us. The realist maintains a balanced view, moreover, steadily adhering to the perspective and evaluations indicated by those facts. In this respect realism includes the kind of balanced and consistent view of things that has been described as perspective (Tiberius 2002).

The treatment setting in psychiatry demands realism in the practitioner, owing both to characteristic symptoms of mental disorder itself and to the nature of the

---

[9] This last point, and a careful evaluation of the moral psychology of professional detachment, are to be found in Oakley and Cocking (2001).

healing project. The value of realism is most obvious in the treatment of severe symptoms of mental disorder. Kant long ago pointed out an important feature of much mental disorder, indeed for him the 'only general characteristic' of insanity: 'the loss of a sense of ideas that are common to all (*sensus communis*), and its replacement with a sense of ideas peculiar to ourselves (*sensus privatus*)' (Kant 1800/1978: 117). If only temporarily, mental disorder often deprives its sufferer of those very capabilities that constitute the trait of realism, indeed severe symptoms of delusion and hallucination have often been characterized as a failure of 'reality testing'. The realistic psychiatrist will play an important part in compensating for those deficiencies in the patient, most immediately by providing a touchstone or 'reality check,' and conveying the *sensus communis* against which the *sensus privatus* can be judged. The everyday prudential virtue of realism will become a role-constituted moral virtue in the treatment setting.

The psychiatric task of changing the self of the patient invites comparison with the somewhat analogous—and certainly analogously profound—task of fostering a child's emotional and intellectual growth and forming its character, which has been described by Sara Ruddick. Among the virtues demanded by this morally significant and culturally essential task Ruddick notes several non-traditional traits including realism.[10] A young child must learn realism as it comes to know and interpret its world, and because realism is a deeply social and relational trait, in which appeal is made to the thoughts, beliefs, and responses of those around us, this requires a nurturer equipped with the trait of realism to act as teacher and guide (Ruddick 1995: 98–101). The analogies between the parenting task and the therapeutic one are not exact, but the social and relational nature of this trait also helps us understand why the practitioner must possess the role-constituted virtue of realism.

Some forms of therapy explicitly presuppose that the practitioner corrects mistaken beliefs and evaluations in the patient. In such cognitive-behavioral modes realism in the practitioner is a cornerstone of healing (Erwin 1978, 2004). The practitioner will likely be required to demonstrate and exemplify realism for the patient in many other forms of treatment as well. Like self-unity and self-knowledge, realism in our twenty-first-century culture represents an honored prudential virtue and mental health norm. As such it will likely be sought in the normative project undertaken by almost all patients.

Is realism, like self-knowledge and self-unity, a role-constituted virtue that fosters other traditional moral virtues, or is it, like unselfing, a virtue limited to the professional context? In her useful discussion of the related prudential virtue of perspective, Valerie Tiberius argues that perspective is a quality that makes people more inclined to value certain moral ends and to honor moral commitments (Tiberius 2002). Possessing perspective involves recognizing and acting on what matters; it predisposes the possessor away from impulsive and unreflective action. It provides the ability and

---

[10] Ruddick also includes delight in the child's accomplishments and pleasures. This extra virtue of delight in the other's achievement might also be called for in the mental health setting where the goal is self or even character transformation, as in the parenting setting where it is formed, though this comparison with child rearing will be apt only to the extent that the psychiatric patient resembles a young child in need of care, rather than an autonomous adult seeking guidance, and psychiatric patients (as of course do children themselves) fall on a spectrum between those two poles.

incentive to appreciate moral values; it also fosters the skill required of moral deliberation, a measured evaluation not overly influenced by the most immediate concerns. In somewhat the same way, arguably, realism is conducive to some of the capacities and habits associated with Aristotelian moral virtues such as integrity, trustworthiness, and justice, which require a measured, reflective, unflinching response to one's experience. Moreover, the realist seems likely protected from some apparently vicious traits, such as the excessive self-love and self-centeredness of narcissism. Realism is not incompatible with vices, as Tiberius recognizes. Nonetheless, like perspective, realism may make practitioners more inclined to acquire some of the other moral virtues called for by the mental health setting.

PART 2: PROFESSIONAL ROLES AND FEIGNED VIRTUES

Paying attention to the way in which professionals inhabit their roles forces us to notice some ethical tensions around professional practice, tensions arguably magnified in the mental health care setting. As a preliminary, we must clarify what is entailed in describing professional conduct as playing or inhabiting a role. Away from the stage and screen, merely acting a part is associated with acting without authenticity, or without the sincerity and wholeheartedness usually deemed appropriate: indeed, 'merely acting' suggests something close to intentional deception practiced for ignoble reasons. Professional roles differ from dramatic performance in at least two important ways. They are identity conferring or even constituting: part of who I am (see Hardimon 1994). In Kronman's memorable phrase, one's profession, 'can't be put on or off like a suit of clothes' (quoted by Oakley and Cocking 2001: 166). And professional roles impose additional moral imperatives, the profession-specific obligations of role morality. Because of these features, doctors generally act the part of doctors in the theatrical sense only when participating in amateur theatricals; otherwise, they are better said to inhabit than to act their roles. There is one notable exception to the identity conferring aspect of professional roles: when the new role is first adopted, through training programs, the fledgling doctor may have to enact it without an accompanying sense of authenticity or identification. She might even think to herself, 'this is not really me,' or 'I'm a fake' (see Rosenthal 2003). This suggests that the identity conferring aspect of professional roles is something acquired with practice. The professional role of doctor will become identity conferring and the role *inhabited*, rather than merely acted, gradually. Adopting the conduct and/or virtues of the ethical doctor may have to precede feeling like a doctor.

The contrast between inhabiting and acting a professional role is one with particular bearing on psychiatric practice. The persona manifested through carefully controlled responses has long received heightened attention within psychiatry, where, as we saw, professional boundaries are observed and maintained with self-conscious vigilance. It is widely accepted that these aspects of the relationship and elements of the practitioner are importantly instrumental in therapeutic effectiveness.[11] Healing

---

[11] Much informal observational support can be found for these claims; in addition they were confirmed in a more rigorous study conducted during the 1980s, the NIMH Psychobiology of

depends on the success of the relationship or alliance, and in developing, protecting, and fostering that alliance, the therapist wields her persona almost as a tool, on analogy with the surgeon's scalpel.

If, with most in psychiatry, we accept these causal assumptions, we will also accept as an implication of those assumptions that the patient 'believes in', that is attributes certain traits to, the practitioner. This means that the patient's belief about the presence of traits X, Y, and Z and not, notice, the presence of traits X, Y, and Z, will affect the outcome of treatment. To take a simple example: the patient's trust in her practitioner to keep her secrets allows the patient to offer those secrets unreservedly. Even if the practitioner is discreet but appears not to be, the therapeutic bond will suffer.

But this raises a problem. If the practitioner wields her persona on analogy with the surgeon's scalpel, we should expect skillfully feigned traits to be as useful as real ones in promoting effective practice. The appearance of honesty, pretended sympathy, a superficial display of trustworthiness, and so on, should be sufficient. Adopting a persona and feigning traits will result in practice whose effectiveness is only limited by the practitioner's skill at dissembling. I want to explore this problem or tension within psychiatric practice by asking several related questions. Is it possible to feign at least *some* virtues? Effectiveness aside, is ethical practice compatible with feigned virtues? Are there different forms of feigning? Can effective healing be achieved when it depends on feigned virtues?

Is it even possible to feign virtues? In everyday settings, it is perhaps less likely that virtues could be successfully feigned (although there, too, can be found 'virtue imposters' (Gehring 2003)). Under normal circumstances, people have access to cues allowing them to discern underlying and real character, and to recognize insincerity and pretense. But the artificialities of the therapeutic setting magnify the psychiatric patient's disadvantage when it comes to verifying and checking traits attributed to the practitioner and provide little access to the cues by which we usually discern real from feigned responses and 'read' another's character. The patient cannot know the practitioner fully because psychiatric engagement is restricted by the rigorous boundaries of therapeutic procedure (themselves apparently required by the patient's other vulnerabilities, especially the vulnerability to exploitation). In addition interaction with mentally disturbed patients is often distorted by the patient's misapprehensions about others due to delusions, projections, and other irregularities of social awareness and response.[12] At least temporarily, such deficiencies serve to limit the patient's capacity for knowing the psychiatrist's true character. These features of therapeutic engagement are part of the psychiatric patient's vulnerability, calling for greater moral integrity in the practitioner. But they also imply that character can be easily feigned in such a setting. (If any further support is required to confirm the epistemic disadvantage

---

Depression study (1982) (see Elkin, Parloff, Hadley, and Autry 1985; Elkin, Pilkonis, Dohenty, and Sotsky 1985; Elkin, Shea, Watkins, and Imber, et al. 1989; Sotsky, Glass, Shea, and Pilkonis, et. al. 1991; and Shea, Elkin, Imber, and Sotsky, et al. 1992).

[12] As the theory of transference suggests, these distortions may not be limited to the patient. A process is theorized by which the patient is motivated unconsciously to influence the therapist toward fitting the misperception (Jackson 1999: 307).

at least temporarily afflicting many psychiatric patients, we need only turn to the sorry history of treatments for mental disorder stretching from the classical era to the eighteenth century, which is replete with references to deceptions, lies, and 'pious frauds', employed to trick the patient into recovery (Jackson 1999: 294–300).)

How successfully virtues can be feigned will also vary with the particular virtue in question. Sincerity, for instance, will be relatively difficult to feign successfully. Virtues are dispositions that manifest themselves in some way, but these manifestations are variously inward states of mind and more outward actions or habits. Some virtue terms are more transparently evaluative and others more descriptive. Some virtues, such as empathy, are closely allied to particular feelings and emotions not immediately subject to self-control. Our inability to direct ourselves to *feel* empathy, may serve to limit our ability to feign empathy. And particular virtues are characterized by more and less easily identified clusters of inner and outer manifestations—actions and behavioral responses. Thus, traits such as benevolence or compassion are identifiable through the combination of their distinctive inner states and outer manifestations. Feigning benevolence or compassion successfully will be relatively easy, involving a display of outer manifestations unaccompanied by the appropriate inner states. It will be harder to feign sensitivity, whose outward manifestations seem to depend for their successful exhibition on a precisely focused exercise of perception, attention, and understanding. Because the attribution of integrity seems to require more evidence than the attribution of many other, more behaviorally based traits, feigning integrity will likely be unsuccessful. Similarly, *phronesis* will not be readily feigned: it is not an inner state that finds expression in particular outward behavior in the way other virtues seem to be. Aristotle says of *phronesis* that because it is a practical virtue concerned with *doing* the right thing, one cannot have it and fail to act correctly or be incontinent with respect to it. Similarly, because it is a judgment *about the right action*, when right action takes place, we can with confidence know it to be evidence of *phronesis,* not a counterfeit. Despite these several hindrances to successful feigning, some virtues can be feigned with a fair degree of success: benevolence and compassion, as we saw earlier, and such traits as kindness, sympathy, and interested attentiveness.

If the goal of treatment is achieved, why would feigning virtues be morally problematic? Several answers immediately present themselves. The patient is manipulated and deceived, manipulation and deception that seem doubly egregious because this patient is already vulnerable to exploitation. This may be an acceptable outcome according to some crude, consequentialist measure (see Szabados and Soifer 2004: 95–120). But such conduct contravenes even Kantian rules on how we ought to treat other people. Moreover such feigning and pretending will corrupt the character of the practitioner, adding to it the vices of deception and dishonesty, if not actual hypocrisy. [13]

---

[13] I am indebted to Roger Crisp for this point. The vice of hypocrisy suggests a pattern of dissembling out of solely self-focused reasons (see McKinnon 1999: 190–4). Although it represents feigned responses more entrenched and more vicious than the responses under discussion, hypocrisy might well be a possible fate of character for those who habitually feign virtues.

At this point, several qualifications seem in order. First, we might need to distinguish different forms of feigning. An intent to deceive is implied in the notion of feigned responses, but some deceptions seem inevitable and blameless. Because acquiring virtues involves habituation and practice, there will be incompletely achieved responses, for example, as when a person strives to convey compassion or sympathy in hopes of becoming a more compassionate and sympathetic character. Indeed, an ethics education based on the idea of a virtuous psychiatrist would presumably depend on the internalization of the virtues often initially adopted in appearance only.

In a tradition found in the virtue theories of both Mencius and Aquinas, real virtues are placed in contrast to two forms of feigned virtues: semblances of virtue (acting virtuously not out of virtue but for some good end) and counterfeits of virtue (affecting virtue for some ignoble end). Semblances of virtue, while they are recognized to be less valuable than the possession of real virtues, are acknowledged to have some moral worth (Yearley 1990: 19–23, 124–9). The practitioner who feigns compassion to deepen the patient's relationship with her, or as an exercise in becoming more compassionate, offers a semblance of compassion, and is different from the practitioner who 'counterfeits' compassion for personal gain (out of a need to feel powerful, for example). Semblances of professionals' virtues will require monitoring, to be sure, but extra vigilance, close supervision of trainees, and consultation among colleagues will perhaps be supposed sufficient to prevent the dangers associated with their misuse.

Attempting to circumscribe the good end for which these semblances of virtue are undertaken, we might venture that as a general rule these feigned responses are acceptable *when undertaken for the sake of therapeutic effectiveness*. Even such broadly paternalistic motives as these contain moral dangers, however, not only in terms of corrupting the character of the practitioner but also in exhibiting disrespect for the patient. As the 'pious frauds' of the past attest, the well-intentioned feigning of responses for therapeutic effectiveness violates and jeopardizes the trust the patient is entitled to feel in her practitioner. The only circumstance in which feigning virtues is unavoidable is the educational one in which the trainee seeks to acquire the virtue through a process of habituation. That alone can be the circumstance under which feigning virtues (by offering semblances of virtue) is entirely acceptable.

But could effective therapy be achieved when it depends on feigned virtues? Interpretations of Aristotle associated with John McDowell (1979) allow us to see a reason to doubt such an outcome. On such a view, only those who genuinely possess a virtue can succeed in manifesting it properly. In a similar vein, Tom Beauchamp has argued that whenever the feelings, concerns, and attitudes of others are the morally relevant matters, only the possession of certain virtues (his examples are human warmth and sensitivity) will 'lead a person to notice what should be done' (Beauchamp 1999). In order to feign a virtue in a particular therapeutic context, and thus to see, as Beauchamp says, 'what should be done', (and we shall want to add, what *should be felt*), a therapist would first need to possess the virtue. To continue with Beauchamp's example, only by being sensitive, or warm, could a practitioner have enough awareness of what responses a particular situation called for to be able to feign the virtues required by that context. We can easily imagine an example: by sidestepping a painful topic out of the misplaced delicacy of insincere or feigned sensitivity, a practitioner misses an important disclosure from the patient. Only a genuine sensitivity and real delicacy could permit the sure-footed response needed here. Or, returning to self-knowledge and self-unity, we might expect that feigned self-unity would leave the practitioner vulnerable to insufficiently integrated aspects of her psyche (surprise, annoyance, or shock registering in non-verbal language, for example). Similarly, if the practitioner does not know her own weaknesses and innermost feelings, those weaknesses and feelings will likely blinker her in the therapeutic encounter and prove a hindrance to effective therapeutic work. For example, she may not remember or attend to some detail of her patient's narrative because of her own unresolved feelings about its content.

It is tempting to invoke the overarching virtue of *phronesis* in this context. Practical wisdom seems capable of guiding us to what should be done in situations such as the therapeutic one. But *phronesis* always ensures right action and response. So it must be concluded that when semblances of virtue prevent right action, as in the examples above, *phronesis* was absent. Only *together with phronesis* do other virtues achieve right action. But *phronesis* requires those other virtues to be real, and not feigned.

Perhaps real compassion, warmth, sensitivity, self-unity and self-knowledge, together with *phronesis*, will always bring about the most effective therapy. Yet virtues are ideals to be striven for rather than rules to be followed (Herman 1993; Crisp 1995; Hursthouse 1999). With that in mind, the qualifications above seem to suggest a professional minimal standard, below which no ethical practitioner can be permitted to fall.[14] Such a standard would require that whenever there is a feigning or semblance of virtues the sole purpose must be to acquire those traits through habituation. Moreover, checks and extra vigilance must be in place to guard against the abuses (of the patient) and corruption (of the practitioner) that feigning might otherwise bring.

A final question about feigned virtues is stimulated by recent work by John Doris emphasizing the situation and role-specific nature of much actual ethical behavior (Doris 2002). Are professionals' virtues feigned at all, or feigned unacceptably, when their manifestations are *limited to* the context of practice? If the trustworthy practitioner shows untrustworthiness in his non-professional relationships, are his professional displays of trustworthiness merely feigned? We can grant that only by possessing the virtue could a practitioner succeed in manifesting it properly in a clinical setting. But we can still imagine someone who is divided or compartmentalized in his responses, capable of manifesting but reluctant to manifest his virtue in every setting: for example, the professionally trustworthy practitioner who cheats on his wife.

There are several points to make here. First, to the extent that this is real trustworthiness, the divided practitioner will likely be a rarity. Because of the identity conferring or constituting aspect of professional roles these roles are not able to be 'put on or off like a suit of clothes'. Because it is constitutive of the practitioner's professional character, trustworthiness will be difficult to divest. Following the Aristotelian model,

---

14 I am indebted to the editors of this volume for the last suggestion.

its presence in the practice setting might be expected to spread, eventually affecting the rest of his non-professional life. Secondly, any divided practitioner must be morally flawed. The professional's virtues are part of his overall character and should harmonize with it; without such harmony, the divided practitioner lacks the virtue of moral integrity.

Are the virtues of the divided practitioner feigned unacceptably when they are thus restricted to the practice setting? Here, too, we may wish to invoke the minimal standards introduced earlier. A supremely or ideally virtuous practitioner will manifest the virtue in every setting, we might admit; even the ethical trainee will strive to do so in every setting. A minimal ethical standard for practice may require only that the virtue is at least consistently manifested in the practice setting.

CONCLUSION

If the effectiveness of psychiatric practice is dependent on certain dispositions in the practitioner, then professional role morality will accord those dispositions the status of virtues within the professional context. I have illustrated such role-constituted virtues using the four qualities of self-knowledge, self-unity, 'unselfing', and realism. Thus, in addition to the other virtues that the ethical practitioner will possess and be required to cultivate—as a professional, as a doctor, and because they are called for by aspects of the mental health care setting—she will possess and cultivate those dispositions that enable her to use her persona, or professional character, in the promotion of the particular good of psychiatry: mental health. I have distinguished among role-constituted virtues between those which are not only valuable in furthering the goal or good of professional practice, but also are conducive to the cultivation of traditional moral virtues; and traits whose value seems to lie solely in their usefulness to the healing process.

I explored some of the moral psychology of feigned virtues because the professional character of the psychiatrist is at special risk when feigning virtues. Feigning is contrary to ideals of professional conduct and character. Yet some kinds of well-intended feigning of responses and semblance of virtue may be compatible with minimal standards below which no ethical practitioner can be permitted to fall. As long as these feigned responses are sought in order to acquire the virtue through habituation, and checks and extra vigilance are in place to guard against the twin abuses of exploitation of the patient and corruption of the practitioner's character, feigning virtue may be at least morally permissible, even if never perfectly ideal.

ACKNOWLEDGEMENTS

I benefited from exploring these ideas with members of the Psychiatry Department at the Massachusetts General Hospital as part of a 1999 program on the Conceptual Basis of Psychiatric Ethics. A version of the present chapter was read at the Bioethics Centre at Monash University where, in 1999, I was a Visiting Scholar. I am grateful for help received from members of that center and of the Philosophy Department at Monash University. For helpful comments and advice on earlier drafts, I must also thank the members of PHAEDRA, Jane Roland Martin, Janet Farrell Smith, Barbara Houston, and Ann Diller, as well as Roger Crisp, Justin Oakley, John Sadler, Adam Beresford, and, last but not least, the editors of this volume.

REFERENCES

American Psychiatric Association (1998). *The Principles of Medical Ethics with Annotations Especially Applicable to Psychiatry*. Washington, DC: American Psychiatric Association.

Applbaum, A. (1999). *Ethics for Adversaries: The Morality of Roles in Public and Professional Life*. Princeton: Princeton University Press.

Aquinas (1945). *Basic Writings of St.Thomas Aquinas in Two Volumes*. New York: Random House.

Aristotle (1985). *Nichomachean Ethics*. Translated by Terrence Irwin. New York: Hackett.

Arpaly, N. (2003). *Unprincipled Virtue: An Inquiry into Moral Agency*. New York: Oxford University Press.

Beresford, A. (2005). *Philosophical Introduction: Plato's Protagoras and Meno*. London: Penguin.

Beauchamp, T. (1999). 'The Philosophical Basis of Psychiatric Ethics', in P. Chodoff, S.

Bloch, and S. A. Green (eds.), *Psychiatric Ethics* (3rd edn.). Oxford: Oxford University Press, 25–48.

Bloch, S. and Green, S. A. (2006). 'An Ethical Framework for Psychiatry'. *British Journal of Psychiatry*, 188: 7–12.

Brown, L. (1994). *Subversive Dialogues: Theory in Feminist Therapy*. New York: Basic Books.

Charland, L. and Dick, P. (1995). 'Should Compassion be Included in Codes of Ethics for Physicians?' *Annals RCPSC*, 28/7: 415–18.

Christianson, R. (1995). 'The Ethics of Treating the Untreatable'. *Psychiatric Services*, 46/12: 1217.

Churchill, L. (1989). 'Reviving a Distinctive Medical Ethics'. *Hastings Center Report*, 19/3: 28–34.

Cox, D., La Caze, M., and Levine, M. P. (2003). *Integrity and the Fragile Self*. Burlington, VT: Ashgate Press.

Crisp, R. (1995). *How Should One Live? Essays on the Virtues*. Oxford: Oxford University Press.

——and Slote, M. (1997). 'Introduction' in R. Crisp and M. Slote (eds.), *Virtue Ethics*. Oxford: Oxford University Press.

Crowden, A. (2003). 'Ethically Sensitive Mental Health Care'. *Australian and New Zealand Journal of Psychiatry*, 17/2: 143–9.

Curzer, H. (1993). 'Is Care a Virtue for Healthcare Professionals?' *Journal of Medicine and Philosophy*, 18/1: 51–69.

De Raeve, L. (1996). 'Caring Intensively', in D. Greaves and H. Upton (eds.), *Philosophical Problems in Healthcare*. Aldershot: Avebury.

Diamond, C. (1992). 'Integrity', in L. Becker (ed..), *Encyclopedia of Ethics*. New York: Garland Press.

Dickenson, D. and Fulford, K. W. M. (2000). *In Two Minds: A Casebook of Psychiatric Ethics*. Oxford: Oxford University Press.

Doris, J. (2002). *Lack of Character: Personality and Moral Behavior*. Cambridge: Cambridge University Press.

Drane, J. (1988). *Becoming a Good Doctor: The Place of Virtue and Character in Medical Ethics.* Kansas City: Sheed and Ward.

Dyer, A. (1988). *Ethics and Psychiatry: Toward Professional Definition.* Washington, DC: American Psychiatric Press.

———— (1999). 'Psychiatry as a Profession' in *Psychiatric Ethics*, Third Edition, edited by Sidney Bloch, Paul Chodoff, and Stephen A. Green. Oxford: Oxford University Press, 67–79.

Elikin, I., Parloff, M. B., Hadley, S. W., and Autry, J. H. (1985). 'NIMH Treatment of Depression Collaborative Research Program: Background and Research Plan'. *Archives of General Psychiatry*, 42: 305–16.

———— Pilkonis, M. B., Docherty, J. P., and Sotsky, S. M. (1985). 'Conceptual and Methodological Issues in Comparative Studies of the Psychotherapy and Psychopharmacotherapy, 1: Active Ingredients and Mechanism of Change'. *American Journal of Psychiatry*, 145: 909–17; '2: Nature and Timing of Treatment Effects'. *American Journal of Psychiatry*, 145: 1070–6.

———— Shea, M. T., Watkins, J. T, and Imber, S. D., et al. (1989). 'NIMH Treatment of Depression Collaborative Research Program: General Effectiveness of Treatments'. *Archives of General Psychiatry*, 46: 971–82.

Emanual, L. and Emanual, E. (1992). 'Four Models of the Physician–Patient Relationship'. *Journal of the American Medical Association*, 267/16, 22/29: 2221–6.

Erwin, E. (1978). *Behavior Therapy: Scientific, Philosophical and Moral Foundations.* New York: Cambridge University Press.

———— (2004). 'Cognitive-Behavioral Therapy', in J. Radden (ed.). *The Philosophy of Psychiatry: A Companion.* New York: Oxford University Press.

Frank, J. and Frank, J. (1991). *Persuasion and Healing: A Comparative Study of Psychotherapy* (3rd edn.). Baltimore: Johns Hopkins Press.

Fraser, A. (2000). 'Ethics for Psychiatrists Derived from Virtue Theory', unpublished lecture delivered at the Fourth International Conference on Philosophy and Mental Health, Florence, Italy.

Fried, C. (1976). 'The Lawyer as Friend: the Moral Foundations of the Lawyer–Client Relation'. *Yale Law Journal*, 85/2: 1060.

Gabbard, G. (ed.) (1989). *Sexual Exploitation in Professional Relationships.* Washington, DC: American Psychiatric Press.

———— (1999). 'Boundary Violations', in S. Bloch, P. Chodoff, and S. Green (eds.), *Psychiatric Ethics* (3rd edn.). Oxford: Oxford University Press.

Gehring, V. (2003). 'Phonies, Fakes and Frauds—and the Social Harms they Cause'. *Philosophy and Public Affairs Quarterly* 23, 1/2: 14–20.

Glover, J. (2003). 'Towards Humanism in Psychiatry'. 2003 Tanner Lectures. Princeton University.

Gutheil, T. and Gabbard, G. (1998). 'Misuses and Misunderstandings of Boundary Theory in Clinical and Regulatory Settings.' *American Journal of Psychiatry*, 155/3: 409–14.

———— Norris, D., and Strasburger, L. (2003). 'This Couldn't Happen to Me: Boundary Problems and Sexual Misconduct in the Psychotherapy Relationship'. *Psychiatric Services*, 54/2: 517–22.

Halpern, J. (2001). *From Detached Concern to Empathy: Humanizing Medical Practice.* New York: Oxford University Press.

Hardimon, M. (1994). 'Role Obligations'. *Journal of Philosophy*, XCI(7): 333–63.

Havens, L. (1987). *Approaches to the Mind: Movements of the Psychiatric Schools from Sects Toward Science.* Cambridge, MA: Harvard University Press.

Herman, B. (1993). *The Practice of Moral Judgment.* Cambridge, MA: Harvard University Press.

Hursthouse, R. (1999). *On Virtue Ethics.* Oxford: Oxford University Press.

Irwin, T. (1985). *Introduction and Notes to Aristotle's Nichomachean Ethics,* translated by Terence Irwin. Indianapolis, IN: Hackett, 430–1.

Jackson, S. (1999). *Care of the Psyche: A History of Psychological Healing.* New Haven, CT: Yale University Press.

Kant, I. (1800/1978). *Anthropology from a Pragmatic Point of View,* Hans H. Rudnick (ed.), translated by Victor Lyle Dowdell. Carbondale: Southern Illinois University Press.

Kramer, P. (1993). *Listening to Prozac: A Psychiatrist Explores Antidepressant Drugs and the Remaking of the Self.* New York: Viking.

Kroll, J. (2001). 'Boundary Violations: A Culture-Bound Syndrome'. *Journal of the American Academy of Psychiatry and Law,* 29/3: 274–83.

Kronman, A. (1993). *The Lost Lawyer: Failing Ideals of the Legal Profession.* Cambridge, MA: Harvard University Press.

Kupperman, J. (1991). *Character.* New York: Oxford University Press.

Lomas, P. (1999). *Doing Good? Psychotherapy Out of Its Depth.* Oxford: Oxford University Press.

Luhrmann, T. (2000). *Of 2 Minds: The Growing Disorder in American Psychiatry.* New York: Knopf.

McDowell, J. (1979). 'Virtue and Reason'. *The Monist,* 62/3: 331–50.

McFall, L. (1992). 'Integrity', in J. Deigh (ed.), *Ethics and Personality.* Chicago: University of Chicago Press.

MacIntyre, A. (1981). *After Virtue.* Notre Dame, IN: University of Notre Dame Press.

McKinnon, C. (1999). *Character, Virtue Theories, and the Vices.* New York: Broadview Press.

May, W. (1994). 'The Virtues in a Professional Setting', in K. W. M. Fulford, Grant Gillett, and Janet Martin Soskice (eds.), *Medicine and Moral Reasoning.* Cambridge: Cambridge University Press, 75–90.

Nussbaum, M. (1996). 'Upheavals of Thought: A Theory of the Emotions'. *Gifford Lectures 1993.* Cambridge: Cambridge University Press.

Oakley, J. (1996). 'Varieties of Virtue'. *Ethics,* IX/2: 128–52.

_____ and Cocking, D. (2001). *Virtue Ethics and Professional Roles.* Cambridge: Cambridge University Press.

Pellegrino, E. and Thomasma, D. (1993). *The Virtues of Medical Practice.* New York: Oxford University Press.

Pincoffs, E. (1986). *Quandaries and Virtues: Against Reductivism in Ethics.* Lawrence: University of Kansas Press.

Plaut, S. M. (1997). 'Boundary Violations in Professional–client Relationships: Overview and Guildlines of Prevention'. *Sexual and Marital Therapy,* 12/1: 77–94.

Postema, G. (1980). 'Moral Responsibility in Professional Ethics'. *New York University Law Review,* 55/1: 64–89.

Radden, J. (2001). 'Boundary Violation Ethics: Some Conceptual Clarifications'. *Journal of the American Academy of Psychiatry and Law,* 3: 319–26.

_____ (2002). 'Notes Towards a Professional Ethics for Psychiatry'. *Australian and New Zealand Journal of Psychiatry,* 36/2: 52–9.

Rosenthal, E. (2003). 'How Doctors Learn to Think they're Doctors'. *New York Times,* November 28.

Ruddick, S. (1995). *Maternal Thinking: Toward a Politics of Peace.* Boston: Beacon Press.

Schauber, N. (1996). 'Integrity, Commitment and the Concept of a Person'. *American Philosophical Quarterly*, 33: 119–29.

Shea, M. T., Elkin, I., Imber, S. D., and Sotsky, S. M., et al. (1992). 'Course of Depressive Symptoms over Follow Up: Findings from the NIMH Treatment of Depression Collaborative Research Program'. *Archives of General Psychiatry*, 49: 762–87.

Sotsky, S. M., Glass, D. R., Shea, M. T., and Pilkonis P. A., et al. (1991). 'Patient Predictors of Response to Psychotherapy and Pharmacotherapy: Findings of the NIMH Treatment of Depression Collaborative Research Program'. *American Journal of Psychiatry*, 148: 997–1008.

Sutherland, A. (1996). 'Integrity and Self-Identity'. *Philosophy*, 35: 19–27.

Szabados, B. and Soifer, E. (2004). *Hypoerisy: Ethical Investigations*. Peterborough, ON: Broadview Press.

Taylor, G. (1985). *Pride, Shame, and Guilt: Emotions of Self-assessment*. Oxford: Clarendon Press.

Tiberius, V. (2002). 'Perspective: A Prudential Virtue'. *American Philosophical Quarterly*, 39/4: 305–24.

Veatch, R. (1991). *The Patient–Physician Relation: The Patient as Partner, Part 2*. Bloomington: Indiana University Press.

Yearley, L. H. (1990). *Mencius and Aquinas: Theories of Virtue and Conceptions of Courage*. New York: State University of New York Press.

6

Trust, Suffering, and the Aesculapian Virtues

Annette C. Baier

Aesculapius, son of Apollo, and pupil of centaur–physician Chiron, son of Chronos, was the Zeus-designated god of healing. What are the Aesculapian virtues, the virtues we want in those to whom we turn to heal and alleviate our ills? Aesculapius was son to serene, expressive Apollo, and pupil of the son of Chronos, god of time, and I shall suggest that both calm communicativeness and right timing are important virtues in healers. I have argued in a recent essay (Baier 2004) that virtues, or at least such virtues as show in our relations with each other, essentially are the wanted attitudes to the realization that we are in one another's power. This combines the Aristotelian view that virtues are what enable us moderately social beings to flourish, or at least not languish, with the Hobbesian reminder that we can have reason to fear each other's power. Virtues, on my analysis, are personal traits that contribute to a good climate of trust between people, when trust is taken to be acceptance of being, to some degree and in some respects, in another's power. The Aesculapian virtues, therefore, will be those found in trustworthy healers, and will include due awareness of the power discrepancy that the doctor–patient relationship involves, the will to communicate appropriately with the patient, and to take timely action of various sorts. As will soon become abundantly clear, I am taking 'healing' to include relief of suffering, as well as restoration of health. In the latter part of this chapter I will discuss the disagreement on euthanasia, and consider what the trustworthy physician will do when her incurable and suffering patient requests that his life be ended.

In addressing these issues I shall be calling on personal experience, consultation with medical care experts, reading, and philosophical reflection on trust, and on life and death. My main concern is with what it takes to be a trustworthy health professional. But since physicians and nurses usually depend on managers and administrators for the conditions in which they work, I will also give some attention to managerial contributions to climates of trust in hospitals. Again, since trust is a relationship that depends on all parties to it, I will also allude to what patients can contribute. Unrealistic demands by patients, and over-readiness to lodge complaints, or, at the other extreme, undue respect for physicians, and reluctance to ask questions of them, just as much as incompetence in caregivers, their failure to communicate, or their inconsiderateness, can contribute to a climate of mistrust that is not only unpleasant for those involved, but unhealthy and dysfunctional.

I take trust to be acceptance of some degree of vulnerability to another's power, in the confidence that this power will not be used to harm or hurt one (Baier 1995). A good climate of trust is one in which the vulnerability is mutual, and people can be encouraged to trust each other. To create and maintain such a climate, some empowerment of the naturally weaker is essential, and recognition of rights is an obvious way to do this. In a medical context, codes of patient rights, and the provision of patient advocates, serve this purpose, since patients are the naturally weaker parties, especially given the fact that their competence to know their own minds and to assert their rights will be determined by their physicians, the very ones against whose possible abuses of power such rights should protect them. This is why third parties, such as patient advocates, are so important. Respect for patients' recognized rights is the first virtue of health professionals, but it needs to be accompanied by other virtues, such as informing them of their rights. Of course physicians too have rights, including rights against patients. If patients survive their medical treatment or mistreatment, and are wealthy enough, they can sue their physicians, and some suits may be malicious. (Physicians now need, and have, their own international Medical Protection Society.)

A trustworthy health professional is, among other things, a properly trained one, competent to do what she undertakes to do, but who is to say what the proper training is, and who should verify that the credentials someone claims to have are genuine? The trustworthy hospital administrator verifies the claimed credentials of applicants for its positions. And what should patients do, if anything, to make sure that their physicians and nurses are properly qualified? How informed should we be about the record and qualifications of our physicians before we trust them to care for us? Obviously if one is taken ill, or is injured, while in a foreign country, one would be foolish to postpone getting medical attention until one has made inquiries about the competence of the local health professionals, but what about one's home town? How many of us do anything whatever to check out the professional record of primary care physicians, surgeons, or other specialists, before becoming their patients? Would we be accepted as their patients if we were known to have done some prior detective work on them? Yet, at the very least, we should be able to know that they are properly qualified for the work they do.

We usually in effect delegate the checking of credentials to regulatory officials, but some sort of check on *their* performance, by someone presumed to be trustworthy, is also in order. To check up on someone is to show some hesitancy about trusting them. And here we are faced with the regress of distrust—the more we insist on checking, the more people there are to be checked up on, and security becomes a vanishing goal. At some point, we just have to trust the checker, and, for the average patient, there is no particular reason to think that the most reliable checker is oneself. We are forced to rely on the medical profession itself, on hospital administrators, and on government agencies, so should be loud in our criticism when any of these fail us in this vital matter. (I am not going to address the question of whom we must trust for a sufficient provision of health-care workers, important as that issue obviously is, but restrict my remarks to trust in those who are provided. But it is very easy to see that if there are not enough of them to meet needs, then they will be overworked, exhausted, possibly resentful, and so less than reliable in their service to those who must rely on them.)

We hope for a sufficient supply of properly trained physicians and other health workers. What sort of training, beyond the obvious, such as training in the recognition of the symptoms of meningitis and other immediately life-threatening conditions, do we want our physicians to have had? And what sort of regular retraining? Most medical schools now put some emphasis on communicative skills in addition to scientific training and clinical know-how. It is fairly obvious that some human-relations skills are part of what it takes to be a good physician, and that these cannot always just be grafted on to a good medical scientist, as an afterthought. Some aptitude for dealing with people should be a minimal requirement, not an optional extra, in a successful entrant to medical school. If fear and distrust are to be avoided in hospitals, there must be something of the human touch in physicians, surgeons, and other experts. (In the nursing profession its importance has long been recognized.) For fear, even terror, is what results when a person is subjected to procedures, sometimes painful ones, that she does not comprehend, for reasons she has not been made to understand. A significant number of the complaints made by hospital patients (about 12% in my local hospital) directly concern poor communication, and a much higher proportion (up to 70%) have been judged to have that as their background cause (data from Denys Court, of the Medical Protection Society, New Zealand branch, and from Ron Paterson, New Zealand Health and Disability Commissioner).

And what sort of training is needed to address the ethical questions I am addressing? I should emphasize that I am a philosopher, not a social scientist nor a person with any special knowledge of the health professions, and I am acutely aware of the limitations this imposes. The interrogative mood dominates in this essay, and not all my questions are rhetorical. I find the issues I am addressing very difficult, and, because of their seriousness, sometimes difficult to address with detachment. (Hence the indignant rhetorical questions, later in this essay.) To prepare myself to write on this hard topic, I have, of course, read books and articles by physicians, and I have consulted with several physicians, including experts in palliative care, with two lawyer–physicians, with a midwife who is a hospital maternity manager, with two nurses, a patient advocate, a government health official, and a hospital manager of clinical services. This consultation gives me, at best, some second-hand knowledge. I did, decades ago, while a student, work for a short while as an unqualified night nurse in a private hospital. I found that experience very stressful, and resigned after the first death that occurred while I was on duty. (So I do not lack sympathy with those health professionals who want, at all costs, not to be thought responsible for a patient's death.) Apart from that brief nursing stint, my only first-hand knowledge of health professionals, with their strengths and their weaknesses, comes from experience as a patient, and as a concerned relative of several patients, with all the limitations that implies. Still, my own experiences in hospitals inevitably influence my views, and the strength of my feelings, so I will mention some of them.

Thirty years ago I was by my mother's hospital bed when she died, choking on her own blood, after two long weeks of post-surgical agony. The surgery had been for cancer of the esophagus. After her death I wrote to her surgeon, saying that his was a terrible profession. I wrote that he had tortured my mother by his refusal to admit that the surgery had failed, and by his consequent unwillingness, despite our pleading, to give much morphine, on the usual grounds that, while relieving her suffering, that would have depressed her breathing. (This man, decades later, was honored by the Queen of England for his services to the hospice movement, but I am told it was surgery he himself underwent, not my charges, nor those of his other patients or their relatives, that led to his change of heart.) Palliative care, I am assured, has come a long way since my mother's death, but part of the problem is of deciding when post-operative care should become palliative care, and when that becomes terminal care. Care of those who have not been cured had not advanced discernibly when my nephew eight years ago died of a brain tumor, after two operations, the second to treat an infection arising from the first. His complaints about his terrible headaches were treated as mere malingering, and it was only when the infection worked its way out to the skin that the second surgery was done. He was a young man in his early thirties, a long distance runner, and of course was depressed at his steadily worsening condition. He made several unsuccessful suicide attempts, before finally, in an emaciated state, dying a morphine-hastened death in hospital. The morphine, of course, was officially given to relieve his suffering, not to give him the death he had for months so desperately sought. For it was deemed unethical, and was in any case illegal, for any physician to administer euthanasia on request.

My experience when I myself was the patient (in Britain, in Australia, in the U.S., in New Zealand), in much less dire circumstances, has been generally good, at the receiving end of excellent care, effective pain relief, and considerate treatment, even from grossly overworked emergency department staff. But one recent unhappy experience made me ponder the question whether individual virtues in health-care workers are enough to ensure good care, if the organizational structure in which they work is defective. Or should I say if the managers are failing in their professional role, and are lacking the special virtues their job demands? For successful care of a patient, including communicative success, requires not merely a physician's will and ability to give appropriate medical treatment, and to explain it to the patient, but reliable access to the means of giving that treatment, and to the means of getting timely information to a patient.

Here is the story of what led me to these thoughts. I had been admitted to my local hospital after a four-hour ambulance trip, following an internal bleed, one that necessitated blood transfusions. Since the bleeding into the stomach was continuing (and maybe because my eighteen transfusions were depleting the blood bank), surgery was planned to investigate the cause of the bleeding, and try to stop it. (A longer than usual gastroscopy, not much fun to undergo, had, because of blood clots in the stomach, failed to disclose the source of the trouble, and had reactivated the bleeding.) I had been given a careful explanation of what surgery was planned, what risk was involved, and what 'discomfort' to expect after the operation. I had signed the consent forms, after a very long discussion with the ward's helpful resident surgeon, in the small hours of the night. I was told to expect surgery during the next night. I lay in the ward waiting to be taken off to theatre, and lay and lay, for an endless and sleepless night. My inquiries to nurse and house surgeon as to what was happening were met with: 'We don't know, there is no response from the gastro-surgical unit.' My initial resolve to be calm and accepting did not extend to being calm enough to forget the matter and sleep, so my night was very unpleasant. It was not until next day that I learned that an industrial accident had led to all operating theatres being needed for emergency surgery on the victims, so that the gastro-surgical team had gone home. And my own blood count in fact improved during that night of waiting, so it was decided to put my surgery on hold until diagnostic tests could be done. I tried to receive this news graciously, but felt some resentment about the anxious waiting that I had already been put through, unnecessarily, or so it seemed to me. For, had I been told of the surgical emergency, and the consequent cancellation of my own operation that night, I could perhaps have slept, or at least lain in less anxious sleeplessness.

Why was I not informed at the time that my surgery that night had been cancelled? Who, if anyone, should have let me know what was happening? Quite possibly there was no one whose appointed task it was to get word to the medical ward about the changed surgical priorities. I certainly did not know whom, if anyone, to blame, and tried not to blame anyone. (It did not occur to me to lodge a complaint, and certainly no one suggested that I consider that, although the New Zealand hospital I was in is governed by an official code of patient rights, whose last-listed right is the right to complain. But no copy of this code lay with the Gideon Bible by my hospital bed, and I was not mobile enough to see the copy posted on the wall by the ward's reception desk.) Hospital procedures may not have given the job of informing patients whose surgery has been unexpectedly cancelled to anyone in particular, especially not in conditions where the surgical services were being taxed to the limit. Proper principles of triage would not assign high priority to this job. Yet it would have taken merely a message to the ward, and this need not have been done by any of the overtaxed workers in the surgical units, but by some porter or telephone worker. The people in the ward, nurses and house-surgeon, did try to find out what was happening, but given the casualty victims with whom the hospital was coping, the surgical units were overwhelmed, and not answering the phone. My interests got lost in the shuffle, as by correct triage principles they should have, if anyone's had to. (I am told that sometimes those awaiting surgery wait as long as three days, on nil-by-mouth, so my unpleasant wait was nothing exceptional. But it was not the delay as much as the lack of information that I felt aggrieved about.) To minimize avoidable anxiety, in such circumstances, different procedures would have to be in place, and that might take initiative and skill in design of procedures at the administrative level. The high incidence, in U.S. hospitals, of death from medical error, making the risk of such death greater than that of death on the roads, was judged to be due not to 'bad apples' among the physicians, but mainly to procedural defects (Gawande 1999). To remedy that, we need initiative and vision at the managerial and administrative level. Their special virtues are vitally important if the virtues of the other experts in hospitals are to deliver their best yield in keeping patients' trust. I trusted my surgeon, later, to operate on me, to remove the by-then-discovered tumor, but it took an effort to do so, since, rightly or wrongly, I could not help thinking that my interests could not have been of great importance to him on the night of the cancelled surgery. This was doubtless unfair, but it is not so easy to be scrupulously fair when one is weak, dependent, and vulnerable, as hospital patients typically are.

That brings us to the patient virtues that are needed if there is to be a good climate of trust in hospitals and other places where health care is given. Is patience a virtue in a patient? Should I just have waited patiently until someone did see fit to tell me that my surgery had been postponed or cancelled, and why it had? And should I have trusted that my real interests were safe, before, during, and after surgery, whether that was planned but cancelled, or planned and carried out? Maybe my anxiety the night I expected but did not get surgery did me no physical harm, and maybe I should have trusted that, if anything really affecting my interests had been at stake, I would been given more attention. But anxiety, just as much as physical pain, is something we hope our physicians will help us to minimize, not increase. It does not seem to me that patience is always a virtue in a patient, especially a suffering patient, and certainly not that implicit trust, rather than vigilance, is in order when one has no choice but to put one's life and well-being in the hands of medical experts. Patients, as well as hospital administrators, have *some* responsibility to protest when things seem to go wrong, and perhaps I should have lodged a complaint about my unpleasantly anxious night, as much for the sake of future patients, as to express my own grievance. Patients have some responsibility to lodge complaints, and to communicate their fears and concerns, not just passively wait for professionals to ask questions of them, and give them information. But equally clearly, some patience, and some trust, is called for, on the part of patients. Threats to sue do not improve mutual trust. Nor is impatience going to get one moved up the triage ordering at an emergency department, or alter the urgency classification of one's awaited surgery. Displays of impatience, by patients, hinder rather than help health-care workers to do their job properly. But even there, as my next little story of another unpleasant night in hospital will show, a person can perhaps be too patient.

On a recent occasion, after accompanying my husband, who was suffering from an acute infection, to hospital by ambulance, I spent twelve hours, from 6 p.m. to 6 a.m., sitting by his bedside in the emergency department, before he was admitted to a ward and I was told to go home. The admitting doctor, seeing my exhausted face as I sat on the hard upright chair where I had spent the night, said: 'They should have sent you home hours ago.' But 'they' were too busy that night to think about me, and I was not their charge. It was for me to ask them if I should go, not for them to look after me as well as their patients. In fact I think they welcomed my staying, since I could do little unskilled things for my husband, things that otherwise they would have had to do. And I stayed, because I wanted to be sure that he was being looked after. But perhaps I overdid the patience and would-be helpfulness that night. Handing over to the professionals, trusting them, and going home to get enough sleep to be able to play my role as hospital visitor next day, might have been better. The virtues needed in those receiving health care, and in their concerned relatives, are those that are functional for the care of patients to go best. And that takes some but not too much patience, some trust but not uncritical trust.

I was not seriously harmed by either of my very unpleasant recent nights in my local hospital. Physicians and nurses have the job of looking after their patients' serious health interests, not making them or their relatives feel good. Relief of pain and other forms of distress is an acknowledged part of their responsibility, but only, it seems, if that does not threaten health or life. It is the prolongation of life, not the relief of suffering, that is the time-honored goal of the medical profession, the main goal recognized in the Hippocratic oath. And even Aesculapius had to be punished by Zeus for finding a way to make humans immortal, so he too seems to have thought life-prolongation to be an important goal, perhaps the main one. This ordering of priorities is the reason why professional medical associations typically oppose the legalization of voluntary euthanasia, and claim that it would be 'unethical' of doctors to end their suffering patients' lives, even when begged to do so. Certainly we would not be able to trust physicians who were overeager to administer euthanasia. Nobel prize winning novelist Coetzee has one of his characters, a helper at an animal rescue center, with the job of 'putting down' animals no one can care for, respond, when asked if he does not mind this task, 'I do mind. I mind deeply. I would not want someone doing it for me who didn't mind. Would you?' (1999: 85). Those whom we can trust to administer euthanasia will indeed be restricted to those who do mind doing what they do. Yet, as the memory of my mother's and my nephew's terrible suffering makes me ask, who can trust a physician who refuses to relieve suffering, however great, if that is thought to interfere with even the faintest chance of success of treatment, or, who, once that chance is gone, refuses to shorten the suffering, even after the wish to end life has been repeatedly expressed by the patient? If anything is 'unethical' behavior in physicians, it surely is letting their patients suffer, refusing their desperate requests for assistance in hastening death, when other ways of ending suffering are failing. The general recognition by bio-ethicists that compassion is a virtue in a healer is accompanied by occasional warnings to physicians against 'pseudo-empathy' with their incurable patients, against empathy that might lead them to a too ready agreement with a patient's expressed view that death may be the best option (Muskin 1998). We find warnings to physicians not to take patients' requests for assistance in hastening death as necessarily anything more than a sign that they are suffering from clinical depression, or even as invitations to be contradicted, as pleas to authoritative father figures for reassurance that their life is still worth preserving (Meier, Myers, and Muskin 2000: 185–8). Suffering is not being taken very seriously, as long as claims to intolerable suffering are treated with such patronizing disbelief. The deck is stacked against the suffering person who wants her life to be ended if her very expression of this wish is likely to be taken to show that she is clinically depressed, and so without power to give or withhold consent to any medical measure.

The relief of suffering, including migraine pain, menstrual pain, and acute arthritis pain, does not seem to be given very high priority in medical research, nor in decisions about government subsidies for medicines. (I have known two migraine sufferers who were driven to suicide to end their pain, one by shooting herself in the temple during an attack.) Must an understanding of the causes of pain be left to torturers, as understanding trust was largely left to con-artists and terrorists (Baier 1995)? Even if suffering is part of the human condition, it is surely the business of the medical profession to understand pain and its causes, and to do whatever can be done to minimize or end it.

Before the advent of anesthesia, physicians had to be capable of inflicting great pain, but now there is no excuse for them to let their patients suffer, and only the excuse of illegality for their refusing to help patients to end their suffering when hope of cure is gone. Would it help enable physicians to speak up for euthanasia, and be personally willing to assist a patient to die, when the patient seriously requests that, if death were reconceptualized as permanent general anesthesia? Anesthesia is the specialty of those who work in pain clinics, and who oversee pain relief after surgery, so it would not be a great extension of their field to make them the ones trusted to administer voluntary euthanasia. Even after the advent of anesthesia, electric shock treatment for mental illness was for decades given without it, so trainee doctors had to steel themselves to witness, and help give, some very cruel forms of treatment.

Labor and childbirth can be extremely painful, and I gather that, although more and more women, especially women physicians, are opting for epidural anesthesia in labor and childbirth, the medical profession is not rushing to make its use routine. A midwife of twenty years' experience explained patiently to me that labor pains are 'natural', and unlike other pain in not being a signal of something wrong. She also explained that the use of epidural anesthesia in labor can weaken muscle contractions, and so lead on to the need for further undesirable 'interventions', to forceps births, sometimes to emergency Caesarian section. And for epidural anesthesia to be even an option, the birth must be taking place in a hospital, with anesthetists available. For all these reasons, most midwives and obstetricians encourage its use only for what are expected to be particularly difficult births, prearranged to occur in a hospital. But not all long labors and difficult births are expected in advance, so many women will still have to console themselves during severe labor pains with the thought that this pain is natural, and with the hope that there is to be a 'happy outcome' (although there is also a not insignificant risk of postnatal depression). Some women, after one experience of 'normal' birthing without anesthesia, now opt for Caesarian section for any subsequent pregnancy, so memorably dreadful is their experience of labor and parturition. Labor can go on for days. Even for gastroscopies, whose length is measured in minutes, patients have to be held down. It is not surprising if many health professionals have had to develop a certain degree of callousness, just to do the job expected of them. But such callousness, however functional in some contexts, surely cannot be deemed an Aesculapian virtue.

Socrates, when about to drink the hemlock, said to his friends that he owed an offering to Aesculapius. Barbiturates of the sort recommended by the Hemlock Society, for use by those who judge they have suffered enough, are not always obtainable by those who want to self-administer them. For example, in New Zealand, even sympathetic physicians cannot prescribe them to patients. So what do New Zealanders do when they judge that their life is no longer worth living, indeed is intolerable? Refuse liquids until they lapse into unconsciousness (about one week), then die (after about another week)? Or, if not willing to keep going for another week (or in ignorance of this method), jump off a roof, or try to drown themselves in a nearby creek, like my nephew? Resort to plastic bags? Desperate people are often entirely dependent on the compassion of relatives, who risk prosecution for manslaughter if they actively assist, or depend on their primary care doctors, who can (and often do) rely on the dubious doctrine of double effect to prescribe lethal doses of painkilling drugs, or on nurses and physicians in hospitals and hospices, who can, in the same way, fudge the line between palliative care and euthanasia without putting themselves at significant risk of legal prosecution.

No wonder there is often despair, and sometimes terror, in sick rooms and hospitals! For we should not expect health-care workers to have to take *any* risk of prosecution, in their surely appropriate role as relievers of suffering. The physician one can trust is the one who will remind one how one can bring about one's own death by exercising one's right to refuse fluids, the one who does not have to risk prosecution if more active assistance in dying is given, and the one who would so assist one, when one unambiguously and repeatedly requests such assistance. (Or when one has in advance made clear the conditions in which one would want to die, and not retracted that directive, or has appointed some trusted person to take the decision for one. For the sad fact is that those most in need of medical assistance in hastening death are those least able to make clear requests, and be deemed in their right mind when they do ask for such assistance.) As the opponents of any law change or change in codes of medical ethics on this matter emphasize, the potential for abuse of the right to euthanasia is great. Anyone who supports such change must have some suggestions to make about how such abuse is to be prevented, or at least made highly unlikely. Or do we just have to accept that ending our terminal suffering is not something we should expect anyone to do for us, nor even help us do for ourselves? That it puts a heavy psychic cost on relatives who do the helping is undeniable, even if they avoid prosecution. But have we no moral right to professional help in hastening death when we unambiguously and repeatedly ask for such help, even when our condition is incurable, our pain or other distress extreme and unrelieved? In New Zealand, where I now live and expect to die, the current list of the rights of the recipients of health care makes no mention of a right to be spared avoidable suffering, let alone any right to be helped to die. There is a right to be treated with respect, a right to dignity, to 'services of the appropriate standard', provided in a manner that 'minimises the potential harm to, and optimises the quality of life of' that person, rights to communication and information, to make informed choices, a right to the presence of a chosen companion for 'support', and a right to complain. But no right to be spared avoidable suffering, unless that is thought to be covered by the right to 'minimized harm and optimized quality of life', or to 'dignity', or to 'informed choice'. (One patient advocate told me that she takes the right to informed choice to license her to inform her clients that Australia suffers less than does New Zealand from what she termed 'paranoia about opiates'.) I suspect that the silence on ending suffering is intentional, in this code of rights issued by the New Zealand Health and Disability Commission. For to recognize a right to be spared avoidable pain and distress would be to run afoul of the existing law on homicide, if such a right could be claimed in cases where the suffering can be ended only by ending the life.

I also suspect that the blank wall I encountered when I tried to get data on complaints about unrelieved suffering is no accident. The categories of patient complaints currently used at my local hospital do not include failure to relieve suffering. The greatest number of registered complaints come under the heading of (lack of) 'skill and competence', that is, violation of the right to services of an appropriate standard, and perhaps some of those complaints took the form 'I was left in great pain'. But I had no success in trying to find out what proportion, and had the same sort of failure when I consulted those with access to wider data. (The Medical Protection Society, and the New Zealand Health and Disability Commissioner.) The medical profession seems to choose not to investigate this matter, or perhaps to think that, since they are asking patients to give their pain a measure, from one to ten, they cannot be charged with ignoring pain. Suffering may indeed be difficult or impossible to quantify, but complaints about unrelieved suffering are as easy to count as any other complaint. The medical profession seems to prefer not to have them counted.

In hospitals some unnecessary pain, and some 'medical misadventures', are due to lack of competence in professionals, rather than to negligence or ill-will. As patients, we must expect sometimes to fall into the inexpert hands of those who are still learning to perform delicate procedures. Lack of skill in learners, as well as superior skill in the senior physicians supervising them, is to be expected in teaching hospitals. For only supervised practice on patients can give the learner the skills that are needed. Since few patients would consent to being such a learner's first try at a dangerous procedure, patients are usually kept in the dark about the degree of experience of the person in whose hands they find themselves. Trust that the supervising senior physicians know what they are doing when they delegate delicate tasks to their junior assistants, whom it is part of their duty to train, may be difficult to sustain, given reports of how those same senior physicians take care to see that their own sick relatives are kept out of the hands of beginners (Gawande 2002: 58). Ignorance on the part of patients is probably best in this matter, since 'in medicine there has long been a conflict between the imperative to give patients the best possible care, and the need to provide novices with experience' (Gawande 2002: 57). But even if a medical learner may unintentionally inflict pain, no very great knowledge is usually needed to relieve it.

A really shocking first-person account of what it can be like to be seriously ill is to be found in *Tiger's Eye: a Memoir,* by Inga Clendinnen, distinguished historian of humanity at its worst (Mayan human sacrifices, the Holocaust, the treatment of the Australian aborigines). She came to suffer from a rare liver disease, active autoimmune hepatitis, which caused great tiredness, an unsteady gait, swollen feet, ankles, and abdomen, a brittle, easily broken skin, and excessive bleeding from any cut, as well as from gums and nose. After it had led to septicemia and liver failure, she was eventually given a liver transplant. The horror of what she suffered was compounded not just by the incompetence and inhumanity of some in the medical profession, but, in the earlier stages, by the inhumanity of some ordinary young people. There were, she writes, 'a cluster of people, all under twenty-five', waiting at a tram stop in the affluent Melbourne suburb of Kew, when Clendinnen, by then diagnosed but not successfully treated, staggered, collapsed, and bled in the street. 'I lay, shocked and winded among my scattered parcels, blood welling out of my knees and arm, rehearsing the brave and reassuring things I would say when someone came to help. No-one moved' (Clendinnen 2000: 11). All looked away disdainfully, presumably taking her to be just an aging drunkard. (Perhaps older Australians would have been more willing to help, since Australians used to be very solicitous of their drunkards, in the days of beer swills before the pubs' early closing. Is it only the yuppie wine-drinkers who are such bad Samaritans?) Clendinnen managed to get herself home, after her fall, but she was, most understandably, 'in a state of serious disaffection from well society' (ibid). Clendinnen experienced the different and lonely world of the chronically ill, and encountered the unkindness of strangers, as well as neglect from some whose special responsibility it was to give her care. (The hero of her story is her dentist, who realized that something systemic was causing the gums to bleed.)

Ironically enough the poor performance of the medical profession in caring for patients and in giving enough attention to the relief of suffering has been invoked by one opponent of legalizing euthanasia as support for his crusade against it. In his emotively titled book, *Forced Exit: The Slippery Slope from Assisted Suicide to Legalized Murder*, Wesley J. Smith asks:

If doctors currently do such a poor job, generally, of relieving the pain and depression of suffering people when doctor-induced death is illegal, what kind of a job would they do if killing a patient were considered just another 'treatment option', and a less expensive and time-consuming option at that? To put it another way, why should we trust doctors to kill us, when too often they don't do an adequate job of caring for us? (Smith 1997: 147)

Compassion is a virtue we all, medical professionals or not, need to cultivate. And the first step we must take before we can think properly about the euthanasia issue is to recognize a right to considerate treatment by others, and, from physicians, relief of pain. Both the proponents and at least some opponents of legalizing euthanasia should be able to agree on that.

Minimizing physical suffering is usually called 'pain management' by health professionals, or at least by their managers. I was told by a hospital manager that patients who complain of not getting enough pain relief (and clearly such complaints are known to occur, even if they are not counted) run the risk of being taken to be 'substance abusers', who may be thought to have themselves to blame if the usual dose of morphine, or whatever, does not work for them. Their complaints, I was given to understand, are not always taken very seriously in our hospitals. Pain thresholds do vary, as does willingness to endure pain, and a good caregiver will try to fit the dose to the need of the individual patient. No one goes into hospital expecting no 'discomfort', and some patients may make unreasonable demands. But that does not mean that complaints about degree of suffering can be dismissed, nor that such complaints as are made about suffering can be ignored. Nor can dealing with them be taken merely as a matter of 'the management of expectations'. If one enters a hospital expecting to suffer excruciating pain, one will feel terror of health professionals, not trust. As my hospital manager put it to me, a balance has to be struck between informing hospital patients of the risks they run of 'adverse outcomes', and keeping patients calm and cooperative. The adverse outcomes which patients risk include infection (10 percent of hospital patients now contract an infection while in hospital), wrong medication, and such things as painful throat burns when oxygen equipment catches fire, or lung collapse when a central line goes in the wrong direction while being put in by an inexperienced learner (Gawande 2002). A conservative estimate of the risk of being harmed rather then helped by what happens to one in New Zealand hospitals is 12.9 percent, and apparently most of these medical misadventures are not admitted to their victims (Davis et al. 2002). (See also Institute of Medicine Report, 'To Err is Human', 1999). An experienced nurse suggested that our public hospitals should have, written over their doors, 'Abandon hope, all those who enter here'. Such a warning might not be a good idea, therapeutically speaking. Yet it is different only in degree from informing each incoming hospital patient of the known risk of 'adverse outcome', and that seems required by the recognized right to information, before consent is sought for treatment.

From a therapeutic as well as a managerial point of view, expectation management has to be geared to mood management, and a trade-off of patient rights is often needed. I was not told, when I had my stomach surgery, that I might lose my spleen, and I am not sorry about that, as I would have been much more worried beforehand had I foreseen the actual outcome of my surgery. Nor was I told, before my first long unsuccessful gastroscopy, just how long that might go on, merely how long such a procedure usually took. Had I known what was coming, I might not have been able to swallow the equipment and cooperate with the procedure. The good healer strikes the right balance between informing the patient what might be involved in the procedure she is undergoing, and keeping her in the frame of mind that is best for her chances of a good outcome. For example, I was told before my stomach surgery that I might lose much of my stomach, and that there might be a need to go further to surrounding areas, but the spleen in particular was not singled out as at risk. (Stomachs can regenerate, but not spleens.) This vague advance warning was probably the best to give me. I do not envy the professionals their decision-making responsibilities in balancing the patient's right to know against the physician's duty not to harm, and to give what reassurances are possible. But lists of patient rights do serve a purpose, even if conflict of rights cannot be ruled out. To include relief of avoidable suffering in our list of patient rights might complicate some decisions, but would also clarify at least some matters, for professionals and for patients. Physical agony is an evil to be avoided or lessened, not just a nuisance to be 'managed'.

Would it be plausible to construe a right to treatment that 'optimizes quality of life' as covering not only pain relief that does not threaten life, but also, in some cases, assistance in dying? The New Zealand code takes optimizing of quality of life to require health workers 'to take a holistic view of the needs of the consumer in order to achieve the best possible outcome in the circumstances'. Could death be such a best possible outcome? Could a timely end to a life optimize its quality? I myself see no reason why we should not say that it could. Death is not the antithesis of life but one of its inevitable limits, and no more necessarily detracts from the quality of the life it concludes than do the facts of conception, gestation, and birth, at the start of the life. A 'holistic view' cannot take life to be endless, but must take its ending, and the quality of that ending, as part of the life. David Hume, dying at sixty-five of 'a disorder in my bowels', wrote in his brief autobiography that 'I consider . . . that a man of sixty five, by dying, cuts off only a few years of infirmities,' and cheerfully records 'I now reckon on a speedy dissolution.' His philosophical attitude to his approaching death, which, since he had no belief in any afterlife, he took to mean his 'annihilation', puzzled and distressed James Boswell. In their famous conversation, Hume raised Lucretius' question why we should feel any sense of deprivation at not living through the time after our death, any more than at having missed living through the time before our birth. This question was given a plausible answer by Samuel Johnson, who, when the disturbed Boswell reported this conversation, gave it as his opinion that Hume either was lying, for effect, or was a fool, since, by his professed beliefs he would at death lose all he had. (He also said that if Hume really did not believe in an afterlife, he had no reason not to lie!) More recently, Thomas Nagel has argued for the asymmetry of reasonable attitudes to the timing of our birth, and of our death. Our birth defines who we are, whose life it is whose length and quality is in question. If we see death as near, we lose the prospect of an open-ended future, in which goods can at least be hoped to outweigh evils. 'Life familiarizes us with the goods of which death deprives us' (Nagel 1979: 9). Even so, how many of those familiar goods is enough? Hume's admired predecessor, the philosopher, Anthony Ashley Cooper, Third Earl of Shaftesbury, who died in 1713 at age forty-two, in Naples (where he had moved because of his weak lungs), mused in his notebook: 'Enough then . . . Pass on, move. You have seen. Now let others see' (Shaftesbury 1900: 261). But Thomas Nagel muses less stoically: 'the fact that it is worse to die at 24 than at 82 does not mean that it is not a terrible thing to die at 82, or even at 806' (Nagel 1979: 9).

The realization that one is having an untimely death may indeed lower the quality of one's life. The last utterance of the German painter, Paula Modersohn-Becker, as she died of childbirth complications after the birth of her first child, when she was thirty-one and at the height of her artistic powers, was, appropriately, 'Schade!' ('A pity!'). But the fact that there can be tragically untimely deaths does not mean that the longer the life, the better. Some short lives may have very high quality, and some very long ones may be filled with a sorry string of fears, losses, pains, and disappointments. To live through two world wars, and on into a century of continuing terrorist threats, as some have, may be to live too long. Just as premature birth does not benefit an infant, who can then be said to have been born too soon, so 'post mature' death may lower the quality of the life it ends. Meier, Myers, and Muskin (2000) tell of the desperate sixty-nine-year-old Mrs C, with a ten-year history of systemic lupus erythematosus, severe osteoporosis, and muscle wasting. She was fed with a gastrostomy tube, which caused acid leakage into the abdominal wall. She was unable to sit, read, or write. She had repeatedly requested assistance in ending her life during the year before she died. She had succeeded in having barbiturates prescribed to her, but expressed anger at her doctor for not helping her more actively, for abandoning her when she needed him most. This doctor had deliberately refrained from telling her that refusal of fluids would accomplish her wish to die, so afraid was he of seeming to advocate a hastened death. With her husband's help, Mrs C finally managed to swallow ice cream containing thirty (crushed) barbiturate tablets, and died. Her death was neither peaceful nor well-timed, but angry and desperate, leaving her husband understandably distressed at his role in her death, which was definitely not a good one. Had her physician helped her to die a year earlier, when she requested that, perhaps just by informing her of the control she herself exercised by her power to refuse hydration, her life would surely have been better, not worse, when judged in terms of overall quality. I say 'surely', but there is no agreement among philosophers, or anyone else, on how much length of life matters, and whether, simply because of mortality itself, 'a bad end is in store for us all' (Nagel 1979: 10). Whether death can be a good outcome, or at least the best possible one in the circumstances, must be left for individual judgment, and both our law and our medical practices should show respect for those who do at a particular time come to judge that, for them, death is the best outcome.

Hume, in his essay on suicide, paraphrased Seneca: 'I thank providence both for the good, which I have already enjoyed, and for the power, with which I am endowed, of escaping the ill that threatens me' (Hume 1995: 583). But this power of suicide, or at least of quick suicide, is not one that always lasts until it is most needed. Seneca himself found that he needed help, to be put into a hot bath, after he had cut his wrists but not bled sufficiently to bring death. And those who choose dehydration as their escape route not only die slowly, but may be foiled, once unconscious, by health workers who insert a drip. To be effective, the power for which Seneca gave thanks needs supplementation by the right to be assisted, or at least to have our last decision respected, should we decide to escape its evils when life becomes intolerable. We are a species who look ahead, and know that we shall die. Epicurus was wrong when he said that death is nothing to us, once we reflect wisely about it. The timing and manner of our death rightly matter to most of us. Our human consciousness of mortality is naturally accompanied both by some natural fear, and some wish to avoid the worse forms of dying. To want the say about when to die is a natural development of our self-consciousness, our wish to plan our lives wisely, and leave our affairs in order when we go. Seneca said that the wise man lives as long as he ought, not as long as he can. Opponents of legalizing voluntary euthanasia might seize on this as showing that the so-called 'right to die', if recognized, would quickly degenerate, with the help of burdened relatives, impatient heirs, and impoverished health services, into a 'duty to die'. But equally, those who oppose euthanasia are in a parallel danger of turning the right to life, especially when construed as inalienable, into a duty to keep living. Seneca and Solomon are surely right that there is a 'time to die', a time when it would be unseemly to struggle to live longer. Of course, physicians too have views about what their rights and duties are. And just as no patient should be forced to live longer than she wishes, no physician should be forced to administer euthanasia against her beliefs. But she should, I believe, be pressured to inform the patient of the lethal effects of refusing fluids, and to refer the patient whom she refuses active quicker help to one who is willing to give it. The autonomy of both patient and physician ought to be preserved, and surely can be, without clash. Medical professionals, especially psychiatrists, are in the dangerously powerful position of being able to declare a patient to be without mental competence, and so unable to exercise autonomy. If suicidal intent is taken as an indication of depression, and so loss of mental competence, then incurable patients are left entirely at the mercy of their physicians. Autonomy that is at one's physician's discretion to deny one is no protection against medical abuse of power.

Doctors are notorious for thinking themselves godlike, and by beginning this essay by noting Aesculapius' divine ancestry, I may myself have been guilty of encouraging such a delusion. The assumption made by some physicians that they have the ability to see beyond the 'manifest content' of their patients' words, when those patients beg for death, to their different real meaning, is of a piece with their insistence, even when they are in favor of legalizing euthanasia, that the license to perform it should be theirs alone. That they alone should be able to prescribe potentially lethal medication is one thing. That they alone can administer a lethal dose to someone who wants it is another. As I write, Lesley Martin, a registered nurse, is in a New Zealand prison after being found guilty of attempted murder, after giving her mother, on request, an overdose of morphine, to end her horrible suffering from cancer of the rectum. (Or is it telling about it, publishing her book, *To Die Like A Dog: The Personal Face of the Euthanasia Debate*, that she is really being prosecuted for?) It may be sensible to require some medical training in those permitted to give assistance in dying. But Martin had such training. And certainly there should be some careful check on whether the patient who requests assistance in dying does really want it, and whether, if he does, that is for his own sake or for his burdened relatives' sake. But an eight-step procedure, such as that advocated by physician and bio-ethicist Linda L. Emanuel, in 'Facing Requests for Physician-Assisted Suicide' (Emanuel 1998), seems excessive and excessively lengthy for the desperate patient. (The first proposed step is to check and if necessary treat for clinical depression. The second is to assess other aspects relevant to the patient's capacity for rational decision-making, and if necessary have a proxy appointed. If the request for assisted suicide is not withdrawn, the third step, repeated in the fifth and seventh, is to engage in structured deliberation, including making sure that the patient is aware of the control he himself possesses through his right to refuse fluids. The fourth step is to try to treat the root causes of the patient's request. If it continues, the physician checks again to make sure the patient has full information, then, in the sixth step, involves consultants. In the seventh, after a third check that the patient knows what his options are, and knows what he is requesting, unwanted intrusive treatment such as intravenous drips are removed. Should the patient still be requesting more active physician assistance, the eighth and final step is to refuse it, explaining that it is illegal.) Must a patient repeat his request for physician-assisted death eight times before he is taken seriously enough to be believed, then only to be definitely refused? Would it not be kinder to stress the illegality of what is being requested at the beginning, and to go on to remind the patient what he can do for himself?

We can turn to the Netherlands, Belgium, and Oregon for help on what checks and monitoring should go on, once assisted suicide is not illegal, and on who should check and monitor the checkers and monitors. These important details have been worked out in their law changes to facilitate euthanasia on request while still protecting a patient against abuse of the new permission. The drafting of any new law on euthanasia needs cooperation between lawyers, physicians, nurses, bio-ethicists, and the public, and study of what can be learned from the pioneering measures already in force in some places. One thing that does already seem to be emerging is that, once there is a recognized right to be assisted to die, many patients who make the initial moves to request such help will not carry through to actually get it. Acquiescence from physicians in a request to die, far from being taken as encouragement to die, is sometimes sufficient to let a patient rest easier, and let death come without finally invoking the special measures that are available to hasten it. To adapt an insight of

Nietzsche's, the thought of physician-assisted suicide can get one through many a bad night.

My very modest input into this collective thinking about what we should want our laws to allow, and to facilitate, is that the patient's primary care physician is usually the physician who is best placed to know if the patient means what she says when she requests death, and best placed to know whether or not she is requesting it mainly for her relatives' sake. Indeed she would often be the one most trusted by the patient to administer euthanasia, or at least to call in the anesthetist. Specialists and surgeons are rarely known as well by the patient as the primary care physician, and, despite their expert knowledge of the medical condition of the patient, they cannot expect to have as much insight into her state of mind, nor to be as readily trusted in such life and death decisions, as the less specialized doctor who has looked after her health for years. Physician Sherwin B. Nuland, author of the disturbing book, *How We Die*, is of the opinion that, in U.S. hospitals, 'the least authoritative member of the team in any good hospital is likely to be the one who has the widest perspective on care' (Nuland 2002), so the not-so-specialized primary care doctor, already known to the patient, is an important person to consult on end of life decisions. And along with this should go a standard disclosure, by primary care doctors, of what attitude to euthanasia they hold, and a standard offer to discuss with patients their advance wishes. At the very least, all terminally ill patients should be informed by their physician how much is in their own control, by exercising their right to refuse fluids. We all need to know whom we can and cannot trust to help us in our final illnesses, and physicians need to know what requests are likely to be made of them. And of course it must be the patient who makes the request for assistance in dying, or appoints someone to act for her, not just her relatives, who may have their own, usually compassionate, but sometimes self-serving, reasons for wanting the dying process to be hastened.

As things are at present, the best relief from suffering, and the easiest deaths, go on in hospices. Many supporters of the hospice movement oppose a law change, arguing that the law changes we need, to improve the quality of life at its end, are those that would enable more people to have access to compassionate terminal care of the sort that hospices provide for some (mainly cancer) patients. It seems that it is not so much that these hospice supporters are against giving patients the dose needed to relieve suffering, even when that hastens death, as that they, like the medical profession in general, are against any law telling them in what exact conditions they may do so. It is the regulation and red tape that legalized euthanasia would bring, not the actual euthanasia, which the medical profession seems to be against. It would indeed be tragic if a law change made it more difficult, not easier, for those who request assistance in ending their life to get that help. (For instance, should the rule that it not be given to those suffering from clinical depression be taken to mean that anyone who has ever had anti-depressants prescribed to them is to be denied the right to euthanasia.)

According to Nuland, and oncologist Charles F. McKhann, physicians, especially specialists, often see their patients' deaths as their professional failures, and tend to abandon their patients once hope of cure is gone—indeed a study by H. Feifel has shown that, as a profession, medicine attracts people with particularly high personal anxieties about dying (Nuland 1994: 258; McKhann 1999: 134, 253). Apart from those working in hospices, and the few who work in (usually understaffed) pain clinics, physicians see themselves as in the business of death-prevention, of rescue and cure, not of relieving the sufferings of those who cannot be cured. So our hope of compassionate physicians, once the time inevitably comes when our chances of cure are gone, may be as faint as any hope of a death with dignity. As Linda Emanuel writes, 'The obligation to provide comfort to the suffering is an ancient professional obligation that is not well implemented in this technologically powerful era' (Emanuel 1998: 647). Nuland approvingly quotes Philippe Aries' comment that death is ugly and dirty, and that we do not easily tolerate what is ugly and dirty. He himself writes, 'I have not seen much dignity in the process by which we die' (Nuland 1994: xvii), and 'By and large, dying is a messy business' (Nuland 1994: 142). Far fewer than one in five, he writes, have a quick, easy, and unconcerned death (ibid). Nor is dirty and undignified the worst of it. He estimates that one in five of the patients whose death he witnessed died in very great suffering (Nuland 1994: 140). The worst indignity the dying can suffer is to have their wishes disregarded. When they wish that their suffering be ended, and have expressed this wish unequivocally, either at the time or in an advance directive, they surely should be helped to die. When they have expressed the wish to live as long as possible, even in great pain (and can afford continued care), that wish too must be respected. Codes of patient rights typically put great emphasis on dignity and autonomy. The highest form of autonomy, as Seneca saw, is to have the say about the timing of one's own death. We exercise this form of autonomy as much when we decide to have our disease treated, in order to prolong our life, or, when treatment has failed, to wait for our disease to kill us, as when we take our own life, or request help in so doing. To be denied this right of decision is the ultimate indignity.

As long as we have to depend on the courage, or even the recklessness, of our physicians and nurses, and have to depend on our own continued communicative powers, and others taking their exercise seriously, to say when we have had enough, we must go into our terminal illnesses either great heroes and heroines, or else in plain terror of prolonged, unrelieved suffering or other intolerable distress, perhaps of 'literally drowning in our own secretions' (McKhann 1999: 156, quoting a neurologist on the sort of deaths some of his patients undergo, unless they are assisted to die). A law change seems clearly called for, both on grounds of compassion to patients, and as protection for decently compassionate health-care workers. It would also help to allow them to be in a position to claim honesty as a professional virtue. As things now stand the humane physician who helps a patient to die has to engage in some form of self-protective doubletalk, to escape prosecution.

Nuland tells of the death by suicide of Nobel prize-winning Harvard physicist, Percy Bridgman, in 1946. Bridgman was seventy-nine, in the final stages of cancer, when, after finishing the index to the seven volumes of his scientific writings, and putting his affairs in order, he shot himself, leaving a letter stating, 'It is not decent for society to make a man do this for himself' (Nuland 1994: 152). Only a law change, enabling physicians to help people in Bridgman's situation, without fear of sanctions, can end this 'indecency' in our society, and make medicine a fully humane profession. James H. Buchanan prefaces his book, *Patient Encounters* (Buchananan 1989), with Jurgen

Thorwald's statement: 'The status and progress of medicine ought always be judged primarily from the point of view of the suffering patient, and never from the point of view of one who has never been ill' (Thorwald 1957). This seems undeniable. Yet we obviously cannot insist that any surgeon first undergo the form of surgery he is to perform on his patients. This would be an especially impractical form of the old advice: 'Physician, heal thyself,' though it did take a physician trying surgery under curare, long used as an anesthetic, before credence was given to patient complaints that the drug merely paralyzed, without anesthetizing (Smith et al. 1947). How, short of doing to them what they do to their patients, can we get the medical practitioner to adopt the patient's point of view? Recognizing compassion as an essential Aesculapian virtue would be a start. If medical professionals are to free themselves of the charge of prolonging the agony of the dying, they must be given the legal power to administer euthanasia on repeated serious patient request. Only then will compassion become a fully functional virtue in the medical profession. But it is sixty years since Bridgman's forced suicide, and we still make those in intolerable final suffering kill themselves, sometimes incompetently, or persuade their relatives to do it for them, as best they can, and be prosecuted for their pains. We shall not have a decent society, nor a humane and trustworthy medical profession, until we follow the lead of the Netherlands, Belgium, and Oregon, and change our laws officially to allow physician-assisted death on patient serious request, along with full protection against abuse of such power. Until such a law change, we patients cannot fully trust our physicians. However many other professional virtues and skills they may possess, if they have not the will and the legal power to end suffering at patient request, so cannot show ultimate compassion, how can we trust them?

I have in this essay spoken as much about rights as about virtues. No personal or professional virtues can do their proper work unless the laws and institutions structuring our lives and our work are in order. When they are not, we need the special virtues of campaigners for law change—vision in designing better laws and codes of rights, and pertinacity and hope in the fight for their acceptance.

ACKNOWLEDGEMENTS

For their generous help with this essay I thank Michael Ashby, Marjolein Copland, Denys Court, Jennifer Galbraith, Tina Gilbertson, Grant Gillett, Cath Leckie, Kristin Kenrick, Frances Matthews, Sarah Naylor, Ron Paterson, Angela Scott, Saul Traiger, and Richard Whitney. I am also indebted to the editors of this volume and to the publisher's readers for constructive suggestions.

REFERENCES

Baier, A. C. (1995). 'Trust and Antitrust'. *Moral Prejudices*. Harvard.
_____ (2004). 'Demoralization, Trust, and the Virtues' in Cheshire Calhound (ed.), *Setting the Moral Compass: Essays by Women Philosophers*. Oxford.
Buchanan, J. H. (1989). *Patient Encounters*. Charlottesville: University of Virginia Press.
Clendinnen, I. (2000). *Tiger's Eye: A Memoir*. Melbourne: Text Publishing.

Coetzee, J. M. (1999). *Disgrace*. Secker and Warburg.

Davis, P., Lay-Yee, R., Briant, R., et al. (2002). 'Adverse events in New Zealand public hospitals: occurrence and impact'. *NZ Med. J*, 115.

Emanuel, L. L. (1998). 'Facing Requests for Physician-Assisted Suicide'. *JAMA (Journal of the American Medical Association)*, 280/1, 7: 643–7.

Gawande, A. (2002). 'The Learning Curve: How do you become a good surgeon? Practice'. *New Yorker*, Annals of Medicine, 52–61.

Kohn, L. T., Corrigan, J. M., and Donaldson, M. S. (eds. (2000)). Committee on Quality of Health care in America, Institute of Medicine. *To Err is Human: Building a Safer Health System*. Washington, DC.: National Academy Press.

Hume, D. (1995). 'On Suicide'. *Essays Moral Political and Literary* (Miller edn.). Indianapolis: Liberty Press.

McKhann, C. F. (1999). *A Time to Die: The Case for Physician Assistance*. Yale.

Martin, L. (2002). *To Die Like a Dog: The Personal Face of the Euthanasia Debate*. Wailuku: M-Press.

Meier, D. E., Myers, H., and Muskin, P. R. (2000). 'When, if ever, should we expedite death?' in Zeman, Adam and Emanuel, Linda (eds.), *Ethical Dilemmas in Neurology*. London: W. B. Saunders.

Muskin, P. R. (1998). 'The Request to Die'. *JAMA (Journal of the American Medical Association)*, 279/1, 6: 323–8.

Nagel, T. (1979). 'Death'. *Mortal Questions*. Cambridge.

Nuland, S. B. (1994). *How We Die*. New York: Knopf.

_____ (2002). *New York Review of Books*, XLIX/20, Correspondence: 89–90.

Shaftesbury, A. A. C. Third Earl of (1900). *The Life, Unpublished Letters, and Philosophical Regimen of Anthony, Earl of Shaftesbury, Author of 'Characteristics'* (Benjamin Rand edn.). London: Swan Sonnenshein & Co Lim.

Smith, S. M., Brown, H. O., Toman, J. E. P., and Goodman, L. S. (1947). 'The Lack of Cerebral Effects of d-Tubocurarine'. *Anesthesiology*, 8/1: 1–14.

Smith, W. J. (1997). *Forced Exit: From Slippery Slope to Legalized Murder*. Random House.

Thorwald, J. (1957). *Century of the Surgeon*. London: Thames and Hudson.

Vincent, C., Young, M., et al. (1994). 'Why do people sue doctors? A study of patients and relatives taking legal action'. *Lancet*, 343: 1609–13.

7

Environmental Virtue Ethics

Rosalind Hursthouse

Environmental ethics is concerned with the articulation and defence of what I shall call 'the green belief'—the belief, namely, that a fairly radical change in the way we engage with nature is imperative. Environmental virtue ethics, then, is concerned with articulating and defending the green belief in virtue ethics terms, rather than in the terms of its two rivals, utilitarianism and deontology. This chapter is about what an environmental virtue ethics might be like. I consider two significantly different versions. First, we might have an environmental virtue ethics that seeks to articulate and defend the green belief in terms of old and familiar virtues and vices that are given a new interpretation when applied to the new field of our relations with nature. The second version goes beyond the first by introducing one or two new virtues, explicitly concerned with our relations with nature. (Note, in the description of both versions, a stress on the 'new'. It is pretty much agreed ground amongst environmental ethicists that the truth of the green belief calls for 'a new ethic', but just how new, and new in just what way remains unclear and extremely tendentious.)

OLD VIRTUES AND VICES

I begin by illustrating (with necessary brevity) how much mileage I think can be got out of the old virtues and vices when they are used to articulate and defend the green belief.[1] One of the earliest modern philosophy books devoted to environmental issues was Passmore's *Man's Responsibility for Nature*. Without explicitly espousing virtue ethics, which barely existed at the time, Passmore argued in defence of the green belief in largely virtue and vice terms, claiming that it is primarily through the vices of greed, self-indulgence, and short-sightedness that we have brought about, and are continuing to bring about, ecological disasters and that what was needed to avert them was 'that old-fashioned procedure, thoughtful action' (1974: 194)—or, as virtue ethicists would say, the virtue of prudence or practical wisdom.

The point that greed, self-indulgence, and short-sightedness are very much to blame is not, I think, questioned by any environmentalist. It can, and frequently does,

---

[1] I wrote the final version of this chapter before reading Louke van Wensveen's (2000) wonderful book, which shows that writers have found it quite natural to invoke over 170 old and familiar virtues in the context of environmental ethics.

form an implicit part of the most straightforward 'human-centred' utilitarian defence of the green belief, and of green economists' and scientists' defences. That some of our practices are, or have been, just plain short-sighted as far as our own interests are concerned is the most straightforward position to defend. No one, no matter how indifferent to environmental issues in general, welcomes air pollution in their city, or the unavailability of uncontaminated shellfish, or being made sick by their water. True, most people believe that 'the government should do something about it' in a way that neither raises their taxes nor prohibits their doing any of the things they have become accustomed to doing, but this response, the defence will plausibly claim, is just short-sightedness all over again. There isn't a quick fix; there is not any way in which the pollution can be halted and turned around without our forgoing a number of practices and activities that we, at least in the 'developed' nations, think of as enjoyments that are part of ordinary pleasant life.

Is it greedy and self-indulgent of us to want to enjoy such things? This is a much less straightforward position to defend, but much of the literature in environmental ethics (by no means just the minute amount that argues in terms of virtue ethics) suggests that convincing others, and ourselves, of the far reaching truth of the green belief, will necessarily involve bringing us all to see that it is. At the moment, a very small number of people have come to see their previous enjoyment of a very small number of 'ordinary' things—the eating of meat and the wearing of fur coats, the acquisition of new mahogany furniture, the owning of several cars—as greedy and self-indulgent, and changed their practices.

However, such a shift in moral self-assessment clearly does not come about just through the recognition that our current practices are short-sighted, if at all. People usually convert to vegetarianism on moral, rather than health, grounds because of some sort of concern about the animals we standardly consume. A change in the many ways in which we use animals, particularly for food, can be defended, in virtue ethics terms, by reference not only to the vices of greed and self-indulgence, but also to that of cruelty and the corresponding lack of the virtue of compassion, without any attempt to defend the idea that animals have rights. [2] Few people nowadays are prepared to deny outright that a great deal of animal suffering is involved in the processes that bring cheap meat to our supermarket shelves. A surprising number still believe that the consumption of meat is necessary for human health, but once that ignorance is dispelled, the animal suffering is revealed to be quite gratuitous and our practices thereby cruel. The fact that I myself, as an ordinary deskbound city-dweller, am not actually out and about inflicting cruelty on chickens, sheep, cows, pigs, and so on, may preserve me from being rightly called 'cruel' but I do not merit being called compassionate, if, knowing about the cruel practices, I still enjoy their fruits, any more than I merit being called just if I knowingly enjoy the fruits of slave labour while congratulating myself on not actually being a slave owner.

---

[2] For a beautifully clear discussion of ancient Greek defences of animals that did not appeal to animal rights (even when maintaining that we owed justice to them) see Sorabji (1993), especially chapter 11.

It has long been recognized that, although the vices do not form a unity, some of them certainly aggravate others. The old, familiar, vices of pride and vanity make us unwilling to acknowledge our greed, self-indulgence, short-sightedness, and lack of compassion; dishonesty, exercised in the form of self-deception, enables us to blind ourselves to relevant facts and arguments and find excuses for continuing as we are (think of the people who are still pretending that global warming isn't happening); cowardice makes us unwilling to go out on a limb and risk the contempt of our peers by propounding unpopular views, and so on.

It seems clear that much of what is wrong about our current practices with regard to nature springs from these familiar and ancient human vices—played out, in environmental ethics, on an unfamiliar stage. And it may well be that if we could find a way of releasing many human beings from the grip of these familiar vices, the change in our current ways of going on would be so extraordinarily radical that it would indeed adequately set the scene for all the changes that environmentalists dream of. After all, no one suggests that we need a new ethic to deal with the human-centred moral problems of poverty, war, and, quite generally, 'man's inhumanity to man'. We suppose that if (and what a big 'if') we could somehow induce many more of ourselves to be truly compassionate, benevolent, unselfish, honest, unmaterialistic, long-sighted, just, patient—virtuous, in familiar ways, in short—the way human beings live would be radically different, and the entirely human-centred moral problems that our own vices create would become things of the past. And if these hitherto intractable human-centred ones, why not the environmental ones as well?

This does not seem to be an unreasonable position, though it perhaps needs to be supplemented by the mention of one more virtue, which, although old, has become somewhat unfashionable in recent decades and thereby unfamiliar, namely humility, which has been emphasized by Thomas Hill Jr. (1983). (Hill calls the virtue 'proper humility' in order to distinguish it from those failings or vices that many people nowadays would find to be connoted by describing someone as 'humble'—obsequiousness, false modesty, wimpishness, and the like.)

Proper humility is the virtue traditionally opposed to the vice of arrogance, the undue assumption of dignity, authority, power, or knowledge, and a constantly recurring theme in environmental ethics—especially in writings that call for a new 'biocentric' approach—has been that we should, indeed, must, recognize and, in recognizing, perforce, abandon our undue assumption of dignity, authority, power, and knowledge—our arrogance in short—in relation to nature. Notwithstanding the surprisingly common belief that Darwinism shows that we are to be dignified as the top species, it gives us no reason to suppose that we are any such thing. As Stephen Clark, early on in environmental ethics, nicely put it, 'We sometimes speak of the dinosaurs as failures; there will be time enough for that judgement when we have lasted even one tenth as long' (1977: 112). The rationality that Western philosophical tradition has made the distinguishing mark of our superiority may well turn out to be, in evolutionary terms, a poor strategy. By the same token, our rationality, whether in its own right, or as the mark of our having been made in the image of God, gives us no especial authority. We do not have 'dominion' over nature; it is not true, as

Aristotle claimed, that plants exist for the sake of animals and all other animals exist for the sake of human beings. We can—that is, it is possible for us to—make use of plants and animals and indeed minerals and other inanimate things, but the old idea that we can do so without restraint, and that bountiful nature would somehow make good our depredations has now been proved to be a fantasy. (It is a notable fact, which might strike one as enragingly arrogant, or heart-wrenchingly innocent, that Aristotle believed that no species could be destroyed.) Our power over nature, we have discovered, is much more limited than we supposed when we first got modern science going, mostly because, as we discovered rather recently, our knowledge and understanding of the biosphere is in its infancy. (I think it is correct to say that the undue assumption of our power over, and knowledge of, nature is comparatively recent. Prior to the dawn of modern science (whenever we might date that) we may have thought that we had superiority and authority, but I don't think we were under any illusion that we had much of the power over nature that knowledge brings until industrialization.)

In that paragraph on arrogance I crudely sum up an extensive body of environmental ethics literature. Most of the literature that emphasizes such points is, polemically, directed towards establishing the inherent or intrinsic worth or value of individual living things or biotic communities but, in the context of virtue ethics, it serves equally well as a convincing condemnation of our arrogance—and thereby as a call to the unfashionable virtue of humility.

It can be seen that defending the green belief in terms of the old virtues and vices involves a particular strategy. Each old virtue or vice mentioned is considered in the context of the new area of our relations with nature, and thereby acquires a new application or dimension. I have briefly alluded to the old virtues of prudence, practical wisdom, compassion, and proper humility, and the old vices of greed, self-indulgence, short-sightedness, cruelty, pride, vanity, dishonesty, and arrogance. We acquire a new perception, or understanding, of what is involved in being compassionate, or greedy or short-sighted or properly humble or arrogant; some of the old virtues and vices get reconfigured. And, we might well say, from the virtue ethics standpoint, this has been a standard strategy for ethical advance. (We might note a parallel strategy in much deontological environmental ethics; you take a familiar old moral rule or duty, such as the duty not to kill, or to harm, and you play it out on a different stage, thereby giving it a new interpretation.)

STILL HUMAN-CENTRED?

Is a virtue ethics thus reconfigured human-centred? Well, it is obviously still concerned with what sort of people we human beings should be and what we should do. But any normative ethics is concerned with the rightness or wrongness of human actions, with what we human beings should do and be and there is nothing in the environmental ethics literature that calls for a new ethic to suggest that there is anything wrong with that. However, there is more than a whiff of a much less widespread human-centredness in Hill which, having noted his views, we should pause to consider.

Hill argues that neither utilitarianism nor deontology can account for the wrongness of wantonly destroying a living thing such as a tree. But when he moves on to account for its wrongness in the virtue ethical terms of proper humility and arrogance, his discussion disconcertingly parallels Kant's account of the wrongness of inflicting gratuitous suffering on animals. And this is notoriously human-centred. Kant held that the animals' suffering was incidental. What is really wrong with cruelty to animals is that it leads to cruelty to one's fellow human beings. Hill, similarly, holds that what is wrong with lack of proper humility in regard to nature is its dangerous tendency to lead the agent to treat other persons disrespectfully.[3]

Most philosophers who deplore the way we use animals have long made two objections to Kant's account. One is that it is based on a false empirical premise. Notwithstanding their enjoyment of watching bullfights, the Spaniards are not notably crueller to each other than members of other European nations. The second, deeper, objection is that Kant's account simply misses the point. Of course the animals' suffering matters. That is why it is right to describe the gratuitous infliction of it as cruel and to deplore it thereby, regardless of whether or not it leads to cruelty to human beings. How manifestly perverse it would be to account for the wrongness of cruelty to small children not in terms of what it did to the children but in terms of how it led to cruelty to rational adults! And most environmental philosophers would want to make the same two objections to Hill. It is quite implausible to say that being humbled before nature promotes humility before persons, and, more importantly, the untoward death of living things matters. That is why it is right to describe me as acting arrogantly if I assume dominion and authority over the lives of non-rational living things, and act as though they were mine to dispose of at a whim, and to deplore my action thereby, regardless of whether or not I am likely to act arrogantly to other humans.

However, it is Hill's Kantian predilections that lead him down this path. He is thinking of virtue (vice) as a tendency to right (wrong) action independently specified, and his paradigms of right (wrong) action involve other human beings. But virtue ethics, as is well known, specifies right and wrong action in terms of the virtues and vices. If cruelty is a vice, then to recognize an act as one of cruelty to animals is thereby to recognize it as wrong, and no further account of wherein its wrongness consists is called for. Similarly, if arrogance is a vice, to recognize an act of wanton destruction of a living thing as arrogant is thereby to recognize it as wrong and no further account of wherein its wrongness consists is called for. So, in particular, no account in terms of its dangerous tendency to lead to the disrespectful treatment of humans is called for. So virtue ethics need not take on the excessive human-centredness of Hill's account.

It is true that neo-Aristotelian virtue ethics holds that the virtues benefit their possessor, that they are necessary and (with a bit of luck) sufficient for *eudaimonia*, for living well as a human being. Does this claim entail that human well-being is the only thing that really matters morally, or that it is the top value, ranked above any other (in an improperly human chauvinistic way)? Some environmentalist philosophers seem

---

[3] '(T)hose who value such traits as humility, gratitude, and sensitivity *to others* have reason to promote the love of nature,' 224, my italics.

to suppose so, but it is unclear why. However, I do not want to dodge this issue, and I shall return to it at the end of the chapter.

Sometimes the disquiet seems to amount to no more than the thought that we should stop thinking about our virtues and vices—and thereby ourselves—and direct our attention to the natural world. And there may be a grain of practical truth in this thought. How, after all, is the reconfiguration of the familiar virtues and vices to be brought about except by a radical change in our ways of thinking and feeling about, and hence acting in relation to, the natural world? Is it not just this change that, for example, Aldo Leopold, Arne Naess, Paul W. Taylor, and Holmes Rolston III have attempted, with some success, to bring about? But a 'way of thinking, feeling and acting in relation to' some field or area of activity is, quite often, an ethical character trait, a virtue or a vice. If what is needed is or are a new way or ways, perhaps what is needed is at least one new virtue, explicitly concerned with our relations to nature.

This brings us to a consideration of the second version an environmental virtue ethics might take.

Before we embark on exploring this, we should note that the introduction—or discovery—of a new virtue is a formidable task. As an ethical character trait, a virtue, say, honesty, is far more than a mere disposition or tendency to go in for certain sorts of actions (say, honest ones). For a start, someone who is honest not only does what is honest but does so for certain reasons, not, for example, simply because they think honesty is the best policy. Further, virtue is also concerned with feelings or emotions; it also involves dispositions to certain sorts of emotional reactions, including finding certain things enjoyable and others painful or distressing. On the more intellectual side, it involves a certain perceptive capacity with regard to the area of the virtue in question (such as, in the case of honesty, an acute eye for occasions on which we are all about to connive unwittingly at dishonesty) and 'practical wisdom'—the capacity to reason correctly about what is to be done—which itself involves reasoning in relation to good ends. And all these apparently disparate elements can form a unity in human nature; that is, they can be recognized as a way a human being, given human psychology, could be.

And finally, if we are not to depart too radically from tradition, this way that we could be should have a recognizable preliminary version; a way that children can be that, although on the right track, still needs to be developed and expanded, and ultimately corrected, by practical wisdom.

Standardly, though by no means invariably, this complex and elusive concept of an ethical character trait is grasped through a noun which names the character trait (e.g. 'generosity'), with an associated adjective ('generous') that can apply to people and to acts—to people as possessing the character trait, to acts that, though not necessarily springing from the virtue, are typical of it. So the introduction or discovery of an unfamiliar, 'new', virtue would, on the face of it, need to involve the invention or coining of a new term or concept, which named a complex unity of dispositions to act and feel for certain sorts of reasons, and to see and respond to things in certain sorts of ways, which we had discovered, or realized, was a way human beings, given human psychology, could be. And this complex unity would have to be the sort of thing we could conceive of as being inculcated in children as part of their moral edu-cation—not totally against the grain, but expanding on and correcting some natural inclination(s) they have.

ONE NEW VIRTUE

Hill himself mentions two features that seem to be involved in being rightly related to nature which proper humility does not capture—some sort of aesthetic appreci-ation of it and some sense of gratitude towards it—and it is noteworthy that finding beauty in nature, and feeling gratitude to it for, not only its beauty, but its abundance, are emotional reactions that are perfectly consistent with proper humility but which rescue one from the proper humility's being crushing or dispiriting. (Could the reflec-tion that human beings and all their works are but an insignificant and fleeting part of the great unfolding of the natural world fail to be crushing if it were not ameli-orated by the joyous thought that we are part of something glorious?) The aesthetic appreciation of nature has, as a topic, its own extensive philosophical literature—in aesthetics—and it is not easy, in this area, to transfer aesthetics talk into ethics talk. However, there are certainly some suggestive lines of thought to be pursued.

R. W. Hepburn (1984), an aesthetician, has at least two important essays which find many echoes in environmental ethics literature. One explores 'the enjoyment of natural beauty as tending towards an ideal of oneness with nature or as leading to the disclosure of unity in nature' (1984: 17) and the other analyses the concept of an emotion, wonder, that, as he says, 'occupies in a paradigmatic way exactly that territory common to the aesthetic, moral and religious' (1984: 7).

Some of the points that Hepburn makes about wonder in relation to nature could well be taken over into an account of (proper) humility, to which he explicitly links it, but he also links it, surely rightly, to openness, to gratitude, and to delight. The interesting question for virtue ethics is whether the emotion of wonder might resemble the emotions of fear and anger in being one whose correct orientation amounts to a virtue. Being rightly disposed with respect to fear amounts to the virtue of courage. Being rightly disposed with respect to anger amounts to a virtue, nameless in Aristotle's time and to this very day. (Following Aristotle, in translation we call it 'patience', while recognizing that this, as he says, 'tends towards describing the deficiency' of not getting angry when one should.) Could being rightly disposed with respect to wonder—i.e. being disposed to feel wonder the right way, towards the right objects, for the right reasons, to the right degree, on the right occasions, in the right manner, and to act accordingly—count as a virtue, a character trait of the required complex sort? It may well be that it could.

There is, one might say, unrecognized by generations of philosophers and psycho-logists, a human emotion as familiar and everyday as fear and anger which is wonder, typically expressed (in English speakers) by the happy cry 'Oh isn't that wonderful!' (or nowadays, with unwitting appropriateness, 'awesome!') that children come up with spontaneously as soon as they have learnt to talk. (In fact it is not quite true that it has always been unrecognized. Descartes has it in the *Passions of the Soul*.) If

Hepburn is right, this emotion can be felt in accordance with, or contrary to, reason just as fear and anger can. Some objects, for instance nature and its works, are proper objects of it; some, such as the merely novel or unfamiliar, are not. And getting this natural human emotion in harmony with reason really matters morally, just as getting the emotions of fear and anger in harmony with reason do. If we think and feel, not that nature is wondrous but that Disneyland or the Royal Family of Windsors are, that the other animals are not, but we are, that the seas are not but swimming pools on the twentieth floor of luxury hotels are, and act accordingly, then we will act wrongly, just as we do when we fear pain to ourselves but not to others, or are angered by justified criticism and not getting our own way but not angered by cruelty to animals or injustice to our fellow humans.

The putative virtue of being disposed to feel the emotion of wonder the right way, towards the right objects, for the right reasons, to the right degree, and so on is, I think, explicitly concerned with our relations to nature (who has written about wonder without talking about the wonders of nature?) and the exploration of this putative virtue, in that explicit connection, would probably form an instructive and inspiring part of an environmental virtue ethic. But it is not uniquely so concerned. Hepburn, after all, discusses it in relation to works of art, and it would be odd for a philosopher to deny that the works of the Great Dead Philosophers are proper objects of wonder. So we might look further, for a putative virtue that takes our relations with nature as its unique concern and incorporates just that part of right wondering which is concerned with recognizing the wonders of nature. (Compare the way the personal virtue of justice incorporates that part of 'patience' which is concerned with being angered by injustice to others.)

ANOTHER NEW VIRTUE

The existing literature suggests the possibility of a further new virtue, one which, unlike the putative virtue of being disposed to feel the emotion of wonder in the right way and so on, has actually acquired something in the way of a name—namely the term 'respect for nature'. The term was originally brought into environmental ethics by Paul W. Taylor, who used it to signify what he calls an 'ultimate moral attitude' rather than a virtuous character trait. However there are at least three, related, problems with Taylor's account, all of which are side-stepped or dissolved if we recognize his 'respect for nature' as a character trait rather than simply as an attitude (even an 'ultimate moral attitude') which I want to spend a little time discussing.

Before I do, I must stress how admirable I think Taylor's introduction and discussion of 'respect for nature' are. I do take him, along with Aldo Leopold, Arne Naess, and Holmes Rolston III, as amongst the really ground breaking, towering, figures in environmental ethics. They, as far as I am concerned, are the people who came up with the real practical wisdom about the subject, so I regard the following points as relatively speaking, mere philosophers' quibbles.

The first problem concerns how it can come about that someone has 'respect for nature' in Taylor's sense.

Taylor begins with the (actually very old Aristotelian) idea that any living thing has a *telos*—a good of its own—and the related claim that, as such, any living thing can be benefited (by that which enables it to achieve its *telos*) or harmed (by that which interferes with its doing so). He then adds the claim that any living thing possesses 'inherent worth', as a member of 'Earth's Community of Life'. This latter claim, he says, is not the sort of statement that can be proved; rather, to regard or conceive of living things as having 'inherent worth' is to adopt the attitude of respect for nature. And he makes his commitment to a Kantian theoretical framework explicit by drawing a parallel between this ultimate moral attitude and that of the attitude of respect for persons as persons. To regard persons as having inherent worth or 'dignity' is, in Kantian ethics, he says, to adopt the attitude of respect for persons *as* persons.

Taylor's construal of Kant (which I think is probably wrong) on respect for persons as persons is instructive, for he says 'When this is adopted as an ultimate moral attitude *it involves the disposition to treat every person as having inherent worth or human dignity*' (1981: 207, my italics). Twenty years ago, such a claim might well have passed without question, but the more recent, fruitful, exchanges between Kantians and virtue ethicists prompt several very awkward ones. The disposition in question is clearly supposed to be much more than a tendency of intention. It is supposed to be an efficacious tendency—a tendency to succeed in treating people as having inherent worth or human dignity. But how does adopting the attitude of respect for persons bring in its train the practical wisdom that enables one to know how to treat a person as having human dignity when, for example, their cultural or social expectations are different from yours and unknown to you? How indeed does it bring in its train the ability to recognize a member of a despised race or religion or sex as a person at all? How does it bring the perceptual capacities and emotional sensibilities needed to appreciate what is called for in particular situations when there appears to be a forced choice between treating one person as having human dignity and another as not having it? How does it bring with it either strength of will or a systematic reorientation of the emotions such that you standardly treat people as having human dignity ungrudgingly and without resentment and moreover with the right light in your eye?

No one gets to have all that just by 'adopting an attitude'. These dispositions and capacities have to be inculcated, from childhood, in the moral training of character.

Taylor always speaks of 'taking up' or 'adopting' the attitude of respect for nature, as though this were something one could do more or less overnight, through a rational process. But as people familiar with his writings will know, adopting the attitude of respect for nature turns out to involve acquiring a set of dispositions and capacities similar to those that would have to be involved in having the efficacious disposition to treat people as having human dignity. What he describes, and explores, brilliantly, is being rightly oriented to nature, through and through, in action, emotion, perception, sensibility, and understanding. What is involved in 'adopting' this attitude would, according to what he says about it, manifestly have to be a complete transformation of character. Really coming to see oneself as sharing 'a common bond' with all living things would involve a radical change in one's emotions and perceptions, one's whole way of perceiving and responding to the world, of one's reasons for action and thereby actions. And that is the sort of change that cannot (for the most part) come about just through, say, reading a philosophical book and deciding to change; it cannot (for the most part) simply be 'adopted' or 'taken up'.

So he has a problem. Can having 'respect for nature', as he describes it, not come about at all, given that it cannot simply be adopted or taken up? The problem is solved if we construe it as a virtue. You can't just decide to have a virtue; virtuous character traits cannot be acquired theoretically by attending lectures or reading books or articles and just deciding to be that way. But they can be acquired through moral habituation or training, beginning in childhood and continued through self-improvement.

The second problem with Taylor's account is his reliance on the contentious notion of 'inherent worth' which, *if introduced in a foundational premise*, notoriously brings standard problems with it. Does it or does it not admit of degrees? Either answer lands one in difficulties, as the ethical literature based on the foundational premise that the other animals share inherent or intrinsic worth or value with human beings illustrates. It seems impossible to allow that it admits of degree without claiming that human beings (or at least all the human beings who are persons) have the highest degree and thereby what promised to be a radical reformation of our old understanding of ourselves in relation to the other animals loses most of its revisionary character. But to the modern city-dwelling philosopher—and her readers—the alternative seems hopelessly impractical. The Jains may command our admiration but we do not go into print saying that that is how we all should live.

From the perspective of virtue ethics, Taylor's introduction of the contentious notion of inherent worth is superfluous. 'Regarding a living thing as having inherent worth' amounts to nothing more (though nothing less) in his account than regarding facts about whether a proposed course of action will benefit or harm a living thing as providing non-instrumental reasons for or against it, and it is his rich and insightful identification of this range of reasons which is significant. For, once they are identified, we can readily see how they might be used to inculcate a character trait—the virtue of 'respect for nature', or, as I would prefer to call it (given the restrictive connotations of 'respect'), 'being rightly oriented to nature'.

This range of reasons not only might be, but in fact *are*, given to children by adults who are beginning to inculcate in them at least the beginnings of a virtuous character trait oriented to nature. The child pokes or hits or tears at the living thing, and the parents say 'Don't do that, you'll harm it.' Or the child swats or slashes at a living thing and the parents say 'Don't do that, you'll kill it.' Or the child is taught how to look after a plant or animal—'You have to do this, because it needs water', 'She wants to go for a walk, take her out.' Or the child condemns some living thing's way of going on as 'stupid' and the parents say 'No, it's not stupid, it's brilliant; what it's doing is this' and then explain how what the living thing is doing results in its achieving its *telos*. And as nature-loving (not yet 'nature-respecting') parents and teachers know, one of the best ways to enable children to get over their disgust and fear, whether instinctive or learned, of various living things is to tell or show the child how the thing in question works—how it achieves its *telos*—and/or how this sort of thing, living in its sort of way, contributes to the life-processes of other sorts of things, including us. Whereupon the children start saying (in effect), 'How wonderful!' rather than 'Yuck!'

Such training begins to shape a particular way of perceiving, acting in relation to, feeling and thinking about, the natural world. We could well say, speaking colloquially, that such training involves teaching a child to recognize the inherent or intrinsic worth or value of at least some living things. (Only some, as things are at the moment, which is why I stressed 'nature-loving' as opposed to 'nature-respecting'.) But there is a very important theoretical difference at issue here. On the one hand, we may start, as virtue ethics does, with the training of children in reasons for action and emotional responses and the colloquial redescription of such training as teaching the child to recognize the inherent or intrinsic worth or value of living things. On the other hand, we may start, as Taylor and many other 'biocentric' deontological ethicists do, with foundational premises ascribing such worth or value to them.

One might bring out the difference as follows. Suppose it is agreed ground that bringing up children to be, at least partly, rightly oriented to nature in fact involves training them through the range of reasons suggested above. (This contrasts with the implausible claim that the training involves no more than 'Don't do this, do do that, look at this, be interested in that, because it has inherent worth.') Then the stance of those who seek foundational premises is that the unity of this practice must be underpinned or guided by something unconsciously or dimly apprehended by the parents and latched on to by the children, namely, the inherent worth of the living things in question, the property that they all share. And, granted the existence of such a property, it is clearly part of the philosopher's task to give an account of it, by working out what the 'worth/value-making characteristic' is that everything with this property has in common. But the stance of those who, following Wittgenstein, regard the search for such foundational premises as a philosophical mistake is that the unity of the practice so far described (insofar as it has a unity) need not be underpinned or guided by anything, let alone by any one thing such as inherent worth somehow apprehended by the parents.

The third problem with Taylor's account is this—he limits his ascription of inherent worth to individual living things (though it seems that these include species' populations and ecosystems). Hence what he has, officially, identified is not so much 'respect for nature' as 'respect for living nature'. According to him, things have inherent worth only because, or insofar as, they are 'members of the Earth's Community of Life'. And he identifies the characteristic outlook of someone with 'respect for nature' as follows:

one sees one's membership in the Earth's Community of Life as providing a common bond with all the different species of animals and plants that have evolved over the ages. One becomes aware that, like all other living things on our planet, one's very existence depends on the fundamental soundness and integrity of the *biological* system of nature. When one looks at this domain of life in its totality, one sees it to be a complex and unified web of interdependent parts. (1986: 44, my italics)

Now what does seem a little odd about that, read strictly, is the insertion of 'biological' before the words 'system of nature'. Do the sun, the moon, and the seas, the minerals in the earth, the ozone layer, have no role to play in maintaining the 'domain of life in its totality'? Is it not nature, animate *and* inanimate, that, in its totality, is seen to be a unified web? True, not much of the inanimate depends on the animate for its existence but why stress interdependence as the all-important feature of unification? Drawing a hard and fast distinction between the animate and the inanimate seems particularly inappropriate in the context of environmental ethics. Some years ago, when the rising of the seas and the consequent higher sea levels at high tide were recognized to be having an unmistakable deleterious impact, I remember reading that someone had brightly suggested we could solve the problem by blowing up the moon. And every environmentalist was (surely rightly) horrified, notwithstanding the inanimate nature of the moon. (Of course I know that the absence of the tides would kill a lot of plants and animals whose survival depends on their occurrence. My point is that many people's horror was, in fact, quite independent of those consequences of the proposed act of extra-terrestrial vandalism.)

Taylor is landed with this problem because of his attempt to provide a foundational premise about inherent worth. Things have inherent worth, when they do, because they share a common feature—being a member of the Earth's Community of Life. This gives the account a philosophically satisfying unity, and one can see that much of this would be lost if one tried to formulate a second feature, common to just the right inanimate things, and claimed that they had inherent worth because of it, yielding a disjunctive premise about what grounded inherent worth. But if we think of being 'rightly oriented to nature', not as an attitude founded on an adult's rational recognition of such a one-sentence premise but as a character trait arising from a childhood training that gives us particular reasons for action (and omission) in particular contexts, and shapes our emotional response of wonder, the hard and fast line he draws between the animate and the inanimate becomes insignificant. (That is why I implied above that the unity of the practice thus far described, which was of inculcating the beginnings of being rightly oriented towards living nature, wasn't much of a unity.)

Environmentally minded parents teach their children not only not to harm and kill the living but also not to despoil or destroy natural inanimate objects. Although a theory-obsessed parent might go to the lengths of teaching a child not to slash at a spider's web just because this might harm the spider, few nature-loving parents find it necessary to do so. The spider's web, notwithstanding its being inanimate, is reconstructed as an object of wonder—so delicate and light but so strong, so intricately patterned—and not to be wantonly destroyed simply because it is such an object. It fits into a spider's achieving its *telos* in such and such a way, and that is also part of what is wondrous about it, but in teaching this to children, who would look around to check that the web-maker was still alive and dependent upon it?

Spiders' webs, like ammonites and other fossils, make it impossible to draw Taylor's hard distinction between the animate and the inanimate. An ammonite is something else that is not to be wantonly destroyed but wondered at—once again so intricately patterned, and also so awesomely old. And, despite being inanimate, it is part of (not the present, or near present, but) the long past domain of life. 'Look,' one says to the child, 'do you know what this is—and *was*?' And the child is thunderstruck. Nor do we find ourselves suddenly talking in distinctively new ways to our children when we come to the Grand Canyon, and similar rock formations. They are so intricately patterned, so old, and so huge, such proper objects of wonder, and have a connection with the domain of life insofar as the geological workings of our planet are inseparable from the workings of life on it, all being part of 'the system of nature', that 'unified web'.

As before, when we teach children not to slash mindlessly at spiders' webs, to look at fossils carefully and try to understand their shape, to be glad rather than sorry that the Grand Canyon is not rimmed with machines dispensing Coca-Cola, giving the reasons that we do, we could, colloquially, redescribe what we are doing as teaching them the inherent worth or intrinsic value of spiders' webs, fossils, and the Grand Canyon. But giving that colloquial redescription simply sidesteps the problem of advancing a foundational philosophical theory which has to start from some (indefinitely?) large set of premises to the effect that these things have such worth or value because or insofar as they are intricately patterned and/or delicate and light (or not delicate but incredibly hard and heavy) or fresh and new (or awesomely old) or tiny and yet still effective (the revelations of the microscope) or huge (the Grand Canyon again) or whatever.

The contrast here is between, on the one hand, trying to ground intrinsic/inherent value/worth/considerability in a few 'x-making characteristics' and, on the other, just starting with an indefinite range of reasons taught for responding, in the broadest sense, to nature, in certain ways. These include, at least, wondering at, looking hard at, finding out more about, rejoicing in, understanding why other people spend their whole lives studying, being anxious to preserve, not dismissing or ignoring or destroying or forgetting or assuming one can always put a price on ... everything in the natural world.

At the moment, as I think we all know, none of us, however committed to environmentalism, has achieved any more than getting a few of our responses to a few of the things in the natural world right. Possession of the virtue of being rightly oriented to nature quite generally is still a long way off. But the green belief does, after all, call for a radical change in us, something rather more radical, one would suppose, than a change in a few theoretical beliefs about intrinsic worth that few people but philosophers are conscious of holding anyhow.

WHAT TO DO?

'But' it might be objected, 'what is the point of thinking of environmental ethics in virtue ethics' terms when it will manifestly fail to tell us what we should do? For whether we talk about reconfiguring the old virtues or recognizing a new one, we don't seem to get any answers to our pressing problems. All we get are some fairly obvious prohibitions against wanton, gratuitous, selfish, materialistic, and short-sighted consumption, harm, destruction, and despoliation.'

True enough. But suppose we turn to any other environmental ethics for guidance about what is morally required of us in detail in the way of actions and changes in life style starting, say, tomorrow. What will we find? Apart from the same fairly obvious prohibitions I think it must be admitted that the answer is 'Not much'.

I am not denying that Taylor, for example, offers principles intended to enable us to adjudicate between the competing claims of human beings and other living things. But the only things such principles clearly yield are the obvious prohibitions that even the palest green environmentalist is already living in accordance with. Has any one of my readers recently bought ivory or a caged tropical bird or hunted a rare wild mammal? One might interpret some of Taylor's principles as, more forcefully, yielding a prohibition against driving a car in, at least, all those circumstances in which one will inevitably kill a number of insects but not save any other lives, but Taylor himself does not construe them as doing so, speaking instead merely of the requirement to use anti-pollution devices on automobile exhausts. And not driving around in a car without an anti-pollution device seems another pretty obvious prohibition.

So if all we find are obvious prohibitions, but no guidance for further detailed changes, the questions arise 'Why not? What's still missing? Is the normative theory incomplete or what?' I don't know whether any non-virtue ethicist has ever answered these questions, but virtue ethics has a straightforward and, I think, extremely plausible answer.

Virtue ethicists seek answers to questions about what we should do and how we should live by considering what someone who really possessed virtue to a high degree would characteristically do, and how they would live. And we have little idea of the answers to such questions in the context of environmental ethics because we have so few exemplars of the relevant virtues, real or fictional, if any.

Suppose that being rightly oriented to nature is pre-eminently, the relevant virtue. (I think, at this stage, that little hangs on the distinction between reconfiguring the old virtues and recognizing this new one. Acquisition of the new would go along with reconfiguring the old, and anyone who had adequately reconfigured the old could be truly described as having acquired the new.) This virtue is not a character trait we see manifested by any academic philosophers who, inevitably, lead lives of standard Western, materialistic comfort, driving to shop at their supermarkets, buying new clothes, listening to opera on their CD players, dining in restaurants, writing their books and articles on computers, jetting to international conferences to present their views on environmental ethics, and teaching them to their students in large, land-occupying, buildings. (This does not mean that environmental philosophers are hypocritical, just that our sincerely held ethical beliefs still leave us far short of possessing virtue, in particular perhaps, the practical wisdom, permeating every virtue, that enables its possessor to know what to do in particular circumstances.)

It is possible, though this is contested, that we have glimpses of what it might *have* been like to live in accordance with the virtue of being rightly oriented to nature in the little we know of the lives of the Australian Aborigines and the Amerindians before European hegemony. But even if we knew a lot more about their lives and even if it were certain that they had possessed the virtue, this would not entail that that is how we should strive to live and be now. Human beings are, essentially, socially and historically situated beings and their virtuous character traits have to be situated likewise. A twenty-first-century city-dweller who possessed the virtue to some degree could hardly manifest it in just the same ways as Australian Aborigines and Amerindians perhaps used to when they lived as hunter-gatherers. What we need to know is what would count as living in accordance with it *now* or in the near future.

One pessimistic possibility is that nothing would count, and that perhaps nothing ever will, because we have already made such a mess of things that there is no virtuous way of sorting them out by human means. In virtue ethics, the (putative) virtue of 'being rightly oriented to nature' is but one virtue amongst many; what one can, morally, do in its name is restrained by other virtues such as justice. Although any environmentalist may well believe that growth is not what we want, justice, if nothing else, restrains what any of us might do to prevent growth while there are still so many people in poorer countries who disagree, because their—and their children's—lives depend on economic growth.

This seems the right juncture to return, as promised, to the question whether virtue ethics is committed to the claim that *eudaimonia* or human well-being is the 'top value', ranked above any other in an improperly human chauvinistic way. The answer is that it is not. If anything counts as the 'top value' in virtue ethics, it is acting virtuously, and the pessimistic possibility envisaged above is not that our choice lies between human well-being and (as it were) the 'well-being' of the natural world, but that our past and present folly has put human well-being beyond our grasp, perhaps forever.

Virtue is an ideal of human excellence, constitutive of *eudaimonia* or living well as a human being. But *eudaimonia* was never something that we could be confident was within our individual grasp. Right back in Aristotle, there is the recognition that it requires 'a complete life' (1101a15) but that there are things one must sooner die than do (1110a27–8) and that it is nonsense to call someone *eudaimon*, however virtuous, if they are being broken on the wheel or surrounded by great disasters (1153b19–20). If I am living under the sway of evil tyrants, then *eudaimonia* may not be possible for me if, for example, they force on me the choice between action contrary to virtue and death by torture.[4]

Limited as this example is, it should suffice to remind us that whatever blocks virtuous activity blocks *eudaimonia*. It might be a few tyrants. It might be the nature of the society into which one was born, unwittingly, as a member of the privileged class whose past horrendous injustice is only just beginning to be righted. Perhaps I can live in accordance with the virtue of justice in such a society, in the vanguard with those bringing about the needed changes at considerable personal self-denial. But perhaps, given my family commitments or some disability which, in my society renders me helplessly dependent on others, I cannot; if I am to live at all, I am forced to live the life of the highly privileged dependent. And then *eudaimonia* is beyond my grasp, for willy-nilly, I shall, perforce, reap the rewards of injustice. Or it might be the nature of the world into which I was born, a world whose societies have become so predicated on despoiling nature that their very existence depends on continuing to do so.

---

[4] Cf. Philippa Foot on the 'Letter-Writers' who died because they refused to go along with the Nazis. She says of them that they were so placed that it was impossible for them to pursue happiness 'by just and honourable means. . . . Happiness in life, they might have said, was not something possible for them.' See Foot (2001).

Perhaps I can live in accordance with the virtue of being rightly oriented to nature to some extent if I leave society. But then I will have cut myself off from the exercise of most of the other virtues. So *eudaimonia* is beyond my grasp.

Virtue ethics is 'about' human beings living well, but it is not committed, in advance, to our living well being a realizable state of affairs regardless of how we, or many of us, are living or have lived up until now. It is possible that we have already made such a mess that we shall not be able to live well, as part of the natural world, for many generations to come, if ever.

More optimistically, the very next generation may start to show us the way. Concern about the environment, and proto-versions of the virtue of being rightly oriented to nature, are currently much more widespread amongst children than they are amongst adults. Many of them have received more training in it than any of us did, and are beginning to have their own ideas about how they and we should live. At the time I began working on this chapter, in 1999, it was reported that 135,000 German schoolchildren had decided to help reduce their communities' emissions of greenhouse gases by 10 per cent, and within seven months had more than reached their target—something that (I believe) no government has achieved in a comparable time. It may be that they will choose to live in ways rather different from our ways, and that their children will choose to live in very different ones. If the deeper green versions of the green belief are true, it is a radical change in human beings' ways of living in the natural world that is called for. If the virtue ethics approach is right, it is hardly surprising that we, currently lacking the relevant virtues, should be unable to imagine, in any concrete detail, how we should live, and we should expect change to come about not primarily through philosophical argument, and not overnight, but through the actions and practical reasoning of people in whom the relevant virtues have been inculcated. Our current task is, thereby, to do what we can to develop those virtues in ourselves and our children, and to adhere to the 'obvious prohibitions' in the hope that we may bequeath to them a world that is not irrevocably spoiled.

COPYRIGHT ACKNOWLEDGEMENT

A shorter version of this essay appeared as Rosalind Hursthouse, 'Virtues', in 'Institutional Issues Involving Ethics and Justice', from *Encyclopedia of Life Support Systems (EOLSS)*, Developed under the Auspices of the UNESCO, EOLSS Publishers, Oxford, UK.

REFERENCES

Aristotle (2000). *Nicomachean Ethics*, trans. R. Crisp. Cambridge: Cambridge University Press.

Clark, S. R. L. (1977). *The Moral Status of Animals*. Oxford: Clarendon Press.

Foot, Philippa (2001). *Natural Goodness*. Oxford: Clarendon Press, 95.

Hepburn, R. W. (1984). *'Wonder' and Other Essays*. Edinburgh: Edinburgh University Press.

Hill Jr, T. E. (1983). 'Ideals of human excellence and preserving natural environments'. *Environmental Ethics*, 5: 211–24.

Leopold, A. (1949) *A Sand County Almanac*. Reissued, Oxford: Oxford University Press, 2001.

Naess, A. (1989). *Economy, Community and Lifestyle*. Cambridge; Cambridge University Press.

Passmore, J. (1974). *Man's Responsibility for Nature*. London: Duckworth.

Rolston III, H. (1988). *Environmental Ethics*. Philadelphia: Temple University Press.

Sorabji, Richard (1993). *Animal Minds and Human Morals*. New York: Cornell University Press.

Taylor, P. W. (1981). 'The Ethics of Respect for Nature'. *Environmental Ethics*, 1: 197–218.

_____ (1986). *Respect for Nature*. Princeton: Princeton University Press.

Wensveen, Louke van (2000). *Dirty Virtues*. Amherst, NY: Humanity Books.

8

The Good Life for Non-Human Animals: What Virtue Requires of Humans

Rebecca L. Walker

The more clearly we see the differences between animals and stones or machines or plastic dolls, the less likely it seems that we ought to treat them in the same way.

Mary Midgley, *Animals and Why they Matter*, p. 14

INTRODUCTION

Most of us have seen giant polar bears lying in the sun behind the high fence of a mid- to large-sized enclosure in a zoo. This zoo could be in nearly any big city in the world. The enclosure has cement floors and a pool for swimming. Or maybe we have seen great apes behind the glass of a viewing cage. In the cage are a few trees and some play equipment. The apes engage one another or look out silently from behind the glass or may even gesture at us as we look in at them. While children are simply fascinated by the sight of these animals, for adults these sights are sometimes troubling. Perhaps we even have mixed feelings about our unease. We are delighted like the children about having the opportunity to see these great creatures without the necessity of traveling to their habitats and pleased moreover about the children learning to appreciate them by getting a chance to see them in 'real life'. Yet there is also something unsettling about the experience. And, to this same extent, there is the additional worry that the children's appreciation of these creatures will be misguided by the experience.[1]

Perhaps the only language that we are able to use to express our unease is, 'It is against the ape (or polar bear's) right to be so confined!' But what if we aren't sure that apes and polar bears have rights like this? Perhaps then we will resort to a claim like, 'Look, it is clear that the animal must be suffering.' But what if we become convinced by the animals' caretaker that the animals are content, fed better there than they would be in the wild and moreover, less likely to suffer from injury or sickness? Are we to go away quietly having all our fears answered? Not necessarily. That is because there is room for a quite different kind of concern.

---

[1] For an argument against zoos that makes a similar point but not specifically about children, see Dale Jamieson's (1994) 'Against Zoos'.

What do we care about when we care about protecting the interests of non-human animals? A significant part of what we care about is whether or not the animals are living lives that are good ones for their kind. It is this kind of concern, I think, that leaves us disturbed by the situation of the polar bear and the great ape. Moreover, it is this same kind of concern that explains why we are less bothered when the zoo is able to replicate the habitat, range, social interactions, and other factors relevant for flourishing for the particular type of animal.[2] The problem is that the usual ways of thinking about the interests of non-human animals cannot fully take account of the concern about species- or kind-specific good lives. These views focus on rights or on suffering, but not primarily on the nature of the good life for particular types of animals.

This chapter is concerned with the good lives of animals, yet it does not argue specifically that we ought to be concerned with animal flourishing *as opposed to* rights or freedom from pain. Rather, it simply offers a theoretical framework for engaging concern about animal flourishing or good lives.[3] In order to offer such a framework, it will be necessary to focus on what makes animal lives good ones as well as why we should care about the good lives of animals. Both issues will be addressed through the lens of a eudaimonistic virtue ethical perspective. By a 'eudaimonistic' virtue ethics I mean generally an approach to ethics that understands the virtues as necessarily tied up with flourishing.[4] This chapter thus develops a specific interpretation of this general type of virtue ethics that accounts for the role of non-human animal flourishing in answering the question how we ought to treat them.[5]

Generally speaking, then, how might we think about our treatment of non-human animals from a eudaimonistic virtue ethical perspective? Initially, the solution seems simple. We ought to treat animals well in so far as doing so is part of *human* flourishing. The explanation goes as follows: if treating animals well is virtuous, and acting virtuously is a necessary condition of human flourishing, then treating animals well is part of human flourishing. Thus it is true on a virtue ethics view that treating animals well is part of human flourishing as long as treating animals well *is* virtuous. Only so far we have made no headway in explaining why treating animals well is virtuous. Solving this piece of the puzzle will thus be a specific focus of this chapter. Moreover, I shall tackle this issue in a way that places emphasis on the flourishing of the non-human animals themselves. As stated above, the answer to the question how we should treat animals emphasizes only a consideration of *our* flourishing. While my

---

[2] For some types of animals an acceptable situation might be a wild animal park where the viewers must enter the animals' own habitat without unduly interfering with it. For other types of animals, zoos with restrictive environments that are nevertheless consistent with flourishing for the kind of animal 'on display' may also be less troubling.

[3] I shall use the terms 'flourishing' and 'good' life interchangeably in both the human and non-human animal case.

[4] Examples include Stoic and Aristotelian accounts. In the modern context, Rosalind Hursthouse's view in *On Virtue Ethics* (1999) offers an excellent example. Non-eudaimonistic virtue ethical views include those offered by Christine Swanton (2003) and Michael Slote (2001).

[5] As discussed in the introduction to this volume, virtue based approaches to ethics may only share a loose family resemblance. Different views of how the virtues are related to flourishing and of the nature of flourishing lead to different versions of eudaimonism. By offering interpretations of each of these factors, in this chapter I support a particular version of eudaimonism.

account will also *begin with* a consideration of human flourishing, it will incorporate, as central, a consideration of animal flourishing.

The structure of the chapter is as follows. First I outline the kind of virtue ethics that I am concerned with. Next I consider whether eudaimonism so understood gives any straightforward recommendation regarding our treatment of animals. Seeing that it does not, I develop an argument for why we ought to care about and act to protect animal flourishing. In so doing I ask why it is that we ought to care about the flourishing of others. Then I investigate whether non-human animals share with us a type of flourishing that we ought to care about for the reasons established.

GROUNDING VIRTUE

A number of contemporary virtue ethical views seem not to depend on any foundation other than the virtues themselves. As with similarly structured rights views, the problem with this approach is that there is no support for the claims made regarding the virtues and vices other than internal consistency and other constitutive features of a good theory—assuming that the view is a *theory*. Given a list of virtues that includes humility while pride is a vice as arguably is found in some Christian views of virtue, and an alternative list of virtues including (proper) pride while (undue) humility is a vice as with Aristotle's view, there is no further principled appeal that can be made for the rightness of one set of virtues over the other. Assuming we don't think that the answer to the question whether pride is a vice is merely culturally relative, this state of affairs is unsatisfactory.

In a sense, of course, all talk about ethics must end (or start) with some fundamental claims. One could say that an attempt to defend which virtues get included in one's view just signals the end of the argument. However, unlike other places where arguments run out, one feels that there must be a reason why something is a virtue. Competing claims about particular virtues are quite different from a claim, for example, that the good is desirable. In that case it may be difficult to say what would even constitute an answer to the question why this is so.

In virtue ethics, the traditional reason for counting something as a virtue has to do with the relationship between this character trait and a flourishing or *eudaimon* human life. I shall take this starting point as basic to my view as well, with the caveat that such a foundational notion of human flourishing may be pluralistic in nature. In this chapter I shall assume for the sake of the argument that some good enough defense of flourishing as our final end is available. Moreover, I shall assume that this defense can give a reasonable account of how it is that the natural can be normative in a sense strong enough to ground the idea of species- or kind-specific flourishing. These issues are in fact highly contested and no clear answer has been given to how we should justify these views at a foundational level.[6]

---

[6] David Copp and David Sobel (2004: 534–8) offer a critique of Hursthouse's (1999) view partly on the grounds that it fails to justify such a foundational story. On my understanding, however, Hursthouse's project is not one of foundational justification. Yet, I do think that such justification needs to be given.

ARISTOTELIAN EUDAIMONISM

Given, then, that flourishing is our final normative end, how specifically should we understand the relationship between the virtues and that end? The view endorsed in this chapter is roughly Aristotelian in so far as our final end of *eudaimonia* is 'mixed'. It is not, as with a Stoic account, reachable with virtue alone, but also requires the satisfaction of other elements.[7] A more detailed account of these other elements and how they relate to virtue on my view is addressed a bit later. To create a backdrop for this discussion, we must first look at Aristotle's account of the relationship between the virtues and the good life.

According to Book One of the *Nicomachean Ethics*, the good life is the complete and self-sufficient end of our actions (1097b5–20). Human virtue as excellence in activity expressing reason is constitutive of the flourishing life since human good activity just is the expression of excellence or virtue (*NE* 1098a15). To put this in terms of our function, virtue as a whole is excellence in the fulfillment of our function, which is activity expressive of reason. The various virtues are individual excellences which, taken together, constitute living well. So in this way, the individual virtues are just particular aspects or activities involved in a flourishing life. The virtues are also instrumental in achieving the good life in the sense that they benefit their possessor. For example, the actions expressing virtue are pleasant to the good person (*NE* 1099a10–15).

However, other external supports will also have to be in place in order to achieve flourishing. For example, not being born into devastating poverty such that the basic necessities of life are hard to come by. On Aristotle's view, without these additional external supports, we shall not be able to become virtuous at all. Alternatively, if we are virtuous and suffer devastating and irredeemable loss of external goods, for example, loss of all of our close friends and family along with financial devastation, we shall also not be counted in the end as having had—all things considered—a good life (*NE* 1099b5–1100a5).

So how should we understand the logical structure of this relationship between external goods, virtue, and flourishing? We might think that a basic set of external goods is necessary for both the development and maintenance of virtue itself. If this is true then an otherwise virtuous person who suffers a devastating loss of external goods will actually suffer a blow to his or her virtue. Yet it seems implausible that a loss of the kind we are imagining would itself interfere with *virtue* rather than only with flourishing. This could be true even if we agree that the lack of certain fundamental goods may be inconsistent with the initial development of virtue. So a loss of external goods does not necessarily undermine established virtue, but rather only flourishing. Moreover, as Aristotle discusses, we praise virtue as an achievement, but to the extent that flourishing has elements that are totally beyond our control, it is a

---

[7] For an excellent discussion of the various problems with Aristotle's view of the mixed nature of our final end as well as of the disagreement between the Stoic view and the Aristotelian view, see Julia Annas's *The Morality of Happiness* (1993: chapters 18–19).

kind of 'blessedness' (*NE* 1101b10–1102a).[8] Since the loss of external goods is also not necessarily in our control, it would make sense that this loss may only interfere with flourishing.

We have opened up a conceptual space between virtue and flourishing such that we could plausibly be said to be virtuous without flourishing (although not flourishing without being virtuous). And if this is true, then being virtuous is a necessary but not sufficient condition of our final end of flourishing. Moreover, it seems right to say that our concept of flourishing is not merely one of activity expressing reason (or virtue), but that other elements are also properly considered central to flourishing. These elements are also not merely the external goods at issue above. As will be seen, although non-human animals do not partake of activity expressive of reason in the sense required for moral and intellectual virtue, they may partake of some elements properly fitted to our concept of flourishing.

EUDAIMONISM AND ANIMALS: IS THERE A STRAIGHTFORWARD SOLUTION?

Once we recognize the centrality of flourishing to a eudaimonistic virtue ethics, we might assume that such a view must also attend to the flourishing of non-human animals. We might think that this is especially true given the gap we have noted between virtue and flourishing. After all, although animals are not virtuous or vicious in the ways that we are, animals do flourish or fail to flourish. The notion of an animal's having a 'good life' is not deeply mysterious. Further, if good lives are what we aim at with virtue, then why would it matter whether these lives are human or non-human animal lives?

If we could jump easily in this way from the significance of flourishing for *us* to an obligation to attend to animal flourishing, working out a virtue ethical approach to our treatment of animals would be mostly a matter of working out details about which kinds of lives are good ones for which types of animals and which kinds of interactions with those animals are virtuous. We might wonder, for example, whether virtue requires that we further, protect, or simply not interfere with animal flourishing in given specific cases. Should we actively work to add members to endangered species with procreative assistance or should we simply stop encroaching on the habitats of such species? We might also wonder which types of character traits are properly brought to bear with respect to which kinds of human–non-human animal relationships and interactions. For example, can we properly feel friendship towards animals or only care? In short, how do we act and feel 'at the right times, about the right things, towards the right [animals], for the right end, and in the right way?' (*NE* 1106b20).

These types of concerns are central to any worked out virtue ethical view of how we ought to treat animals. Yet they are not central concerns for this chapter because a

---

[8] According to Annas (1993: 44), '*eudaimon*' (she translates as 'happy') and '*makarios*' (blessed) are interchangeable terms for Aristotle.

consideration of the good lives of non-human animals by itself does not straightfor-
wardly tell us *why it is* that virtue requires that we care about and attend to the good
lives of animals. Thus we must focus on answering this question before we could hope
to offer a rich practical view of how we ought to treat animals.

So what must be resolved in order to know why it is that a virtuous person must
care about and attend to animal good lives? One obvious issue is what kind of 'good
life' we ought to value. Within a traditional eudaimonistic virtue ethics the focus is on
the capacity for reason. It is the proper exercise of this capacity that constitutes living
well. As long as no one is arguing that non-human animals are themselves capable
of the relevant kinds of intelligence, the sense in which their lives are 'flourishing'
or 'not flourishing' is one that may seem far removed from the application of this
concept to our lives. A similar idea is expressed by Aristotle when, after describing
eudaimonia as consisting in 'activity of the soul expressing virtue' (*NE* 1100a25) he
concludes, 'It is not surprising, then, that we regard neither ox nor horse nor any other
kind of animal . . . [*eudaimon*], since none of them can share in this sort of activity'
(*NE* 1100a). It would seem, then, that in order to establish that we should care about
non-human animal flourishing we must first establish that there is a relevant notion
of flourishing at issue.

In order to see whether this is the case, we need to look more closely at why it is
that we ought to care about the flourishing of other human beings. Once we have the
answer to that question, we shall be able to see whether these same kinds of reasons
apply to the flourishing of non-human animals. We shall do so by considering what
kinds of flourishing animals aim at and by investigating the relationship of these types
of flourishing to that of human beings. Since, on my view, a resolution to this set of
issues formulates a necessary backdrop to a more detailed virtue based picture of how
we ought to treat animals, I shall have only limited points to make about particular
implications. That is, I shall have little to say about those issues that are the primary
topics for the virtue ethicist who starts with the assumption that virtue requires that
we attend to animal flourishing.

CARING FOR OTHERS

So far we have said of human flourishing that this is both what we aim at with virtue and that it is also constituted, at least in part, by virtue. In this sense, flourishing
grounds our ethical aims in life by giving us an end for which there is no further
justification and that alone—as self-sufficient and complete—is our ultimate end as
human beings. But it is quite clear that we cannot act virtuously if we do so merely
for the sake of achieving our own flourishing. Actions are only successfully virtuous if
done for their own sake (see, e.g., *NE* 1105a30). So we are left with a familiar question. Since I cannot act virtuously if I do so only *for the sake of* gaining some good
for myself (my own flourishing, in this case) what is it that gives me reason to act,
through being virtuous, in a way that *in fact* furthers my own flourishing? Further,
and this is the significant question for our concern, what gives me reason to act in a
way that aims at the flourishing of others?

The obvious response is to point out that flourishing is not something that we gain instrumentally by our virtue, rather it is *constituted*, at least in part, by virtuous activity. Virtuous activity, for its part, must be done from the motive proper to the virtue and not egoistic reference to one's own good life. Further, part of what it is to have some virtues is that we do aim at the good of others. Yet, correct as this response may be, it doesn't so much answer the question as simply restate the problem. We are still left with our primary worry, namely, why is it that I *should* care about and act to support the good lives of others whether the lives at issue are human or non-human animal?

The practical answer to the question, 'why care about others' flourishing?' is that we ought to because that is just what we learn to do when learning to be virtuous. And, at an even more basic level, caring about others simply goes hand in hand with our nature as social beings, whether we manage to be virtuous (to care properly for the right others in the right way at the right times) or not. From this practical point of view, asking for a further explanation of *why* it is that I should care about the good lives of others is absurd. In this practical sense as well, the story of why the flourishing of others should be normative for us, is a story that can be told with the same subtle detail for our interactions with non-human animals and the environment generally.

Yet it might well be pointed out that our answer so far only indicates *how* it is that we end up caring about and acting to further others' flourishing, not yet why it is that we have reason to do so. Ancient eudaimonistic virtue ethicists were not so worried about this question as such. Rather they simply incorporated concern for other (humans at least) into their theories as an obvious element of virtue.[9] Yet in the modern context it is hard to take concern about others as simply a given. I wouldn't for example want to claim that we have reason to care about others just because we've been taught to do so as part of our character training or conversely that we would not have reason to do so had we not been so taught.

Still, a consideration of how it is that we come to care about others does some significant work. It makes vivid the necessity of distinguishing between the question why we should care about others at all and why we should care about those that are not the natural objects of our affection. The question why we should care about *any* others is not our question. That is a question about why we should be moral beings at all. Our question has to do with what sort of care and for what types of others is consistent with virtue. To answer this question we must know why it is that we should (if we should) cultivate care about the good lives of others who are not necessarily the natural objects of our affection. This is an especially important question for both those animals and faraway humans with whom we may have no natural affinity.

So how might we approach the question why we should care about the good lives of others from this narrower perspective? We might simply state that we ought to care about all others (human or non-human animal) for their own sakes because they are ends in themselves. This seems correct in general but does not give an explanation for why they are ends in themselves or of what sort of ends. We won't, for example,

---

[9] For a rich discussion of this topic see Annas (1993), chapters 10–13.

want an explanation according to which all beings cared about for their own sake have absolute value. So then what shall we say? To begin, we need an explanation for the human case. Then we can see whether this explanation also provides reasons to care about animal flourishing. We need to know why the good life, as the in fact ultimate human end or telos, is something that we, as virtuous, must love for its own sake not only for ourselves, and those other humans for whom we have natural affection, but also for all who aim at the same end.

Since, according to any eudaimonistic virtue ethics, a good life is our proper end, when we recognize it as such in our own case we do so rightly. Moreover, duly to appreciate this end, we must love it because of the kind of good it is, and not simply because it is our *own* good end. This does not mean that we love it simply *by itself* since it is valuable (and intelligible) only as manifested as an end of particular humans. But it is also true that a good life is the proper end of every other (at least) human *person* as well (leaving aside the issue of which humans are persons). If we recognize the good life as our end, but fail to recognize that it is also the end of others, we also fail to appreciate what kind of good it really is. In other words, we fail properly to appreciate what it is for us to flourish if we fail to recognize the way in which a good life is also the end of others. So fully to recognize good lives as good in the way in which they are good is to recognize them as good for each one of us. But then to pursue it only in our own case (and in the case of those we naturally care about), but not in the case of others, also seems to fail to take seriously just what kind of end this is. How much so and in what ways virtue requires us to contribute to the good of others (as opposed to simply not interfering) I leave for some other discussion.

It is important that the claim is not that we should care about other humans *because they are like* us. Rather, they have a feature in common with us, which is that they also aim at their own flourishing. It is this feature that we ought to care about, but as a feature that cannot be valued independently of valuing those whose good lives are at issue. The good life is then a shared end in so far as it is a good for humans as such (and thus has certain generally shared elements as will be discussed below), but it is also a good for each individual in so far as good lives can be coherently manifested only by particular individuals.

This view may start to sound strangely familiar, yet not in a way comfortable to virtue ethics. It will be good, therefore, to differentiate it from two views in the neighborhood. In particular, I make no claim here as a utilitarian might that we must maximize the good aimed at or that we must count the good of each equally. Further, unlike on the Kantian view, on the view offered here, there is no rational necessitation in the claim that we ought to care about the flourishing of others. That the good of others *is* normative for us if we happen to latch on to virtue properly does not imply that it is rationally required of us to find that good normative.

But even if all this is true, why does it give us reason to support the good lives not only of other humans, but also of non-human animals? After all, non-human animal lives are not good in the *same way* that human lives are good. At least not in so far as they are made good by the exercise of the virtues. An answer to this question begins with the ways in which human good lives are, after all, not so different from non-human animal good lives. To expand, we should start by going back to Aristotle and his explanation for why activity expressive of reason should count as the characteristic human function.

THE CHARACTERISTIC HUMAN FUNCTION?

Aristotle seeks our characteristic human function in order to determine which function, if fulfilled with excellence, is constitutive of a flourishing human life. He considers, and discards, the possible answers: living itself (as nutrition and growth) and sense-perception. The fundamental reason why these functions are not to be counted as the characteristic human function seems to be that we share them with, in the first case, plants, and in the second case all sentient animals (*NE* 1098a). Instead, the proper characteristic function for humans must be activity of the soul expressive of reason, for this is the sole function that is unique to humans (*NE* 1098a5–15). Excellence in this function, then, must define our end.

However, being a unique function is not required in order to be a characteristic function. How odd it would be to discover that intelligent aliens exist, or that dolphins, chimps, or elephants do in fact share the capacity for reason of the sort required for virtuous activity and thereby claim that reason is not, after all, the characteristic human function. Sharing the other functions with plants and/or other animals, does not itself imply that the excellence of these functions is not our particular end as well. Nor is it true that sharing the function of practical reason with other kinds of beings would diminish its role for us unless we are strangely constituted indeed.

Moreover, there is no good reason why our function should be monistic in nature. It is more plausible that our characteristic function should be a combination of all those functions that are characteristic of us as a kind or species. These functions could be described in the manner Aristotle outlines or perhaps with a modern assay more akin to functional capacities. In so far as a flourishing human life is constituted by the excellence of characteristic functioning, then, it would be constituted by excellences in our many different types of functioning, however understood.

A WIDER SCOPE FOR HUMAN GOOD LIVES

If we understand the human function as activity of the soul expressive of reason, then the good life is one in which excellence in this function is achieved. If we do not limit the human function out of hand to that function unique to humans, then how should we view the good human life? To get a thorough answer to this question, we would need to know what role reason plays in flourishing and what role other functions play. In addition, we would need to look in detail at the other factors that contribute to human flourishing including the external factors that Aristotle mentions. For our purposes a thorough understanding of human flourishing is not necessary; we need merely to get enough of a picture of human flourishing to see where it overlaps with animal flourishing. To do this, we should review briefly both some aspects of the role of reason in human flourishing and virtue as well as some other aspects of human flourishing.

To begin with the connection between reason and virtue, it is possible that the proper exercise of reason, although necessary, is not a sufficient condition of virtuous action. When one's health is failing or one is consumed by pain it can be very difficult, if not impossible, to behave virtuously and certainly difficult to develop virtue initially under such circumstances. Indeed, the fact that we admire very much those who manage to be virtuous despite gross physical difficulties implies that these deficiencies in general good human functioning compete in at least some cases with the goals of reason. Having a healthy body and generally high spirits will help greatly with both the development and maintenance of virtue, and thus with achieving flourishing, and lacking these things in the extreme may make virtue difficult if not impossible to achieve.

Yet, even if it is not true that the development and/or maintenance of *virtue* depends on capacities other than properly functioning reason, surely flourishing is so dependent. It is quite unlikely that flourishing depends only on reason and its excellent functioning in virtue and not also on other additional functions and, as already discussed in the section on Aristotelian eudaimonism, on at least some basic external goods. As mentioned at the end of the last section, 'functions' may be understood in different ways appropriate to this context. What is important is that they include characteristic human capacities and activities significant for human flourishing such as the ability to communicate with others, to have sympathy for others, to feel empathy for others, to engage in physical exercise, to engage in 'nesting' activities such as homemaking, to sleep restfully, and so on.

This does not mean all of a person's capacities must function fully (or at all) in order to have a good life. Humans are amazingly adaptive creatures and can lean heavily on the capacities they do have in filling in for whatever capacities they may lose or lack. Indeed, it can happen that loss of some particular capacity may make a human life better overall if this loss leads a person to flourish in a previously neglected, but perhaps more significant, life aspect. For example, if a person highly obsessed with physical activity finds his physical abilities limited by an impairment, he may instead put more of his energy into enriching personal relationships that end up contributing more to his overall flourishing. Similarly, in the case of external goods, it is clear that many deprivations can be borne and can in some circumstances promote rather than undermine flourishing. Further, apparent external goods may in fact undermine flourishing. For example, newly found wealth may lead some families to distance themselves from less wealthy relatives and friends whom they wrongly fear will want to get at their money.

Despite all this, it is clear that our notion of flourishing is one that carries with it an assumption of both a certain level of basic external goods and basic levels of human capacities and activities (or functions). With respect to external goods, for example, human beings without enough food to maintain sustained focus on activities other than food procurement, and without decent shelter suffer, thereby a blow to their potential to flourish. Similarly, in terms of capacities and activities, human beings without the capacity for interpersonal relationships are thereby incapable of activities central to human flourishing. Of course, there is a distinction to be drawn between those things that contribute to and those things that constitute our flourishing. I leave aside the question exactly which elements are actually constitutive of flourishing, and additionally leave aside the question which constitutive elements may be properly reduced to the function of reason. What is important is only that what constitutes flourishing is broader than activity expressing reason alone and also includes elements (functions and the obtaining of some external goods) that are shared with animals, as will be discussed in the next section.

The response to the expanded view of human flourishing that I support here might be that these so-called additional elements of human flourishing are actually only background conditions of virtue. That is, they are elements of flourishing only by way of being conditions of virtue itself and so not properly separate aspects of flourishing. This leaves logical room for virtue as both necessary and sufficient for flourishing. However, it is less plausible that those additional elements (external goods or functions other than practical reason) are required for either the development or maintenance of virtue than it is that they are required for flourishing. In the section on Aristotelian eudaimonism we made the point that external goods seemed not to be required for the maintenance of virtue although they might plausibly be required for the development of virtue. In the current section it seemed at least plausible that physical health should contribute to the maintenance of virtue, although it might not be required. Yet in both these cases it is clear that the relationship between these elements and virtue is less straightforward than the relationship to flourishing which obviously requires both (some basic physical health and external goods).

To make the point a different way, we have conceptual reasons to differentiate between the requirements for virtue and those for flourishing. Even if external goods and functions other than practical reason are required for both the development and maintenance of virtue, they still do not seem to be conceptually part of virtue. Alternatively, elements other than the excellent functioning of practical reason are clearly part of our concept of human flourishing. Finally, as also mentioned earlier, the view that I support allows us to escape from the worry that virtue and flourishing are too tightly explanatorily related.

INCORPORATING ANIMAL GOOD LIVES

If we accept the general view I have outlined regarding human flourishing, where does it get us in answering the question how we ought to treat animals? In so far as animals flourish in ways that partake of elements of our own normative end in *eudaimonia*, we have the same kinds of reasons for caring about and acting in accordance with their flourishing as we do with respect to the flourishing of other humans. But do animals flourish in ways that partake of the elements proper to human flourishing? We should begin with the obvious. As already noted, animals do not themselves have or lack moral or intellectual virtues of the sort that Aristotle describes for humans. Certainly some animals are 'smarter' than others and some exhibit extraordinarily complex social interactions, but even sophisticated animals do not exhibit the forms of virtue and vice at issue. To say otherwise, strikes me as putting our theoretical eggs in the wrong basket. It is also true then, that in so far as human good lives are constituted by moral and intellectual virtue *alone*, animal flourishing is not in the same general category. As already argued, however, one shouldn't think that is the proper picture of human flourishing.

While animals may not flourish in the sense required for the exemplification of moral and intellectual virtue, we can make good sense of an animal's having a life that is a good one for its kind. The fact that animals can't *tell* us which kind of life they prefer does not hinder our ability to perceive which type is good. The good life for an animal will depend on its characteristics and the environment to which it is best suited, but flourishing for it will be of a type that is both good for it as an individual and as a normal member of a particular kind.[10] To return to our zoo example, animals normally ranging over wide tracts of land may not be suited to life in a zoo, but this may not be true of animals normally occupying a narrowly circumscribed habitat. Animals having a keen consciousness of, and negative reaction to, being monitored or watched also should not be held in captivity. As Rosalind Hursthouse points out, 'There are few things more sad than the notice that used to appear on the cages of certain animals in zoos, "Does not breed in captivity" ' (1999: 200). When such a basic biological function is eroded this serves as a strong warning that the possibility of flourishing for this type of animal is deeply undercut in captivity. This is consistent with the claim that, for any individual animal, it may turn out that it is better off not breeding (because, e.g., it would pose a threat to its health or because it happens to have no paternal or maternal sense—even where it is characteristic of the species to have such a sense).

In a way it is much easier to say what counts as a good life for non-human animals than for the human animal.[11] The human animal is an odd one in that it has the capacity itself to determine, at least in part, what kind of life will count as a good one for it. The squirrel, on the other hand, who manages to 'squirrel away' a good haul of nuts for the winter, avoids the wheels of our cars, builds a particularly plush leaf nest in a nice high nook of a tree, has a healthy litter of young, and so on, just does have a good year. A package of these good years of the length that is normal for a squirrel makes it true of that squirrel that 'she has had a good life of the kind appropriate for a squirrel.' When a squirrel dies after having led that sort of life, it can be rightly said, 'she had a good life.' This is quite different from the case of a very young squirrel that ends up under the wheel of a tire on the first trip out of the nest. This one did not manage to have a good life. It did not flourish. Further, this kind of story may be made more interesting as we portray the lives of animals with more complex social relationships and intellectual capacities like those of dolphins, great apes, elephants, pigs, dogs, and so many others.

But do these ways in which animals flourish or fail to flourish provide normative ground for our care in the way that human flourishing does? If human flourishing is something like what I have described above, then human and non-human animal

---

[10] For a more thorough description of flourishing for both plants and animals, see Hursthouse (1999: 197–205). Hursthouse's description is part of an argument about naturalism, which is an issue that I will not be able to address in this chapter.

[11] Philip J. Ivanhoe (1998) makes a similar point. He points out that we often have a more reliable sense of what animals (and plants) *need* than of what other humans need even though other humans can tell us what they *want*.

flourishing are more similar than appears to be the case when one focuses only on the role of moral and intellectual virtue in human flourishing. In so far as we are all animals of some sort or other, the same kinds of things that make our lives good also make the lives of non-human animals good. Not in the capacity for moral virtue or of abstract theoretical thought, but in having, to give a few examples, a safe and comfortable place to sleep, enough to eat, appropriately satisfied sexual urges, sufficient room for exercise, clean water, sunshine (or darkness), appropriate social relations and hierarchy, physical health, and positive psychological states.

We have said already that non-human animals do not seem to have the capacity for moral virtue. Yet, it is a quite familiar phenomenon to be impressed by the virtue-like characteristic activities of both individual animals and species of non-human animals. In this way certain traits of cognitively and socially advanced animals appear to mirror human virtues and vices and even to share in rudimentary elements of actual virtue and vice. Stories of elephants that gather in support of a dying member of their group or of apes that refuse to eat for long periods after the loss of their young tend not just to bring up fellow feeling with these animals but in some cases bring us to wish that humans would be so caring. These actions may seem even more like the virtue of care when they are the actions of individual members of a certain species rather than characteristic activities of most members of a particular species. This is likely because the actions then seem even more like the results of individual character traits. So the dog who 'heroically' saves her human companion from a burning building serves as a model of courage for us in a very real way. If the dog was also trained to be a rescuer, this in no way diminishes our admiration. After all, no human becomes virtuous except through proper training and habituation (although admittedly of a different sort). These types of examples are easily contrasted with a purely anthropomorphized symbolic projection of virtue or vice. The spider that 'wickedly' entices victims into its web is not thought by any reasonable observers actually to share in anything other than a symbolic representation of wickedness.

So even though we cannot properly say that non-human animals are either morally virtuous or vicious we can say that some of their activities partake in rudimentary elements of moral virtue (and vice). Furthermore, the ways in which animal activities parallel these human character traits reveal important parallels between the ways that we, and they, flourish in a social environment. Just as our expression of courage in the face of danger constitutes part of our flourishing, the rescuer dog's flourishing is in part expressed through her loyalty to her human companion in the face of danger. I am not claiming that animals 'really do' have the capacity for moral virtue and vice after all. There are important aspects of rational reflection that are simply missing for them—such as knowing that the action is virtuous or choosing an action for its own sake. However, animal activities that parallel human virtue in a way that is not purely symbolic, but rather reflect more advanced animal dispositions, are likely also to share some of the rudimentary elements of what for us becomes virtuous and vicious action. For example, they might spring from a rudimentary motive of care.

Along with the ways in which animal lives mirror and inspire moral virtue, they also share subsets of the functions that are important for human flourishing. Contrary to what may appear to be the case from what has been said so far, many types of more cognitively developed non-human animals share with us the use of various forms of practical reason and in particular agency, even if not moral agency (Degrazia 1996: 140–72). Not in the least due to the fact that the nature of the emotions is itself controversial (see, e.g., Sherman in Ch. 12), the extent to which various non-human animals have emotions is a matter for dispute. However, it does seem implausible to claim that the ape who suffers loss of appetite and general motivational depression because of the death of her young is not experiencing emotion of a familiar sort. There are many such cases of non-human animal feelings. That is not to say that simple sensations or basic responses such as the 'fight or flight' response would constitute emotions, but rather that some of the more advanced animals are likely to have feelings that are very similar to, if not just like, our emotions.

So the lives of some non-human animals are like ours in ways that partake of some part of even our highest types of characteristic functions. Non-human animals that do not share with us some capacity for reason or emotion will share with us some of those other functions that contribute to our flourishing. In the most general sense, to return for simplicity's sake to Aristotle's classification, flourishing animal lives depend on nutrition and growth and, for many, sense perception. Animals also share with us requirements for external goods necessary to flourishing, although their specific needs are often very different (in a generally species-specific manner) from ours. But if it is true that what it is for non-human animals to flourish is in some core respects the same as what it is for us to flourish, then it is false that we can fail to care about and act in accordance with their flourishing without undermining proper commitment to our own constitutive end.

In response to the view that I support here, it may be argued that animals such as squirrels have no awareness of their lives *as* either good or not good and so, although there may be similarities between human and squirrel flourishing in such things as having a fine place to sleep, there is no corresponding subjective similarity. While it is true that, as a conscious being, the squirrel may in fact experience the positive benefit of a flourishing life, the squirrel is not self-conscious and so she fails to recognize *that* her life is either good or not good. For human beings, on the other hand, the having of a good life is partly dependent on the recognition of the nature of that good life and thus a proper recognition of our own good end. Thus it may seem that although there are parallels in the ways that we describe good human and good squirrel lives, the nature of the good life for them is so different as to make them wholly different in kind.

The question at the root of our inquiry has been whether or not animal lives can be good in ways that partake in some of the same elements that are significant for our flourishing. In answering this question, the issue of whether animals are self-conscious, merely conscious, or indeed unconscious is not *the* deciding factor. After all, even plants can either flourish or fail to flourish in ways that partake of *some* features that are significant for our flourishing—namely nutrition and growth. The question is an objective one: Is the plant, animal, or person in fact flourishing? For a human being the answer to this question will depend to some extent on whether they experience their lives *as* flourishing and may depend also on whether they are *aware that* they are flourishing. For plants this question is totally irrelevant since flourishing for them does not include any kind of consciousness.

On the other hand, whether something is the type of thing or being that is non-conscious, conscious, or self-conscious will make a significant difference for what virtue requires of us in our interactions with it. We cannot act cruelly towards wheat by cutting it down at harvest time although we might act wastefully by carelessly harvesting it in a way that ruins a large portion of the crop.[12] Similarly it is not necessarily callous to kill an animal with the capacity for pain and pleasure, but without a sense of itself as continuing over time, although doing so in a way that imposes unnecessary suffering is cruel. Thus the squirrel's lack of self-conscious awareness of the nature of her flourishing life does not diminish her flourishing as such, however it does change the nature of our responsibilities with respect to that flourishing. The specific nature of those responsibilities and how they may be shaped by the nature of the flourishing life in question cannot be developed any further in this context. Clearly such an account will require, among other things, a thorough understanding of the nature of the flourishing life for the animals in question.

CONCLUSION

In this chapter, a view of the normative role and nature of human and animal flourishing has been developed as a way of offering a particular virtue ethical framework for addressing the ethics of how we ought to treat animals. A fundamental issue has been the role of considerations of animal flourishing in virtuous interactions with them. Given the apparently very different nature of human and animal flourishing, how is it that their flourishing should be normative for us? To answer this question we first recognized a broader problem for virtue ethics, namely why we should pay heed to the flourishing of other human beings. To explain why we should be so concerned we turned to the idea that a flourishing life is the value that constitutes the complete and self-sufficient end of our actions. As such, flourishing grounds what we value ethically speaking. Properly aiming at this value includes recognition and pursuit of it not only for ourselves, but also for others who share this end. Yet this answer left open the question why we should also place value on animal flourishing, which is so different from ours. We then saw that human and non-human animal flourishing are closer in kind than appeared to be the case when we focused more narrowly on the human capacity for reason. To the extent that this is true, we have a subset of the very same general kinds of reasons for caring about and furthering non-human animal flourishing as we have for caring about and furthering the flourishing of our fellow humans.

I have thus argued that animal good lives are of a kind with our own good lives, giving us the very same kinds of reasons for caring about and acting in accordance

---

[12] I will not discuss in very much detail how my picture would apply to environmental virtues. For two excellent discussions of virtues and the environment following somewhat different lines see Hursthouse's essay in this volume and Tom Hill's now classic paper 'Ideals of Human Excellence and Preserving Natural Environments' (1983).

with their flourishing as we have with respect to one another's flourishing. Of course, even when the good-making aspects of the lives of non-human animals seem quite foreign to our own, they will still share some relevantly similar general features (even the elements of plant nutrition and growth share some relevantly similar features). In that respect, then, there will be some ethical reasons, on the picture I have given, for caring about and acting in accordance with the flourishing of all kinds of plants and animals. As already discussed, however, that does not mean that it would be wrong to destroy some plants and animals. These judgments are contextual and the virtuous actor takes into account the kind of being at issue, but also the relationship or relevance to others (including other animals and even ecosystems), the manner of acting, and the reasons and motivations for action.

Yet some might worry that I have not left sufficient resources for the protection of animals, plants, and aspects of the non-biological environment that either do not flourish at all or do not flourish as we do. It is thus important to make explicit that I claim only that partaking of a subset of the elements of our flourishing provides a sufficient, but not a necessary, underpinning for such care and activity. This view is thus consistent with a consequentialist argument that virtue requires protection of the environment—biological or non-biological—and non-human animal species of all sorts in so far as doing so supports human flourishing and that of non-human animals whose flourishing is independently a proper object of concern. The ways in which animals, plants, and things directly support human flourishing should be construed broadly to include not merely human interests such as health and longevity, but also such interests as enriched aesthetic appreciation. The (to us) sometimes very strange and wonderful creatures, plants, and ecosystems that make up our planet fill us with wonder and respect and in that way contribute to our flourishing. To return to Mary Midgley whose words opened this chapter, 'That eager reaching out to surrounding life and to every striking aspect of the physical world, which in other species belongs only to infancy, persists in human beings much longer, and may be present throughout their lives' (1983: 119). This includes that trait of children to seek in particular what is different from them (Midgley 1983: 118). Even more broadly, one can argue that traits that are basic to human flourishing such as self-respect are somehow bundled up with care about or respect for the environment and animals of all sorts (see, e.g., Schmidtz 1998; Hill 1983).

Yet a focus on human flourishing alone should not offer the primary virtue ethical resource for care about animals for two reasons. First, the result of such an interpretation is not clear. Dead animals also can be said to contribute greatly to our flourishing (because, among other things, they are tasty to eat, a good source of protein, and building on their habitats may give us wonderful homes). While virtue may require that we attend to animal flourishing for its own sake, the reasons for this are lost when we focus only on the moral significance of human flourishing. Secondly, a focus on human flourishing alone obscures a primary benefit of a virtue ethical analysis of how we ought to treat animals, namely that such an analysis offers the theoretical tools for understanding the ethical significance of animal flourishing as such. While the view offered in this chapter does place great significance on human flourishing, it does so in a way that opens up the notion of 'flourishing' to encompass the moral significance of the animals themselves.

ACKNOWLEDGEMENTS

I owe many thanks to those who read and commented on earlier drafts of this chapter. In particular, thank you to Philip J. Ivanhoe, Jennifer Baker, Heather Gert, Thomas Hofweber, Susan Wolf, participants in the Research Triangle Ethics Circle, and the anonymous external reviewers for Oxford University Press.

REFERENCES

Annas, Julia (1993). *The Morality of Happiness*. Oxford: Oxford University Press.
Aristotle (1985). *Nicomachean Ethics*. T.H. Irwin (trans.). Indianapolis: Hackett.
Copp, David and Sobel, David (2004). 'Morality and Virtue: An Assessment of Some Recent Work in Virtue Ethics'. *Ethics*, 114: 514–54.
Degrazia, David (1996). *Taking Animals Seriously: Mental Life and Moral Status*. Cambridge: Cambridge University Press.
Hill, Thomas E. (1983) 'Ideals of Human Excellence and Preserving Natural Environments.' *Environmental Ethics*, 5: 211–24
Hursthouse, Rosalind (1999). *On Virtue Ethics*. Oxford: Oxford University Press.
Ivanhoe, Philip J. (1998). 'Early Confucianism and Environmental Ethics', in M. E. Tucker and J. Berthrong (eds.), *Confucianism and Ecology: The Interrelation of Heaven and Earth*. Cambridge, MA: Harvard University Press, 59–76.
Jamieson, Dale (1994). 'Against Zoos', in L. Gruen and D. Jamieson (eds.), *Reflecting on Nature*. Oxford: Oxford University Press, 291–9.
Midgley, Mary (1983). *Animals and Why They Matter*. Athens: University of Georgia Press.
Schmidtz, David (1998). 'Are All Species Equal?' *Journal of Applied Philosophy*, 15 (1): 57–67.
Slote, Michael (2001). *Morals from Motives*. Oxford: Oxford University Press.
Swanton, Christine (2003). *Virtue Ethics: A Pluralistic View*. Oxford: Oxford University Press.

9

Law, Morality, and Virtue

Peter Koller

In recent times, the concept of virtue has regained a prominent role in public discourse and in academic ethics as well, by contrast to previous decades in which this concept was widely deemed as old-fashioned and conservative. This turn does not only manifest in a huge proliferation of popular publications on virtues, but also in a renaissance of 'virtue ethics' in philosophy, that is, ethical theories in which virtue plays a central or constitutive role (Chapman and Galston 1992; Crisp and Slote 1997; Stratman 1997). Even if this fact may mirror, to some degree, a trendy fashion in the cycle of intellectual tides, there are good reasons to believe that it also reflects a proper demand: the insight that virtue is an indispensable element of morality and good life.

In my view, virtues play a significant role in ethics because of their importance for moral practice, although I doubt that they can provide a sufficient ground for the justification of morality. I would like to demonstrate this with respect to the relationships between law, morality, and virtue. With this aim in view, I am going to proceed in three steps. First of all, I'll try to work out the notions of virtue and morality more precisely in order to illuminate the functions of virtue in morality. Secondly, I'll discuss the relationship between morality and law in regard to the questions whether and to what extent the law may be used as a legitimate means of enforcing or fostering moral virtues. Thirdly, I'll deal with the problems whether and to what extent a well-functioning legal order itself is dependent on moral virtues on the side of its citizens and officials.

1. THE ROLE OF VIRTUE IN MORALITY

The concept of virtue refers to the *character traits of persons*, their practical attitudes or dispositions, which have some motivating force for their conduct. There are, however, lots of attitudes which are widely regarded as virtues, as well as there are a great number of dispositions that count as vices. As to virtues, I want to mention just the most prominent examples: prudence, courage, moderation, and justice (these are so called cardinal virtues); reasonableness and truthfulness; honesty and sincerity; goodness and benevolence; helpfulness, generosity, and politeness; open-mindedness and tolerance; fidelity and loyalty; reliability and punctuality; sensibleness and expertise; diligence and carefulness; humility and modesty; piousness, obedience, and the like. It seems obvious that it highly depends on the respective viewpoint and context, whether or not a certain disposition is deemed a virtue. Sometimes it is even possible that a human attitude may be regarded as a virtue in one context, whereas it appears as a vice in a different context.

In order to put this variety of possible virtues in a systematic order, it is helpful to make use of some traditional distinctions that enable us to differentiate between different types of virtues. The most fundamental distinction is the one between *intellectual* and *practical* virtues (Aristotle *NE*: 1103a, 14ff). Whereas the intellectual virtues, such as reasonableness and truthfulness, are aiming at correct theoretical insight or true knowledge, the practical virtues are directed to right conduct, for example, justice, prudence, and reliability. In the present context, I am interested only in practical virtues which themselves can be divided up into two different sorts, namely *non-moral* and *moral* virtues (Höffe 1998: 47).

Non-moral virtues are character traits that motivate individuals to behave in a way that is good for themselves or fellow beings for whom they feel sympathy, such as diligence, modesty, and obedience. So these virtues are instrumental to the pursuit of particular interests of certain individuals or collectives. By contrast, *moral virtues* are directed to moral conduct, a conduct that seems desirable from a general and impartial point of view, such as justice, benevolence, and honesty. There are, however, borderline cases which cannot be easily assigned to one category or may belong to both sorts. For instance, prudence, understood as the pursuit of one's reasonable self-interest, is a controversial case: Some authors advocate the view that its proper exercise is always in accordance with the basic demands of morality, while others think that it can also be directed to immoral ends. But this question is of no importance for the following considerations that will deal with moral virtues only.

A *moral virtue* can be conceived of as a character disposition that motivates to a certain conduct which, in the light of the accepted moral standards, appears desirable, be it approvable or even laudable. This definition, which is in accordance with the usual understanding of virtue from Aristotle (*NE*: 1105b, 19ff) to Rawls (1971: 192), is sufficiently narrow in order to understand virtue as a specific aspect of moral life, and it is also wide enough in order to be compatible with different conceptions of morality. This leads to the question of the role of virtue in morality.

In order to decide whether a character disposition is a moral virtue, morally indifferent, or a moral vice, we need a more fundamental conception of morality that tells us whether the corresponding conduct is morally laudable, approvable, permissible, or unacceptable. Accordingly, it is impossible to reduce a sound conception of morality completely to the idea of virtue, as some advocates of virtue ethics believe, since, without any prior moral standards, we could neither identify moral virtues nor determine their content (Gert 1998: 277ff). This insight is clearly manifest in most modern moral theories (e.g. by Hobbes, Locke, Hume, Kant, Mill, and Sidgwick), whose basic elements always consist in certain standards in the form of general principles on which all other moral notions depend. But this also applies to Aristotle's theory which counts as the paradigm case of virtue ethics because of the central role that it attributes to virtues in achieving *eudaimonia*, a human life that is intrinsically good from the individual's viewpoint and the general perspective as well. For it is hardly possible to define the goodness of such a life completely in terms of virtues without any reference to additional features of *eudaimonia* that make it desirable both from an individual and a general viewpoint (Ackrill 1995: 39ff). So a conception of moral virtues can never provide a complete account of morality, since it presupposes further normative standards that cannot be reduced to virtues.

This, however, does not imply that virtues are of minor significance in morality. To be sure, virtues are extremely important, because a moral practice can never rely on the insight in moral norms alone, but also requires appropriate human attitudes and dispositions that motivate people to behave according to those norms (Baier 1995: 7ff, 89ff). Nevertheless, the standards of morality, be they principles or rules, represent the primary elements of morality, since they are necessary to determine the content of moral attitudes. For delimiting moral standards from other practical standards, like those of prudence, social etiquette, or law, I want to characterize them by three features (Koller 1997: 255ff).

First of all, moral standards are *autonomous standards* in the sense that they have binding force only for those persons who accept them freely and voluntarily. This feature distinguishes them from the heteronomous norms of law and social etiquette, but not from the standards of prudence, and personal taste. Secondly, moral standards *claim universal validity* in the sense that people who accept them regard them as binding also for other people. This distinguishes those standards from personal desires, the recommendations of prudence, and social habits, but not always from legal norms. And thirdly, moral standards have a *special weight* in the sense that they are deemed to be more important than other guidelines of human conduct, in some cases even so important that they take absolute priority over other guidelines, such as those of personal taste and prudence. On the basis of these features which leave room for a great variety of different conceptions of morality, it is possible to introduce two more specific concepts of morality, namely the concept of a *conventional* morality on the one hand, and the idea of a *rational* morality on the other (Körner 1976: 137ff).

A *conventional morality* is a set of moral norms that have effective validity in a certain aggregate of people, be it a social group, a society, a culture, or even humankind in general, because they are acknowledged by a vast majority of its individual members as supreme standards of their conduct. Such moral norms create, within the respective social aggregate, a certain degree of social pressure which results from the interplay of the individuals' positive or discouraging reactions to the behaviour of others. Consequently, a conventional morality, though it is based on autonomous individual moral attitudes, always develops some heteronomous force too, because its norms are connected with corresponding social sanctions that enforce them even vis-à-vis those people who do not accept them. Of course, the mere fact that moral norms are widely acknowledged by the members of a social aggregate leaves completely open the question as to the reasons for their recognition. Thus, a conventional morality may be more or less rational, arational, or even irrational. However, when people enter into a critical consideration of their received moral attitudes, they transcend conventional morality and engage in the enterprise of rational morality (Baier 1995: 214ff).

A *rational morality* is a set of moral standards that are based on good reasons rather than mere convention or non-rational beliefs. Moral standards are based on good reasons if there are sufficient reasons to assume that these standards should be unanimously acknowledged by all individuals possibly concerned as generally binding guidelines of human interaction from an impartial viewpoint and in consideration of all relevant information. And I suppose, without entering into a discussion of the various conceptions of moral justification, that this is the case if the general observance of those standards, according to all available knowledge of the relevant facts, would result in outcomes that, regarded from an impartial point of view, accord with everyone's fundamental interests better than any alternative (Habermas 1996: 59f).

Yet, we can never be completely certain whether or not a moral standard is rationally justified. This is true even of those moral standards which are commonly accepted for the best reasons we know, because it may be that there are reasons that question these standards. This fact, however, provides no reason for moral scepticism. For moral discourse is, like any other rational discourse, an ongoing enterprise in which we have to consider any moral standard in the light of all reasons for and against it, in order to accept those standards which seem to be based on the best reasons available. So the idea of a rational morality can play a very important role in moral life, since it provides a critical viewpoint for individual moral consideration and public moral discourse as well, a viewpoint which helps us to reflect on our individual moral attitudes and scrutinize the standards of conventional morality. Accordingly, the public moral discourse in a society can be understood as an ongoing interplay between its received conventional morality and the quest for a rational morality.

Now I want to turn to the various sorts of norms of which a morality usually makes use in order to guide human conduct. For a first approximation to this matter, it is helpful to recollect two well-known distinctions that differentiate between moral norms according to their respective normative force.

The first distinction, which can already be found in the classical theories of natural law, but is better known from the works by Kant and Mill, differentiates between perfect and imperfect moral duties. *Perfect duties* are understood as strictly binding moral demands that have absolute normative force under certain circumstances and, therefore, ought to be complied with without exception under these circumstances. Paradigm examples are the widely accepted negative duties of not harming others. By contrast, *imperfect moral duties* are conceived of as moral demands that leave us a certain degree of discretion as to the circumstances and the extent of their fulfilment, and, therefore, are not strictly binding in the same way as perfect duties. According to common opinion, these duties include certain general duties to positive action which would ask too much of us if we had to fulfil them in any particular case (Kersting 1989).

The second distinction is the differentiation between *moral duties* in the sense of compulsory moral demands and *supererogatory ideals* that exceed proper moral duties. Unlike moral duties, which include both perfect and imperfect moral duties, supererogatory ideals refer to ways of conduct that, from an impartial point of view, are valued as highly good or desirable, but do not appear morally obligatory, because their fulfilment would require sacrifices that cannot reasonably be expected from every-one. When we face violations of moral duties, we are in the habit of responding with disapproval and censure, since we regard their fulfilment as a matter of course. In con-trast, we do not blame people who fail to pursue supererogatory ideals, but rather praise and applaud those persons who distinguish themselves by acting in a com-mendable way.

By combining these two distinctions, which are partly overlapping, we come to a classification of *three kinds of moral guidelines* that differ in the degree of their norm-ative force. I want to name them 'strict moral demands', 'restricted moral demands', and 'commendable moral ends'.

(1) *Strict moral demands:* These demands express strict moral duties requiring a certain conduct under certain conditions, duties that have priority not only over con-siderations of prudence, but also over weaker moral guidelines. There are good reas-ons to assume that these sort of moral demands include the widely accepted moral duties of not harming other people, such as the duty not to kill or to hurt others, to refrain from deceiving others, to respect the property of others, and to keep promises. Furthermore, it appears reasonable to strengthen some of these demands by ascribing to each individual certain basic moral rights of non-interference, such as rights to life and physical integrity, to liberty and free movement.

(2) *Restricted moral demands:* These demands require a certain way of acting which is directed to a morally acceptable state of social affairs that can be achieved by a sort of moral division of labour only. Therefore, the individual duties cannot be determ-ined completely for any particular case in advance, and must be restricted to the extent to which their fulfilment can be reasonably expected from an impartial perspective. It is widely agreed upon that this sort of demand contains most of those general moral duties that require positive action in favour of others to whom one has no special obligations, especially the duties of charity, such as the duty to help people in need; and some people seem to think that no further moral norms belong to that set. In my view, however, imperfect moral demands do also include all those moral require-ments that result from a reasonable account of distributive social justice, since these requirements can only be met by a particular assignment of moral duties and rights to special people or institutions.

(3) *Commendable moral ends:* These are guidelines recommending ways of acting, the performance of which appears highly desirable, but cannot be generally required of individuals, because such a requirement does not appear rationally acceptable from an impartial point of view. Examples are beneficial activities for people in need that entail significant sacrifices, or heroic actions of political resistance against a despotic regime.

This classification of moral guidelines enables us to determine the function of virtues in moral life more precisely. Moral virtues, understood as character dispositions to morally guided human conduct, have, first of all, the *general function* to strengthen the weak motivating force of moral norms, which often compete with our self-interested preferences and, therefore, are highly susceptible to defection.

By creating 'internal' sanctions, namely feelings of good or bad conscience, our internalized moral attitudes provide us with some additional, though often rather weak, incentives to comply with acknowledged moral norms even in cases where external sanctions are insufficient or missing. In this way virtues contribute to the effectiveness of morality. Since such moral attitudes, however, will flourish only in a supportive social environment that is reinforcing and fostering them, it is necessary that we pay appropriate tribute to their appearance. That's why we are in the habit of acknowledging and praising persons of whom we learn that they have behaved or are still behaving in a morally desirable way beyond the degree that can be expected of average people as a matter of course.

When the general function of moral virtues is applied to the three sorts of moral rules mentioned previously, it can be differentiated in three *special functions*.

(1) As to *strict moral demands*, which, in general, are not only rather clear, but also not very demanding, virtues have the function to motivate individuals to a regular and lasting compliance with these rules. For although it may be regarded as a matter of course that one complies with one's strict moral duties in particular cases, it is certainly not a matter of course that one behaves in such a way all the time, even in cases where one could easily violate such duties without risking any social sanction.

(2) In regard to *restricted moral demands*, which are even more susceptible to defection than strict moral duties, because, in general, they are more demanding and less precise, virtues can help to counteract the permanent and significant temptation to an insufficient compliance with the duties stated by these demands. So we may feel moral shame, when we are confronted with the social injustices and evils that result from the fact that the uncoordinated behaviour of individuals fails to achieve a morally acceptable state of social affairs, a moral shame which itself may lead us to contribute to social reform.

(3) As far as *commendable moral ends* are concerned, moral virtues serve the purpose to motivate individuals to act in ways that exceed their moral duties, but are desirable from a general point of view (O'Neill 1993; Gert 1998: 285ff).

So much for the role of virtues in the context of morality. Now, I turn to the relationships between law and virtue. In the next section, I want to deal with the questions whether and to what extent the law may legitimately urge people to be virtuous by enforcing or fostering the respective character dispositions.

2. THE MORAL FUNCTIONS OF LAW

Morality and law have, essentially, the same object, namely the social interaction of people, and they serve a similar function, namely making a just and efficient social life possible. Yet, they refer to that object in different ways, and they fulfil this function by different means. In contrast to morality, law is a system of heteronomous norms which are based on authoritative enactment rather than voluntary acceptance and made effective by formal enforcement rather than informal social pressure. And this fact also explains why legal norms, in general, are mainly concerned with the external behaviour of people rather than their internal convictions and traits (Hart 1961: 163ff).

In spite of these functional differences, any law is connected with morality in the sense that it requires a moral justification. It needs such a justification for two reasons. First of all, under social conditions where a conventional morality alone cannot secure a just and peaceful social order, establishing an appropriate system of law is itself a moral imperative that is directed to the ultimate aim of any law: to ensure a just and generally advantageous social life. Insofar as the law demands strict obedience to its norms and threatens with the use of force in cases of their non-observance, it actually does claim moral legitimacy. Secondly, any law must take the moral convictions of its addressees into account in order to gain their acceptance without which it cannot achieve sufficient effectiveness. A legal system that deviates too far from the moral attitudes of its addressees drives them permanently into moral conflicts which will motivate many individuals to refuse not only the acceptance of legal norms, but also their obedience whenever they can.

Although every legal system claims moral bindingness and, consequently, needs moral justification, the legitimation of law differs from the rational justification of moral standards in several respects. First, the formal and organized force connected with the law makes its legitimation more complicated: since the existence of this force not only represents a bad as such, but also includes significant dangers of misuse, its negative consequences and side-effects must always be balanced with its utility. Furthermore, the legitimation of legal norms is not only based on moral arguments alone, but must also take into consideration the viewpoints of efficiency and practicability, with the result that the consequences of such considerations often differ from moral justification.

These two features of legal legitimation explain why some strict moral demands, for example, the duty of truthfulness, appear much less important within the law: the costs of the legal enforcement of these demands would heavily outweigh its utility. And they also explain why the law is not an appropriate means for enforcing inner convictions, attitudes, and virtues: using it for this purpose unavoidably would turn it into an instrument of terror. Notwithstanding, a legal system must enforce the most fundamental and well-founded rules of morality to a certain degree, so that it can claim moral legitimacy. Understood in this way, it is certainly not wrong to characterize the law as an 'ethical minimum' (Radbruch 1999: 47). This characterization, however, is not very illuminating, since it leaves the moral content of law too indeterminate. So it is necessary to investigate a bit further wherein the minimum of morality consists that the law ought to enforce.

A possible approach to this question is perhaps Kant's distinction between 'duties of right' (*Rechtspflichten*) and 'duties of virtue' (*Tugendpflichten*) which, in his view, is coincident with the previously mentioned differentiation between perfect and imperfect moral duties. According to Kant, *duties of right* are all those moral duties which may and must be enforced by the law, because other persons have a right to their fulfilment; and he was of the opinion that such duties could only be perfect moral duties. By contrast, he regarded *duties of virtue* as imperfect moral duties that are not connected with correlative rights, with the result that their legal enforcement appears neither necessary nor permissible. Furthermore, Kant thought that duties of right are always negative duties commanding the omission of some acts, whereas all duties to positive acts are mere duties of virtue which could never justify the use of legal force. Consequently, his conclusion was that only negative duties would be capable of being enforced by the law (Kant 1968: 347ff, 519ff).

This conception, however, is not convincing. In view of the significant costs of organized legal force, it seems hardly plausible that all perfect moral duties ought to be enforced by the law, even if they are connected with correlative moral rights, for example, the duty of not telling lies to others. Furthermore, it is not acceptable that all imperfect moral duties should be left legally unregulated, for the law provides an effective means for coping with the insufficiencies of such duties as, for example, the duty to render help to people in need. Law can establish special institutions which are responsible for their fulfilment which cannot be achieved by the uncoordinated behaviour of individuals. Finally, the view that only duties of right, or perfect duties, may be legally enforced would also make it impossible to use the law in order to pursue *collective goals* that are in the common interest of the citizenry without being morally required, such as the provision of public goods like public roads, means of transport, parks, or museums. As a result, a legitimate legal order has many more aims than Kant would admit. I think that these aims are the following.

First of all, law has to determine and enforce those fundamental rights and duties of individuals which flow from well-founded and widely acknowledged *strict demands* of morality, insofar as their enforcement serves the protection of essential interests of people which outweigh the negative consequences of legal force; in my view, these rights and duties not only include the familiar *negative duties* of non-interference and their correlative rights, but also a few modest *positive duties*, such as the duty to render help in the case of emergency, if such help can be reasonably expected. Secondly, a legal order should aim at establishing and enforcing an arrangement of individual rights and duties that makes possible the cooperative fulfilment of those *restricted moral demands* whose realization is in the essential interest of individuals, but can only be achieved by coordinating their behaviour in an appropriate way; this is obviously true of those *positive rights* and their correlative duties that flow from the requirements of social justice, such as the rights to democratic participation, equal opportunity, and economic justice. And thirdly, law should issue and enforce individual rights and duties which are necessary for achieving *collective goals* that need cooperative interaction, if their pursuit has been decided on in an appropriate way, even though these goals are not morally required in themselves; so law may establish rights and duties in order to provide public goods to the citizens' common benefit.

On the other hand, a legitimate legal order has *definite limits* that are also set by rational morality. First of all, law must not enforce eccentric moral ideals that are not aimed at the protection of essential human interests common to all people concerned. Secondly, it is not its function to enforce commendable moral ends that exceed the duties generally acceptable to all people concerned from an impartial point of view.

And thirdly, law is also not a legitimate means of enforcing inner moral convictions or moral virtues.

That the law must not enforce *eccentric moral ideals*, such as the prohibition of soft drugs or the prevention of homosexual relationships, results immediately from its ultimate aim to guarantee a just and generally advantageous social order. The legal enforcement of such ideals creates significant costs to those individuals who do not share them without serving the realization of generally acceptable aims. But even when certain *commendable moral ends* may appear generally desirable, it is not the law's job to enforce them if they exceed the moral duties whose fulfilment can be reasonably expected of average individuals, such as donating a kidney to somebody who needs one for survival, or rescuing a person by risking one's life. By enforcing such commendable conduct, a legal order would ask too much of its subjects and, thereby, create social affairs which appear even less desirable than the continued existence of the dangers that could possibly be diminished through the enforcement of that conduct. Neither is legal force an appropriate means to bring forth *moral virtues*, since any attempt at achieving this goal unavoidably leads, at best, to public hypocrisy, or, even more likely, to a total repression of free thought.

This does not mean, however, that law cannot contribute to stimulating moral virtues at all. Quite the opposite: moral virtues will hardly flourish without a legal order that encourages them. Yet, its contribution consists in the *indirect support* rather than the direct enforcement of virtues. There are at least two options.

First of all, the legal system may contribute to the flourishing of moral virtues by setting a framework of conditions of social interaction under which moral conduct is beneficial to the individuals rather than to their disadvantage. This becomes particularly obvious when such a framework of conditions does not exist: In a state of social affairs which is dominated by corruption, lawlessness, and injustice, individuals have little incentive to develop moral dispositions, such as honesty, reliability, justice, trust, and benevolence, since these dispositions would be to their detriment. Conversely, a legal order which, by and large, succeeds in preventing people from perpetrating dishonesty, injustice, exploitation, and the like will support the diffusion of moral virtues by making them beneficial to its subjects. Thus, a legitimate and functioning legal order is a necessary precondition for the emergence and continuing existence of moral virtues, even though it is not its job to enforce them.

Secondly, a legal order may foster moral virtues by providing appropriate *positive incentives* in order to support them. It can pursue this goal in various ways that include the application of suitable methods of education, the encouragement of desirable social activities, and the provision of special awards for people who distinguish themselves by laudable conduct. So, for example, a legal order may support private activities of charity by the tax system, contribute to a climate of tolerance and solidarity through the regulation of public education, encourage public spirit and democratic commitment by a suitable arrangement of political decision procedures and civil rights, and the like. It is true that the provision of such positive incentives also requires expenditures which must be raised from the members of the respective community by the use of legal force. As this legal force, however, takes a rather indirect and weak form, it can be justified by the argument that the moral virtues which it promotes have the character of a valuable public good that eventually is to the benefit of all members.

So much for the relationship between morality and law in general and the questions whether and to what degree law may enforce or foster moral virtues in particular. As far as the enforcement of virtues is concerned, my conclusion is, not very surprisingly, *negative*. Now, I turn to the questions whether and to what degree a legal order needs moral virtues on the side of its officials and addressees in order to operate in a sufficient way.

3. THE SIGNIFICANCE OF VIRTUE IN LAW

An influential approach in modern social philosophy, an approach which can be traced back to Thomas Hobbes and today is represented by the so-called *Rational Choice Theory*, begins with the premise that human beings, in general, are rational egoists who pursue only their own self-interest and, therefore, always attempt to act in a way that maximizes their individual utility (Elster 1986).

If this approach is applied to the question how to achieve a peaceful and well-ordered social coexistence among individuals, it recommends the view that such an order needs nothing more than a legal system which, by setting appropriate negative and positive sanctions in the form of penalties and gratifications, induces its addressees to behave in their own self-interest in a way that leads to the desired result. In other words: A peaceful and well-ordered social order is possible if, and only if, the law provides framing conditions of human interaction which make it advantageous for any individual member to act in a way that contributes to bringing about such an order. Consequently, a well-functioning legal system ought to be arranged to the effect that it is appropriate even for individuals who seek only their own benefit and have no moral scruples.

This view seems plausible to me, if it is understood in the sense that a legal order should not rely on the virtuousness of its subjects, but create framing conditions of social interaction that encourage individuals with regard to their own self-interest to behave in a way which leads to the desired social state of affairs. Understood in this sense, it is certainly expedient to reckon with the worst case and design legal rules and institutions in a way that they meet their goals even in the case when people usually pursue their own benefit without caring about morality.

Yet, the view mentioned above has been interpreted by many advocates of a strict rational choice approach—from Hobbes and Spinoza to Gary Becker and James Buchanan—in a much stronger sense, namely in the sense that a peaceful and advantageous social order may be guaranteed by the means of legal regulation alone without the support of corresponding moral attitudes of the individuals (Becker 1976; Buchanan 1975). Understood in this strong sense, the view implies not only the modest and highly plausible recommendation that, when designing the rules and institutions of law, one should reckon with the worst case, but rather the strong position that a well-functioning legal order could emerge and persist even then, when all people concerned were mere egoists without any moral motivation. This position, however, seems completely wrong to me. I think, there are at least five objections that can be raised against it.

First of all, the sanctions that can be used by a legal system in order to influence the conduct of its subjects, especially its threats of force and punishment, are certainly not sufficient to provide the individuals with appropriate incentives to abide by the law, when everybody only pursues his or her self-interest. For whatever means of force the legal order may use, there will always remain many opportunities to violate its commands without risk, and the more means the law mobilizes in order to diminish such opportunities, the more restrictive its rules and the higher the costs of legal force become. If the fear of legal force were the only incentive for individuals to comply with the law, the enforcement of a legal order would not only be extremely weak and incomplete, but also so expensive that it would forfeit any legitimation. As a result, a legal order cannot sufficiently function without the support of corresponding civil virtues of its subjects supplementing the legal threats, such as a sense of justice, fairness, honesty, and public spirit (Baurmann 1996: 261ff; Höffe 1999: 195ff).

Secondly, an effective and extensive enforcement of law requires that individuals are willing to cooperate with the law-enforcing institutions, for example, the police and the courts. But why should people do that? It is certainly true that, in many cases, some individuals are immediately interested in rendering such assistance, because the enforcement of legal rules serves their own benefit; and it may also be true that most people, even when they are not themselves immediately concerned, have an indirect self-interest in the existence of a well-functioning legal order, since such an order is also to their own benefit in the long run. The cooperation with legal institutions, however, causes some costs and disadvantages, too: in any case, a loss of time, often also certain financial costs, and sometimes even a danger to life and limb. Since these costs will frequently exceed an individual's expected utility of legal enforcement, which is especially probable in those cases in which one does not have an immediate interest in it, the question arises how legal prosecution can work at all. This question cannot be answered satisfactorily on the assumption that all people actually pursue only their self-interest. Consequently, an effective legal enforcement can only be achieved if there are a sufficient number of individuals who, at least in some cases, are willing to contribute to legal enforcement for the sake of justice rather than their own benefit (Pettit 1990).

Thirdly, any legal order stands or falls with the sense of justice of its highest office bearers, including the leading politicians, judges, and officials, since there is no way to induce these persons to comply with the law by means of legal threats alone. It is true that there is an appropriate method of diminishing the risk of misuse of legal power by distributing it among different independent institutions who control each other. Yet, this method can neither completely prevent any corruption of legal powers nor create an affirmative attitude of its bearers towards the existing legal order. Thus, a legal system will not function properly without the inclination of its rulers to comply with its principles and defend it against corruption (Hart 1961: 107ff). And it is pretty obvious that this inclination does not flow from their self-interest alone, but must be backed by moral dispositions, since otherwise it could not be explained why, all other things being equal, some officials misuse their powers unscrupulously to their own profit, while others resist all temptations to corruption and strive to exercise their powers as correctly as possible. As a consequence, a legal order will operate in a proper way only under the provision that at least a part of its officials—judges, civil servants, government members—are, to a certain extent, motivated by moral virtues, including loyalty to the law, justice, integrity, impartiality, correctness, and truthfulness.

Fourthly, a functioning legal order requires some organized authority which, in developed societies, takes the form of the state with a monopoly of power. This fact, however, creates significant dangers, particularly the danger of corruption of power which increases in proportion to the concentration of power that lies in the hands of that authority. In order to counteract this danger, there is need for an effective control of power which, to a certain extent, may be exercised by special legal institutions, but also requires the commitment of the citizenry (Baurmann 1996: 176ff). Although one can assume that citizens have a rational self-interest in the public control of state power, this self-interest is hardly sufficient to lead them to appropriate activities, because, in most cases, the individual costs of such activities will override their individual utility. Consequently, people are confronted with a *cooperation problem* by which they unavoidably fall into a trap, if each of them is seeking only his or her individual utility. As a result, public control of power will not take place, unless there are a sufficient number of citizens who are led not only by their self-interest, but at least to a certain degree by moral attitudes, such as political commitment, benevolence, truthfulness, and courage (Höffe 1999: 208ff).

Finally, moral virtues are also necessary for a process of legal development that is directed to produce a just and efficient legal order. Such a process includes two elements: first, an appropriate procedure of legislation which itself must be accepted by most members of the legal community in order to guarantee the acceptance of its results, and secondly, an ongoing public debate in which citizens seek to form their opinion and reach an agreement on the legal regulation of their common affairs. Both the legislative procedure and the public debate, however, will lead to acceptable results only under the provision that participants are prepared to distance themselves from their particular interests to a certain degree, in order to consider the common interest of all people concerned (Habermas 1996: 277ff). But this would certainly not be possible if all individuals were always acting as pure egoists. Thus, a successful process of law-making also rests on the condition that the participants are capable of balancing their own interests with the interests of others in an impartial way and acknowledge legal regulations that are generally acceptable. And this requires that a sufficient number of citizens and politicians have internalized supportive moral attitudes, of which tolerance, fairness, public spirit, and devotion to the commonwealth are of particular importance (Höffe 1999: 199ff).

If these considerations are, by and large, correct, then it follows that a well-functioning legal order requires the support of moral virtues on the side of its subjects and officials for several reasons. In summary, such virtues are required for the following aims: (1) for compensating the weak and insufficient incentives of legal sanctions, (2) for making possible an effective and complete enforcement of legal norms, (3) for leading legal officials to comply with the law, (4) for guaranteeing the necessary control of legal power, and (5) for enabling an appropriate process of legal development. So a legal order cannot function in a proper way without moral virtues of the individuals involved. This result raises some problems which I want to address very briefly at the end.

I have argued that a well-functioning legal order needs the support of moral virtues which, however, cannot be produced by means of legal force. So law is dependent on moral resources that must be provided by *civil society*, the social community of the people concerned. This somewhat paradoxical result leads to the question how civil society may produce the moral virtues that are required in order to guarantee a well-functioning legal order. This is a very complex question which I cannot answer satisfyingly, if there is a satisfying answer at all. Yet, I want to mention three features which, in my view, are important for the formation of moral dispositions: moral empowerment, public discourse, and social solidarity.

By *moral empowerment* I mean the creation, encouragement, and reinforcement of basic moral capacities through a supportive social practice rather than preaching moral values and norms. These capacities, that combine cognitive and emotional attitudes, mainly include the following: the inclination to empathize with other human individuals and sentient beings; the willingness to consider the interests of others and balance them with one's own desires from an impartial point of view; the capacity of acting on social rules and orders that appear generally acceptable; and last but not least, the habit of activating appropriate emotions vis-à-vis good and bad, such as, for example, satisfaction, guilt, shame, compassion, and indignation. These capacities are neither inborn nor emerging naturally. Rather, they develop and flourish preferably in social surroundings in which they are conveyed to individuals from birth through a loving and understanding guidance, and reinforced by an ongoing social practice (Rawls 1971: 453ff).

Even if most members of a legal community have the basic moral capacities, it may be that they do not share a common conception of a just and efficient legal order. Such an order, however, requires a *public* morality, a set of widely shared fundamental moral standards. The only acceptable means to generate and renew a public morality is an ongoing process of *public discourse* that must be open to all people concerned and sensitive to any intelligible concern. Such a discourse can foster a moral consensus because it does not only provide the participants with better information about the relevant facts and aspects of the issues under consideration, but also create a situation in which they must respect each other as equals and attempt to reach an agreement on the regulation of their common affairs. And to the degree to which such an agreement can be reached, the agreed-on moral norms will gain increasing force, for it becomes more probable that their observance or violation will cause appropriate social reactions, be they positive or negative (Habermas 1992: 399ff).

The motivating force of moral norms, however, has its limits, too. In general, its strength depends on the extent of reciprocity of human interaction. Therefore, a public morality needs a social world in which individuals feel bound together by ties of *social solidarity*, a shared interest in mastering their problems of existence cooperatively, based upon an effective social practice. Without such an idea, we shall hardly

succeed in establishing a widely acknowledged political and legal order, since the voice
of morality will not be strong enough to gain attention against the parties' selfish
interests in their struggle for power and benefit. It is, therefore, an important task
to create and preserve a climate of social solidarity in order to bring forth the moral
virtues without which a well-functional legal order cannot exist.

ACKNOWLEDGEMENTS

I wish to express my thanks to Philip J. Ivanhoe, Rebecca Walker, and Edith Zitz for
their helpful comments on an earlier draft of this chapter.

REFERENCES

Ackrill, J. L. (1995). 'Aristotle on Eudaimonia', in Otfried Höffe (ed.), *Aristoteles: Die Nikomachische Ethik*. Berlin: Akademie Verlag, 39–62.
Baier, K. (1995). *The Rational and the Moral Order. The Social Roots of Reason and Morality*. Chicago: Open Court.
Baurmann, M. (1996). *Der Markt der Tugend*. Tübingen: J. C. B. Mohr.
Becker, G. S. (1976). *The Economic Approach to Human Behavior*. Chicago: University of Chicago Press.
Buchanan, J. M. (1975). *The Limits of Liberty*. Chicago: University of Chicago Press.
Chapman, J. W. and Galston, W. A. (eds.). (1992). *Virtue*. New York: New York University Press.
Crisp, R. and Slote, M. (eds.). (1997). *Virtue Ethics*. Oxford: Oxford University Press.
Elster, J. (ed.). (1986). *Rational Choice*. New York: New York University Press.
Gert, B. (1998). *Morality: Its Nature and Justification*. New York: Oxford University Press.
Habermas, J. (1992). *Faktizität und Geltung*. Frankfurt/Main: Suhrkamp.
——(1996). *Die Einbeziehung des Anderen: Studien zur politischen Theorie*. Frankfurt/Main: Suhrkamp.
Hart, H. L. A. (1961). *The Concept of Law*. Oxford: Clarendon Press.
Höffe, O. (1998). 'Aristoteles' universalistische Tugendethik', in Klaus Peter Rippe and Peter Schaber (eds.), *Tugendethik*. Stuttgart: Reclam, 42–68.
——(1999). *Demokratie im Zeitalter der Globalisierung*. München: C. H. Beck.
Kant, I. (1968). *Metaphysik der Sitten* (1797). Werkausgabe vol. VIII, ed. by Wilhelm Weischedel. Frankfurt/Main: Suhrkamp.
Kersting, W. (1989). 'Pflicht'; 'Pflichten, unvollkommene/vollkommene'; 'Pflichtenlehre'; 'Pflichtethik, deontologische Ethik', in *Historisches Wörterbuch der Philosophie*, vol. 7. Basel: Schwabe, 405–39, 456–60.
Koller, P. (1994). 'Moral Conduct Under Conditions of Moral Imperfection', in Herlinde Pauer-Studer (ed.), *Norms, Values, and Society*. Dordrecht: Kluwer Academic, 93–112.
——(1997). *Theorie des Rechts: Eine Einführung*. 2nd edn. Wien: Böhlau Verlag.
Körner, S. (1976). *Experience and Conduct*. Cambridge: Cambridge University Press.
O'Neill, O. (1993). 'Duties and Virtues', in A. Phillips Griffiths (ed.), *Ethics*. Cambridge: Cambridge University Press, 107–20.

Pettit, P. (1990). 'Virtus Normativa: Rational Choice Perspectives'. *Ethics*, 100: 725–55.

Radbruch, G. (1999). *Rechtsphilosophie* (1932). Studienausgabe, ed. by Ralf Dreier and Stanley L. Paulson. Heidelberg: C. F. Müller.

Rawls, J. (1971). *A Theory of Justice*. New York: Oxford University Press.

Stratman, D. (ed.). (1997). *Virtue Ethics: A Critical Reader*. Edinburgh: Edinburgh University Press.

10
Virtue Ethics, Role Ethics, and Business Ethics

Christine Swanton

(I) THE META-ETHICS OF VIRTUE ETHICAL ROLE ETHICS

Much has been written in substantive moral philosophy from the perspective of the 'big three' theories: Kantianism, Virtue Ethics, and Consequentialism (Baron, Pettit, and Slote 1997). Considerably less has been written about the nature of a Kantian, virtue ethical, or consequentialist role ethics. Part of the explanation for this neglect lies in scepticism about role ethics itself, or at least scepticism about its importance or centrality.[1] In this chapter I remedy the neglect by elaborating my own conception of a virtue ethical role ethics, showing how my view handles apparent role conflict, and conflict between role ethics and 'ordinary morality'.

I apply my views to business ethics, which is a paradigm example of the supposed tension between role ethics and ordinary morality. Sections (II) and (III) show that there is characteristically no such tension, without falling into a range of errors where there is failure adequately to recognize that business has a distinctive purpose, not reducible to leading or fostering the good life in general. Meanwhile, in the current section, I outline the meta-ethics of role ethics from a virtue ethical point of view.

Standard virtue ethics entails belief in role ethics for the following reason. Standards of goodness will vary according to the point, function, or nature of roles, so standards of goodness will vary across roles.[2] Hence standard virtue ethics entails that what is demanded by virtue will vary across roles. That is to say, virtues are role-differentiated. For example, as R. E. Ewin points out, a lawyer acting qua lawyer cannot be generous to the community at large by sacrificing his client's legal rights—such 'generosity' is not expressive of the virtue of generosity *in that role*. Rather it is expressive of vice, 'something like arrogance'.[3] Lawyers can be generous, but not in that way.

---

[1] See further, and a defence of role ethics, Michael O. Hardimon, 'Role Obligations', *Journal of Philosophy*, 91 (1994).

[2] For a good discussion of goodness and roles, see Bernard Williams, *Morality: An Introduction to Ethics* (Cambridge: Cambridge University Press, 1972).

[3] 'Personal Morality and Professional Ethics: The Lawyer's Duty of Zeal', *International Journal of Applied Philosophy* (1991), 35–45 at 39; discussed and cited in Tim Dare, 'The Role of Law and the Role of Lawyers', in Tom Campbell and Jeffrey Goldsworthy eds., *Judicial Power, Democracy and Legal Positivism* (Aldershot: Ashgate Dartmouth), 371–90.

The question arises: what determines the goodness of a role? In Aristotelian virtue ethics, the answer to this question lies in a hierarchical approach to goodness, with the hierarchy terminating in goodness qua human being. The goodness of a role is determined by reference to its place in the life of a good human being, and there is no conflict between role virtues and 'ordinary' (role-undifferentiated) virtues: namely those making one good qua human being.

There is another, non-Aristotelian, possibility for a virtue ethical role ethics. Role virtues make one good qua role occupier, and those roles must themselves be worthwhile or valuable. However, it is not necessarily the case that such virtues, for example, the virtues of an artist or a business person, contribute to one's goodness as a human being. For there is no hierarchy of ends such that role virtues are always subordinated to virtues making one good qua human being. This non-Aristotelian position allows for two broad views about possible conflict between being good in a role and being a good human being. According to the first, there is characteristically conflict between many role virtues and ordinary virtues, and this conflict is not necessarily resolvable in favour of being good qua human being. For example, it may be thought that artistic passion is a (role) virtue in a talented artist, and this virtue is conceptually connected to a tendency to act indecently towards, for example, friends and family (Slote 1983). Furthermore, it may be thought that where the artistic stakes are sufficiently high, the role virtue trumps ordinary virtues of, for example, constancy, or loyalty. According to the second possibility, there is characteristically no conflict between role virtues and ordinary virtues, so the fact that there is no complete hierarchy of ends—that there is a genuine pluralism of ends—is not a serious problem. On this view, though artistic passion is a role virtue in a talented artist, that passion is tempered or modified by other demands. [4] Such emotional/cognitive wisdom is part and parcel of a *virtue* of artistic passion. In this chapter I shall argue for the second of these options within a non-Aristotelian role ethics.

The two broad versions of a role ethics of virtue were offered as answers to the question: 'what determines the goodness of a role?' But it should be appreciated that accounts of the various role virtues need not be directly derivable from an answer to this question. For example, one might say that business roles are good because the institution or practice of business as a whole increases prosperity, and is therefore worthwhile. It does not follow from this that the target or aim of a business role virtue is to promote the overall prosperity of society as a whole, or the prosperity of the worst off. For the nature of a role virtue in an individual agent is determined by the purpose or function of individual business organizations, and it is not necessarily the case that the purpose or function of *individual* business organizations is to increase the overall prosperity of society, or the prosperity of the worst off. I shall have more to say below about this distinction, and the dangers of ignoring it.

Whether or not a virtue ethicist is or is not Aristotelian in role ethics, all virtue ethicists will claim that possessing virtues is the basis of being good as a human being. There will be differences about what being good qua human being amounts to, and

---

[4] For a defence of this view, against Slote, see Marcia Baron, 'On Admirable Immorality', *Ethics* 96 (1986), 557–66.

the relation between virtue and that goodness. For eudaimonists, to be (fully) good qua human being, it is necessary that one flourish. Furthermore,

(a) it is a necessary condition of her flourishing that a human being possess and exercise at least the core virtues, and

(b) it is a necessary condition of a trait being a virtue that it characteristically (partially) constitute (or contribute to) the flourishing of the possessor of the virtue.

For non-eudaimonists, to be a virtue it is not necessary that it characteristically be partially constitutive of (or contribute to) personal flourishing. According to Michael Slote (2001), it is a sufficient condition of a trait being a virtue that it be an admirable trait of character even if that trait does not serve some further good or end (such as personal flourishing). The possession of a sufficiency of such admirable traits makes one good qua human being. On my non-eudaimonistic view (2003) a virtue is a disposition to respond to or acknowledge items in its field or fields in an excellent or good enough way. We need to know what kinds of response to items in a virtue's field constitute virtuous responses and they include excellence in, for example, promoting (good), producing, appreciating, loving, respecting, creating, being receptive or open, using or handling things. Excellence in loving responsiveness, for example, includes not just excellence in loving actions, but also excellence in loving feelings, emotions, and motivations. This account of virtue, which I call pluralism, does not entail that virtues are characteristically good for one, that is, tend to, or are partially constitutive of, the flourishing of their possessors. It entails only that virtues make one excellent in responding to what I have elsewhere called the 'demands of the world' (2003) which includes of course the demands of self.

In this chapter I shall apply my view of virtue to role ethics. What implications does the non-Aristotelian picture have for the meta-ethics of role ethics? It cannot claim that goodness qua human being is entirely extractable from a theory of human nature. If goodness qua human is dependent on the goodness of an agent's responsiveness to the demands of the world, then we need not only a theory about what are characteristic human responses (such as bringing about, respecting, loving, creating, appreciating) but also a theory or view about the nature of items other than the agent, and characteristic human relations to those items. We would need to know whether those items are worthy of bonding to, conserving, preserving, creating, respecting, and so forth, in an excellent way, even at the characteristic cost of an agent's flourishing. The goodness of roles would be understood in terms of their point or function in institutions whose value lies in their function in enabling us to produce, bond to, preserve, create, respect, appreciate items worth bonding to, preserving, creating, and so on.

(II) THE ROLE PROBLEM

I claimed above that all virtue ethicists believe that possessing virtues is the basis of being good as a human being. It does not follow from this claim that:

(a) being good qua human being is able to be integrated into being good-in-a-role, or

(b) given that there is some conflict between being good qua human being and being good in a role, goodness in-a-role is always to be subordinated to being good qua human being.

Indeed, business ethics provides a challenge to claims (a) and (b). First we need to ask: is claim (a) true of business? That is, can a human being who is good qua business person be good qua human being?

Call this problem of the compatibility of being good qua human being and being good in a role the role problem. Let me first pose the problem in general terms. Any work on professional ethics needs to supply a view about the point or function of the institutions in which roles are embedded. For, as claimed above, the point or function of those institutions determines the nature of the roles which individuals in those institutions occupy, and the nature of those roles determines what counts as ethical behaviour of individuals occupying those roles. Right here, however, lurks a central problem of professional ethics. The purpose of many institutions such as business, it may be thought, seems not to contain an ethical dimension, and indeed may appear amoral or contra-moral. Yet individuals occupying roles supposedly serving that purpose are expected to behave ethically.

Faced with the role problem, the theorist may offer one of several broad solutions. We illustrate with business.

1. She may expand the proper role of business to embrace clearly moral ends such as social responsibility to stakeholders.

2. She may say that business in capitalist society is intrinsically immoral since it cannot be part of the life of a good human being.

3. She may maintain that (individual) business organizations have a distinctive purpose such as promoting or maximizing (within limited constraints) owner value over the long term by selling goods and services,[5] claim that this aim is a moral aim but not reducible to the 'expanded' aim of 1, and argue that, nonetheless, there is characteristically no conflict between pursuing this aim in a business role and being a good human being.

4. She may maintain that business has a distinctive purpose along the lines suggested by 3, claim that this purpose is good, but argue that there is characteristic conflict between pursuing this end and being a good human being.

Of these options, I shall argue for the third. First, it should be mentioned that virtue ethics is particularly vulnerable to the role problem. For an account of business virtue is extractable from a correct theory about the purpose of individual business institutions. But being disposed to serve the point or function of business—being

---

[5] See Elaine Sternberg, *Just Business: Business Ethics in Action*, 2nd edn., (Oxford: Oxford University Press, 2000), 6. Note that she insists that the defining purpose of business is to *maximize* owner value (discussed below).

good qua business person—is arguably at odds with possessing character traits required for being a good person. Given that character traits are relatively robust, it may be claimed, one cannot switch at an instant from being a decent, caring, just, loyal individual, to being a person possessing traits designed to serve the distinctive purpose of business.

I shall now argue that characteristically there is no conflict between being good in a business role and being a good human being. For, I shall argue, it is both the case that (A) being good as a human being is itself shaped by role demands, and that (B) role demands are constrained by requirements of being good as a human being. I argue for (A) by claiming that what I shall call prototype virtues are themselves too vaguely specified to give *specific* requirements about what it is to act well as a human being—rather, such virtues need to be contoured by, inter alia, role considerations. I argue for (B) by claiming that though prototype virtues are vague they are not empty. They provide constraints inhibiting the unfettered pursuit of institutional goals.

For this strategy to be seen as plausible we need to emphasize that on a virtue ethical view, some conceptions of being a good human being—conceptions which would invite conflict between role requirements and being good qua human being— are ruled out. It is clear that being good as a human being, on a virtue ethical reading, would not pose the role problem in the manner of Charles Fried's formulation (1976). In Fried's formulation of the problem, being a good person is tied to an 'ideal of moral purity' (1976: 1061) which in turn is given an impartialist understanding of devotion to the greatest good for the greatest number. From *within* a virtue ethical perspective that particular understanding of the role problem is ruled out *ab initio*, but this is not to say there is no role problem.

In order to show how a business virtue can be both role-differentiated and manifested in ways compatible with being good as a human being, we need to introduce a virtue ethical conception of goodness as a human being via the notion of a prototype virtue. Three things need to be explained: first, what is a prototype virtue; secondly, how is a prototype virtue contoured or shaped to yield a role virtue; and thirdly, how does a prototype virtue provide constraints on role- differentiated virtues, so that possession and exercise of the latter are characteristically not incompatible with being good as a human being.

(III) PROTOTYPE VIRTUES AND ROLE VIRTUES

Prototype virtues are virtues specified at a very high level of generality, where aspects of the surrounding contexts such as the agent's role, her actual relation to specific other agents, her social circumstances, cultural conventions, and the narrative particulars of her life, have not been supplied, or have been abstracted away. [6] In this

---

[6] The notion of a prototype virtue (Churchland 1998) is associated with work on the connectionist model of mind which suggests that the mind works through the recognition, refinement, and extension of 'prototypes' rather than knowledge of precise rules, readily applicable to the world in a determinate way, by calculative reasoning. As Andy Clark puts it, 'one way to think of the way knowledge is encoded in a neural network is to think of the experienced network (the network

chapter, prototype virtues are contrasted with professional role virtues, but the distinction between prototype virtues and, say, role-differentiated virtues, is not hard and fast, but is relative to context. Let me illustrate this point with an example.

For some, such as Robert Solomon, love is a virtue. However, as C. S. Lewis points out in *The Four Loves* (1977), love is able to be differentiated into types: affection, friendship, eros, and charity or agape. Love, as such, would be a prototype virtue on this view. However, friendship, one of the loves, and in a sense a role virtue, can also be seen as a prototype virtue relative to *professional* role virtues. That is, it may be (not without controversy) further differentiated in terms of these roles, such as friendship qua teacher. We shall illustrate some of these controversies below.

Sometimes it is not easy to see how a professional role virtue is connected to a prototype. It has been argued for example that the doctor–patient relationship and the lawyer–client relationship should be modelled on the (prototype) virtue friendship. This view is vehemently opposed by Justin Oakley and Dean Cocking (2001). The protagonists' views might however be integrated as follows. Yes, it is wrong to think of these relationships as friendship understood simply in terms of the prototype virtue friendship. Nonetheless, it can be argued, one might think of them in terms of professional role-differentiated friendship, insofar as certain notions of partiality, or concern, may apply in these relationships. On the other hand, this conciliatory view is itself controversial. Since friendship as a prototype virtue is also characterized by intimacy, mutual affection, shared interests, and devotion to the overall welfare of a friend, the conciliatory strategy poses difficulties, for these aspects of the prototype are not present in the putative professional role virtues. Either we need to learn connections to a different prototype (such as the loyalty prototype), or we have to develop a new prototype, or we have to extend (or diminish) the prototype of friendship in ways which are very stretched indeed. There is no easy answer to this conundrum.

What the above shows however, is that the title of Charles Fried's article—'The Lawyer as Friend: The Moral Foundations of the Lawyer–Client Relation'—should not mislead us into thinking that Fried is likening the lawyer's relation to the client to friendship proper. He is using friendship as a prototype, and speaking of a role-differentiated form of that prototype. In this role-differentiated form, only one aspect of the friendship prototype—partiality—is salient. The other aspects, for example, mutual affection and shared interests, drop out. For Fried's main target is the tension between the lawyer's role and the supposed impartialist moral requirement to promote overall good.

after extended training on example cases of input and desired output) as commanding a rich and context-sensitive battery of prototypes ready to be deployed in response to incoming stimuli'(2000: 270). However, as Clark emphasizes, the idea of a prototype can be accessed in part by sentential devices such as rules, provided those rules are understood in a sufficiently flexible way to be presently explained. (Professional) role virtues can be seen therefore as refinements and extensions of the relevant prototype virtues.

Although I am favourably disposed towards the ideas of Clark, I do not intend the basic idea of a prototype virtue as explained here to imply commitment to any specific theory of concepts, such as all the features of prototype theory (a species of 'similarity-based' accounts). (See further, Prinz 2002.)

I myself would use a different prototype (namely loyalty) to accommodate Fried's points about the legitimacy of zealous advocacy of client interests. The reason Fried uses friendship as the relevant prototype is that he regards as the 'classical definition of friendship' adopting the friend's interests as one's own (1976: 1076). Since the lawyer does this with respect to a limited range of interests, Fried regards the lawyer as a 'special purpose friend' (1976: 1076). By contrast, I prefer loyalty rather than friendship, as the relevant prototype virtue, since I disagree with Fried's 'classical definition' of friendship, and think that mutual affection is a salient aspect of friendship as a prototype virtue. And mutual affection is certainly not necessary or even desirable in the lawyer–client relation.

Another theorist, concerned with the putative coldness of lawyers (or doctors) perhaps, may focus on a different aspect of the friendship prototype—namely caring. Again, the prototype has been extended in a certain direction to provide another account of the relevant role-differentiated virtues. In this case one may argue, the relevant prototype is seen not as friendship, or loyalty, but friendliness or caring. In any case there would be no suggestion that the way the relevant prototype is extended accommodates all aspects of the prototype.

Another area of debate concerns the application of the prototype friendship to academics in their role as teachers. According to Peter J. Markie, friendship necessarily involves shared activities, mutual affection, and acknowledgement of mutual affection through expectations and commitments (1990: 136). Because of these features, he argues, friendship is not a role virtue in a university teacher, for it conflicts with the required impartiality of justice to students. On the other hand, one may wish to argue that prototype virtues should not be understood as possessing features which are necessary conditions: though the above features are important, none is necessary, and indeed may lose salience when the prototype virtue is extended into role virtues. In particular, it may be argued, the partiality which is at the core of the features deemed necessary for friendship by Markie may lose salience, and be replaced by other important features such as caring, concern, sensitivity, and a friendly demeanour. My own view is that friendship is a poor prototype for the relevant academic role virtue, since Markie is right to emphasize the damaging consequences of important aspects of friendship for the required impartiality of teachers. The prototype virtues that need to become role-differentiated in the university teacher are arguably friendliness and caring, rather than friendship itself.

Having illustrated the importance of the claim that extensions and applications of prototypes are not determined by precise rules and are controversial, we describe how a prototype virtue is specified. The specification of a prototype virtue has two stages: first what Martha Nussbaum calls the thin account, and secondly, what she calls the thick account (1988). The thin account gives the specification of the field of a virtue (its domain of concern) and states that the virtue is being well disposed in relation to that field. The thin account is important because even at the level of prototypes it is very easy to go wrong in the specification of a virtue, since many of the so-called virtue terms in the English language do not have the notion of excellence built into them, but are rather descriptive. Thus 'loyalty', 'trust', and even 'honesty' must be treated warily as virtue terms. For example, loyalty as a virtue must be contrasted with non-virtuous forms of loyalty. So to define a prototype virtue, it is best to begin with the thin account. This is done as follows. The virtue is individuated by the following type of description: being well disposed in relation to its field (or fields). Thus the thin account of loyalty (as a prototype *virtue*) is being *well* disposed with respect to sticking to and 'going in to bat for' relevant individuals or institutions. Trust (as a prototype virtue) is being *well* disposed with respect to believing, supporting, and so forth relevant individuals. Hence, right at the level of the thin account of a prototype virtue we are in a position to distinguish loyalty as a virtue from for example blind loyalty, trust as a virtue from for example gullible trusting.

A full account of a prototype virtue—the 'thick' account—is given by so-called 'mother's knees' rules and basic accounts of relevant emotional and motivational dispositions (Hursthouse 1999). What is characteristic of such rules is that they are unsophisticated and vague, but they provide, as we shall see, some sort of guidance on what are acceptable accounts of role virtues. Though thick accounts of a prototype virtue such as loyalty provide saliences and paths to assist the development of appropriate emotional and cognitive takes on the world, they are still vague. Not only do they not provide universal principles, they do not even provide rules that are specific enough to provide guidance of the form: 'Characteristically you should do thus and so.' For example, the prototype virtue loyalty does not prescribe that, characteristically, you should stick with your employer for several years. The prototype virtue honesty does not prescribe that, characteristically, you should state the bad features of your product and not overhype or exaggerate its good features when advertising or selling it.

The claim that prototype virtues are vague is central to the idea that role demands do not characteristically conflict with those of being good as a human being. For if we think that acting well as a human being requires that we act in accordance with prototype virtues, what it is to act well as a human being would then be vague. For example, insofar as honesty is a prototype virtue, it does not mean something specific like telling the truth and not lying here and now. 'Mother's knee' rules such as 'Tell the truth!', 'Don't lie!', 'Don't exaggerate!' are not to be given universal or precise readings. So in business ethics, the substantive question is what counts as excellence in the field of divulging and disseminating information, and one has to consider such questions as the legitimacy of bluffing in certain contexts, overhyping products in advertising, and the non-divulgence of trade secrets. Only when more specific requirements are determined by role-differentiation do we know what it would be to act well as a human being. However, given that honesty is a prototype *virtue*, an agent with that virtue will have emotional and cognitive dispositions which make her not ready to lie or distort the truth (and certainly not for her own convenience, or to exact revenge); which ensure that she is not economical with the truth out of moral cowardice, and so on.

Again, given that benevolence is a prototype virtue, that virtue's associated 'mother's knee' rules such as 'Do good for others!' and 'Be helpful to others!' are not to be interpreted universally or in specific ways. What counts as excellence in regard to the field of promoting others' welfare in business virtue requires that we consider such specific questions as the legitimacy of undercutting competitors by buying in bulk from cheap sources, and predatory pricing. Elaine Sternberg for one argues that given the business purpose and its nature as competitive, predatory pricing is legitimate

(2000). But, again, the emotional and motivational dispositions of someone with the prototype virtue will ensure that pleasure is not gained by harming others, nor will one harm others out of malice, or desire for power and superiority.

I have claimed that prototype virtues are vague. Here lies the common complaint that virtue ethics is too vague to be of use in applied ethics. However, an account of prototype virtues is but the first stage to a full understanding of virtue. Prototype virtues must be contoured by several features if a more or less complete account of virtue is to be supplied. We shall concentrate on role features, but other contextual features are also needed. Here are some examples of the ways in which prototype virtues are contoured:

(1) Politeness as a prototype virtue needs to be contoured by cultural features if a full understanding of the virtue is to be gained. As a virtue, politeness (like hospitality) has considerable but not indefinite cultural latitude: what is required by politeness in one culture may be considered rude and disrespectful in another.

(2) Generosity as a virtue is heavily contoured by the narrative structure of an individual's life. However, this latitude is not boundless. In particular, the personal latitude given to an individual in her generosity is sharply curtailed when she acts in a role, such as managing director of a business firm. A managing director whose charitable business donation mirrors a personal desire to reward a local organization that saved the life of his father-in-law may legitimately be chastised by his overseas boss.

(3) Loyalty as a virtue is strongly contoured by role contexts. Indeed it is claimed that in some roles loyalty as a virtue ceases to exist. John Mitchell, the (ex) coach of the All Blacks rugby team, was quoted as saying after dropping an icon of New Zealand rugby, 'loyalty is a great word but it does not exist in professional sport' (*New Zealand Herald*, July 2003).

In a sense this is correct. Merit (understood along various dimensions) is the only criterion of international selection. However, it is not true that the prototype virtue of loyalty ceases to exist in this role context. Rather it is contoured according to the exigencies of the role. It does not affect selection, but it affects emotional and cognitive dispositions possessed and expressed on dropping a player who has served brilliantly over a long period, and the manner of approaching the dropping of the player. The virtue demands proper communication to the player, compassion and consideration in the approach, and, assuming the player is no longer available for selection, public recognition of past glories instead of simply a public exposé of current faults.

The danger of loyalty dropping out altogether as a virtue, occurs also in other areas of business. In 2003 there was consternation in many quarters about the fact that the Guardians of the New Zealand Superannuation Fund were investing only 7.5 per cent of their massive fund in the New Zealand Share Market, and 62.5 per cent in overseas share markets. For comparison, we might say that UK investors generally invest almost entirely in their domestic market, and American and Australian investors invest similarly, with only a slightly greater offshore investment proportion. There is no doubt that the lack of domestic investment over a long period has had serious negative consequences on local ownership, interest rates, exports, and the New Zealand economy generally. There are two issues of loyalty which arise from this example. Loyalty (and moral courage) as role virtues in politicians arguably require that they do not (contrary to what is now happening) stand back and let the Guardians make their (totally) independent judgments qua financiers. Loyalty to their country's interests demands that they put the interests of their country's economy first (compatible with the demands of other (role-differentiated) virtues). The second issue concerns individual decisions by the financiers of large national companies. Should they act in the best interests of shareholders only, or should loyalty to the interests of their country play some role in their decision making? These issues are complex and controversial; my point, however, is that we should not confuse the refinement or extension of prototype virtues with their non-existence in role contexts.

Let us now discuss further the notion of a role virtue, and show in more detail how prototype virtues are contoured to yield role-differentiated virtues. A role virtue in its thin account is differentiated according to its distinctive field (field of concern) and target (its aim or aims) in regard to that field. In a prototype virtue the field is relatively broad. In a role virtue the field is further delineated by appeal to the point and purpose of the role, which itself is understood in terms of the purpose of the institution in which the role is embedded.

Recall the basic account of a virtue as a disposition of excellent responsiveness to items in its field. Given that there is a plurality of types of response, an account of a role virtue needs to supply a view about the appropriate modes of response for the role virtue, be that mode love, respect, appreciation, creativity, or promotion of good. A thick account of excellence of responsiveness in a role virtue requires then a view about how the various responses are role-differentiated. For example, love as a mode of moral response is role-differentiated according to whether the role is that of, for example, a parent, friend, nurse, spouse, or salesperson. Love will be the love of a parent, the affection of a friend, the caring of a nurse, the eros of a spouse, or altogether absent. Alternatively, one may believe that agapeic or universal love is present in all virtue, including all role virtues, and that the forms of love specific to roles are founded on a base of agapeic love.

Appreciation of employees by a boss will not be as demanding as the appreciation of one's children, but this may well leave scope for admiration of managing directors who appreciate their employees to a high degree (taking an interest in personal details) provided that this appreciation is not tainted by vice. For example, there should not be inefficiency due to tendencies to displacement behaviour (there is a preference for attending to employees' private lives rather than doing boring administration or number crunching), or invasion of privacy associated with injustice. In the former case, love (as a kind of affection) may border on the pathological; in the latter case, there is a failure of respect. Creative thinking, though part of virtue in business, has to be characteristically constrained by prudence, and respect and care for colleagues whose working lives may be disrupted. Creativity is part of vice in business if it constitutes inefficiency, self-indulgence, or grandiosity, but in a very talented artist what may be called grandiosity and self-indulgence in the business world may be virtuous creativity.

(IV) PROTOTYPE VIRTUES AS CONSTRAINTS

Recall the role problem, and the strategy of integrating goodness in roles with goodness qua human being. To argue for (A)—being good as a human being is shaped by
role demands—I claimed that prototype virtues are vague, needing to be contoured
by role considerations. I now want to show (B)—that prototype virtues provide constraints, inhibiting the headlong pursuit of institutional goals.

Given that prototype virtues are vague and need to be precisified by role- differentiation for example, how do they provide constraints on role virtues? We might say that
they provide anchors for moral thinking in role contexts, alerting us to possibilities of
excess and other forms of wrongness. Such anchors are traits of character whose emotional and cognitive features are deeply rooted through early training. If a role virtue
appears to cause an agent to dirty her hands by the lights of a prototype virtue, she will
do this with compunction, distaste, perhaps with difficulty. She will react viscerally to
expressions of vice which egregiously violate the demands of a prototype virtue, even
when that display of vice is commonly (though mistakenly) thought to be required or
permitted by role demands.

Thus prototype virtues are not empty—they provide constraints which inhibit
the untrammelled pursuit of the institutional goal. For example, in a defence lawyer,
loyalty (to client) manifests itself in the role virtue of zealous advocacy, but that zeal
is not unfettered. In order to prevent excess, zealous advocacy is contrasted with
what has been called 'hyper-zeal', [7] in which loyalty as a virtue descends into vices
of excess: excessive partialism in the interests of the client. Loyalty descends into a
vice of excess because basic features of prototype virtues such as justice and efficiency
are seriously compromised. For example in rape cases, hyper-zeal leads to injustice
to defendants; in other cases, it may lead to endless delays in court proceedings. In
business ethics, the parameters of loyalty as a business virtue are similarly determined.
Though loyalty of employees to firms does not make the same demands as loyalty
in friendship, there are limits if the prototype virtue is to have some bite in business
behaviour. For example in New Zealand, advertisements for an Internet job-search
web-site advocated that people keep pre-written resignation notes in their top drawer
ready to send to their boss the moment a better looking job turned up on the web.
The active undermining of loyalty as a virtue encourages 'the grass is greener over
the fence' mentality, high staff turnover, and consequent business inefficiency. Faced
with these problems, management may refuse to re-employ good staff begging for
their jobs back, in order to help create a climate where loyalty is seen as an important
virtue.

The idea that a role virtue is constrained by prototype virtues overcomes scepticism about role virtue, a scepticism that may appear to allow vices as 'virtues' in role
contexts. My notion of a prototype virtue appears to have been questioned by Judith

---

[7] For the distinction between 'mere zeal', and 'hyper-zeal', see Tim Dare, 'The Role of Law and
the Role of Lawyers'.

Shklar who claims in 'Bad Characters for Good Liberals' that 'we have no need for simple lists of vices and virtues' (1986: 249). Her reason for this claim is that there is a place for what we might call socially or culturally differentiated vice in pluralistic and role-differentiated society. As a result, we need to be fine-grained in our accounts of virtue and vice, for there may be a place in a society for a character such as one whom we would now regard as possessing the vice of snobbery. For example, a person who is 'ceremonious—so cold and polite that no familiarity is thinkable' (1984: 246) is claimed by Shklar to have his place in the *ancien régime*. Given that my account of prototype virtues allows for them to be differentiated according to such features as the nature of society, culture, or role, Shklar's view is inconsistent with my own only if she means by simple virtue and vice something like my account of prototype virtue (and vice). But I am not sure her view is inconsistent with mine. She would recognize limits to differentiation in order to avoid cultural relativism. It would be odd to think that the prototypical requirement of respect (understood by Kant as 'keeping one's distance') (Kant, Gregor trans. 1996), and which is appropriately role-differentiated in contexts of ceremony and deference, might not allow for any warmth or familiarity in any role or context. The need for respect-based virtues to recognize some forms of closeness, love, or affection is an anchor for our moral thought recognized by such (prototype) virtues as friendship. The notion of a prototype virtue, contoured to yield role virtues, allows us to recognize Shklar's point without our being forced to claim that vice may be good.

(V) ADEQUACY OF VIRTUE ETHICAL BUSINESS ETHICS

In the last section, I showed how prototype virtues, which provide ethical constraints on the institutional goal, and role virtues, which serve role functions within distinctive institutions, are characteristically not in conflict but are integrated. This section shows how my account avoids two mistakes common in role ethics. The mistakes are these:

(1) the constraints of prototype virtues are incorporated into institutional goals in such a way that the distinctive function of an institution is lost or undermined; and

(2) the constraints of prototype virtues are so stringent that they routinely override the realization of institutional goals.

This second mistake comes in two forms:

(a) the internal goals of institutional practices are thought to be not properly part of the domain of morality, but are merely 'practical', and since the moral is thought to override the non-moral, the constraints provided by prototype virtues are regarded as highly stringent; and

(b) though institutional goals may be seen as part of the moral domain, the constraints are understood as part of a deontological ethics, functioning as absolute or near absolute 'side-constraints' on the realization of goals.

Let us now discuss each of these mistakes, and consider how my virtue ethical conception of role ethics avoids both. In business ethics, the first mistake is made by some versions of stakeholder theory. The stakeholder theory of business can have a strong or a weak form. The strong version is characterized by Sternberg thus: 'The stakeholder theory of business typically holds that business is accountable to all its stakeholders, and that the role of management is to balance their competing interests' (2000: 49). She interprets the idea of 'balancing' to mean that business 'ought to be answerable equally to all' stakeholders (2000: 50). She rightly criticizes this view as losing sight of the distinctive business purpose, and operating with a confused idea of accountability, namely that one is accountable to all that are affected. A weaker conception of the stakeholder view is compatible with my own view. It claims merely that, first, ethical constraints on the business goal extend beyond the interests of the owners, and secondly, that those constraints embrace more than the rights-based concerns of justice. In the words of Robert C. Solomon, this view may be described as follows: 'the point is precisely to replace the overemphasis on the rights and demands of the stockholders with a more general regard for all those constituencies who are involved with and affected by the corporation' (1997: 208).

Such a view must be elaborated in a way which avoids the first mistake. It may be thought that Solomon himself in various writings on business ethics has failed to do so. He claims 'The good life is the goal of business—not profits, not competition, not management or the work ethic' (1997: 87). In *Ethics and Excellence: Cooperation and Integrity in Business,* Solomon has another account of the purpose of business, which is also very broad: 'The purpose of business is to promote prosperity, to provide essential and desirable goods, to make life easier' (1993: 118).

Does Solomon make the first mistake? Not necessarily. It seems to me that Solomon's and Sternberg's accounts of the purpose of business are answers to different questions. Solomon's is an answer to the question: What makes business as a whole a worthwhile practice or institution? Sternberg answers the question: What is the purpose of individual business institutions? It is not the purpose of an *individual* business organization (directly) to promote prosperity, the good life, or to make life easier. If one thinks this, one will have made the first mistake, like the strong version of stakeholder theory. The ethics of role occupiers in an individual business organization cannot be derived directly from an answer to the question: What is the purpose of the institution of business as a whole? For the ethics of the part cannot necessarily be derived from the point or function of the whole of which it is a part. For example, individual businesses are competitive; they do not cooperate in order to secure prosperity or the good life for all. The point is made by Sternberg as follows: 'however much kindness and generosity may be virtues, exercising them and helping the opposing side to win is incompatible with playing properly' (2000: 65). This recognizes that business is competitive: a business is aimed at its own advantage and not that of others. This is not to deny that generosity and kindness are not virtues at all in the business role. They are appropriately contoured in line with the function of individual business organizations.

The point that the ethics of the part cannot be derived from the ethics of a whole applies also to the relation between the individual agent and the organization for which he works. In *Above the Bottom Line* Solomon says 'business ethics is essential as a reminder to people in business that they are, after all, in it for the good life' (1994: 9). Again, it looks as if the first mistake has been committed. However, in this passage, Solomon is speaking of individuals' goals. We should distinguish between the goal of a business organization and the goal of an individual working in that institution. The goal of every person should be to lead the good life on Solomon's view, but it is not necessarily the goal of a business organization to ensure that this is so. Nonetheless, one's working life should be integrated with what is required to lead the good life as a whole. As Solomon argues, one's personal life should not be that of a workaholic or directed solely at amassing money, even if this best serves the business purpose.

It may be thought that my own account makes the first mistake described above, failing to acknowledge that the institutional goal must be distinctive and not be tantamount to the promotion of, or instantiation of, the good life as a whole. For, it may be thought, I failed to claim that role virtues are designed to *maximize* the realization of the function or purpose of the institution in which the role is embedded. One may think that the first mistake is avoided only if we first define a role virtue by reference to its distinctive (worthwhile) role function, and then claim that the virtue enables their possessors collectively to maximize the realization of the institutional function which the role is designed to serve. So we may say that the goal of medicine is to promote health, and claim that medical role virtues maximize health promotion. Indeed in business ethics, it is claimed by, for example, Elaine Sternberg that the distinctive function of business is to maximize (and not merely promote) owner value in the long term by selling goods and services (2000: 6). By 'owner value' Sternberg means the following: 'Owner value consists of the present value of the future cash flows that the owners will obtain from the business. Those cash flows are normally of two kinds: Distributions from the business, in the form of dividends or other payouts, and the capital gains or losses that are realised when (the owner's financial interest in) the business is sold' (2000: 48). Certainly, if a connection is made between role virtue and *maximizing* the realization of the purpose of the institution in which the role is embedded, the first mistake is avoided but at the cost of conflict between role virtue and prototype virtues. On a virtue ethical view, I shall claim, the first mistake can be avoided without incurring this cost. Role virtue should not be understood in terms of 'best serving role function' if 'best' is understood in terms of maximization as opposed to excellence. 'Best serving' should be interpreted as 'serving excellently', where excellence recognizes the constraints of prototype virtues.

It may be claimed that my strategy waters down the role function so that its distinctiveness is lost. Sternberg claims that:

> It is essential that the objective be to maximise owner value, not just to increase or promote, secure, or sustain it. Less stringent objectives than maximising fail to differentiate business from other activities. If there were no requirement for owner value to be maximised, any activity or association that increased owner value through occasional sales would thereby qualify as a business. Hobbyists making casual sales would constitute business as would families selling their houses. (2000: 54–5)

Sternberg's point could be preserved by conceiving of excellence not simply in terms of 'increasing, promoting, securing, or sustaining', but in terms of maximizing subject to the demands of prototype virtues. It is important to appreciate however that these prototype virtues are many and varied, extending well beyond justice and minimal decency. These virtues may in certain contexts directly militate against maximization. For example, a woman may conduct a private business, but eschew maximizing on the grounds that caring, demanded by her role as parent and spouse, precludes maximization within her business role. Indeed, a self-regarding virtue such as self protection may also demand this. A woman's successful horticultural business growing and selling peonies for export to the USA may offer unlimited opportunity for expansion. But she limits herself, and this does not turn her business into a mere hobby, even if she greatly enjoys admiring her peonies.

My claim that a number of prototype virtues may inhibit maximization points to another way in which my strategy may be thought to make the first mistake: that of undermining or losing the distinctive role function. It may be thought that the mistake is avoided only if a limited number of prototype virtues are relevant to an institutional purpose, and to the roles of that institution. For example, it may be assumed that the only prototype virtue relevant to nursing is care; the only virtue relevant to the business purpose is justice. Sternberg claims that business ethics concerns merely distributive justice understood as requiring that 'organisational rewards should be proportional to contributions made to organisational ends' (2000: 80), and 'minimal decency', which is also justice-related, requiring the exclusion of 'lying, cheating, stealing, killing, coercion, physical violence and most illegality' (2000: 79). No mention therefore of kindness, friendship, loyalty (not connected with justice), environmental soundness (not impacting on human justice-related issues) as prototype virtues needing to be shaped by, and constraining, the business purpose.

Would the inclusion of these and other virtues result in a business losing its distinctive point and function? This seems to be Sternberg's view. She claims that as a consequence of the limited role of business, justice and ordinary decency are the ethical values essential to business (2000: 110).

On my view, to the contrary, all virtues are liable to be in play in business ethics, without the business purpose being compromised. Both mistakes described above can be avoided. But how? By extending the scope of business virtues well beyond the confines of justice, but contouring them appropriately. Sternberg herself identifies unkind and even callous ways of dismissing employees by, for example, leaving a black plastic bag by their chair as 'callous', but this behaviour does not reduce to a form of injustice. Caring, which may approximate the prototype friendship, may also be warranted. For example, the treatment of Samoan and Tongan employees beyond the demands of justice has been publicized and lauded as effective business practice, by a cereal manufacturer, and by the coach of the New Zealand Warriors rugby league team who attended the church of one of its stars in order to gain further understanding, and the confidence of the players. However, the caring is contoured by business-related values of effectiveness, and not by the intimacy and closeness of personal relations. This does not entail that the exercise of this role virtue is purely instrumental.

A virtuous agent acts *out* of the virtue (sometimes misleadingly ex-pressed as 'for the sake of' the virtue). The claim that a prototype virtue must be appropriately contoured in a role virtue is not tantamount to a claim that the exercise of the role virtue is merely instrumental.

We turn now to the second mistake. The constraints of prototype virtues may be seen as so stringent that the business (or other institutional) purpose is seriously compromised. I identified two reasons for this mistake. The first is a spurious separation of the moral from the practical, with the pernicious consequence that the 'merely practical' is downgraded in significance relative to the moral. However, doing one's (worthwhile) job properly is a moral requirement, and if problems such as a printer not getting course books ready in time for the first class are seen as 'merely practical problems', then they may not be attributed to the moral failings of individuals, as opposed to, for example, 'systems' failure where no one takes responsibility for contributing to the failure. The mistake of reducing many morally important features to the merely practical is not always made, but it is still common nonetheless to think of many institutional goals such as business goals as amoral (Sternberg 2000: 57–8). It is harder to make this mistake with respect to other worthwhile institutions such as medicine. It would be very odd indeed to regard the saving of life and the reduction of health-related suffering to be an amoral (or a 'merely practical') goal. Yet if deontological constraints have not been properly contoured in the kind of virtue ethical way described in section (II): if, for example, justice, informed consent, privacy, and prohibition of donation of organs with racist and other conditions have been understood in ways which have seriously compromised the medical purpose, then philosophical confusion (on e.g. ethics committees) can cost lives.

The question arises: How severe are the constraints on maximization provided by the prototype virtues? In particular, what is to prevent the constraints that are enshrined in the prototype virtues from undermining the ethical requirement to pursue institutional ends served by role virtue? The mistake is avoided by having a firm grasp of the distinctive function and importance of the institution in which the role is embedded, and contouring the prototype virtues properly, in the light of that goal. It is avoided by appreciating that such goals are *morally* important goals and that the 'moral' or ethical is not confined to *constraints* on those goals (such as privacy, informed consent, racial and other forms of equity or justice).

(VI) CONCLUSION

I have argued that role virtues do not characteristically conflict with those of ordinary morality. The argument may be summarized as follows using loyalty as an example:

(1) Loyalty as a prototype virtue is defined in the thin account as being well disposed in regard to sticking with relevant individuals and institutions.

(2) Loyalty as a role virtue is defined in the thin account as being well disposed with respect to sticking with relevant individuals and institutions in ways suitable to one's role as, for example, friend, defence lawyer, sports team selector, investor. Sticking with—a vague concept—is precisified in role virtues. 'Sticking with' a player

in selection is not interpreted to mean continued selection despite prolonged loss of form. A defence lawyer's 'sticking with' a client permits zealous advocacy. 'Sticking with' a friend permits certain sorts of preferential treatments of friends not afforded to acquaintances or strangers.

(3) The thick accounts of prototype virtues provide the limits of what is permitted by role virtues. The thick accounts of prototype virtues such as benevolence, honesty, justice, kindness are vague, but provide markers for excess and other forms of wrongness. So zealous advocacy cannot extend to hyper-zeal. Sticking with one's friends does not permit sharing their immoral ends. Loyalty does not permit dropping players capriciously or because one no longer likes them. But one may drop a friend for the latter reason.

(4) As a result, the thick accounts of role virtues do not allow for the untrammelled pursuit of role functions. Saving life does not allow for saving life at all costs, pursuing profit does not allow for maximizing profits without ethical constraints, defending clients in court zealously does not allow for injustice to victims and gross inefficiency. However, the requirement of role-differentiation which gives due weight to the importance of the role function will ensure that constraints do not undermine the role purpose, but make for excellence in that pursuit.

It may be thought that my strategy of integration is excessively sanguine. It should be realized however that I have not claimed that there is never conflict between manifestations of various role-differentiated prototype virtues. I have claimed only that conflict is not characteristic. The notion of a prototype virtue and its role-differentiations allows for a powerful virtue ethical response to a claim that, when the business purpose is taken seriously, one cannot be both good as a human being and good as a business person.

REFERENCES

Baron, M., Pettit, P., and Slote, M. (1997). *Three Methods of Ethics: A Debate*. Oxford: Blackwell.

Baron, M. (1986). 'On Admirable Immorality'. *Ethics*, 96, 557–66.

Churchland, P. M. (1998) 'Toward a Cognitive Neurobiology of the Moral Virtues'. *Topoi*, 17, 83–96.

Clark, A. (2000). 'Word and Action: Reconciling Rules and Know-how in Moral Cognition', in R. Campbell and B. Hunter (eds.), *Moral Epistemology Naturalized: Canadian Journal of Philosophy*, 26 (suppl. issue), 267–89.

Dare, T. 'The Role of Law and the Role of Lawyers', in Tom Campbell and Jeffrey Goldsworthy (eds.), *Judicial Power and Legal Positivism*. Aldershot: Ashgate Dartmouth, 371–90.

Ewin, R. E. (1991). 'Personal Morality and Professional Ethics: The Lawyer's Duty of Zeal'. *International Journal of Applied Philosophy*, 6, 35–45.

Fried, C. (1976). 'The Lawyer as Friend: The Moral Foundations of the Lawyer–Client Relation'. *Yale Law Journal*, 85, 1060–89.

Hardimon, M. O. (1994). 'Role Obligations'. *Journal of Philosophy*, 91, 333–63.

Hursthouse, R. (1999). *On Virtue Ethics*. Oxford: Oxford University Press.

Lewis, C. S. (1977). *The Four Loves*. London: Fount.

Kant, I. (1996). *The Doctrine of Virtue: The Metaphysics of Morals*, trans. and ed. Mary Gregor. Cambridge: Cambridge University Press.

Markie, P. J. (1990). 'Professors, Students, and Friendship', in Steven M. Cahn (ed.), *Morality, Responsibility, and the University: Studies in Academic Ethics*. Philadelphia: Temple University Press, 134–49.

Nussbaum, M. (1988). 'Non-Relative Virtues: An Aristotelian Approach', in P. A. French, T. E. Uehling, Jr., and H. K. Wettstein (eds.), *Midwest Studies In Philosophy*, 12, 32–53.

Oakley, J., and Cocking, D. (2001). *Virtue Ethics and Professional Roles*. Cambridge: Cambridge University Press.

Prinz, J. J. (2002). *Furnishing the Mind: Concepts and their Perceptual Basis*. Cambridge, MA: MIT Press.

Shklar, J. N. (1984). 'Bad Characters for Good Liberals', in Judith N. Shklar, *Ordinary Vices*. Cambridge, MA: Harvard University Press, 226–49.

Slote, M. (2001). *Morals from Motives*. Oxford: Oxford University Press.

—— (1983). *Goods and Virtues*. Oxford: Clarendon Press.

Solomon, R. C. (1993). *Ethics and Excellence: Cooperation and Integrity in Business*. New York: Oxford University Press.

—— (1994). *Above the Bottom Line: An Introduction to Business Ethics*, 2nd edn. Fort Worth, TX: Harcourt Brace College.

—— (1997). *It's Good Business: Ethics and Free Enterprise for the New Millenium*. Lanham, MD: Rowman and Littlefield.

Sternberg, E. (2000). *Just Business: Business Ethics in Action*, 2nd edn. Oxford: Oxford University Press.

Swanton, C. (2003). *Virtue Ethics: A Pluralistic View*. Oxford: Oxford University Press.

Williams, B. (1972). *Morality: An Introduction to Ethics*. Cambridge: Cambridge University Press.

11

Racial Virtues

Lawrence Blum

Race, or the racial domain of life, presents a very rich context of value. There are many different kinds of things that can go wrong and right in the area of race, and race and racial identities can play an important role in understandings of a just society, a good society, a good individual life, and a good life for groups. Yet, by and large, moral philosophers have given race scant attention, apart from social justice concerns such as discrimination and affirmative action. Although love, friendship, family, civic relationships, and other aspects of our interpersonal lives have increasingly drawn the attention of moral philosophers, the racial dimension of this complex domain has not. In this respect moral philosophy has not kept pace with public concern. Popular understandings of race are shot through with evaluative takes on various aspects of our relations with one another—being offended in a manner relating to one's racial identity, exhibiting an adequate grasp of the character and importance of others' racial identities, showing an adequate moral understanding of the role race plays in one's own life, shows respect or disrespect to racial others, evincing subtle forms of exclusionary behavior and attitude, and so on.

Virtue theory in particular has been an untapped resource in this area. Yet virtue theory provides a rich psychological framework for encompassing the complexity of emotion, perception, motivation, imagination, and behavior implied in our evaluations in the racial domain. Perhaps one reason for the general lack of engagement between virtue theory and race is that race is seen as a primarily negative evaluative domain—one in which the moral task is primarily to avoid doing wrong, for example, to avoid being 'racist'. By contrast, virtue theory, while of course encompassing vice as well, has a primary focus on positive qualities of character. Even if virtue theory were able only to help articulate the myriad ways things can go wrong or badly in the racial domain, it would still provide essential understandings. I will argue, however, that there are also genuine positive virtues or sub-varieties of virtue of a race-related character, and that race presents opportunities for value as well as disvalue, where the value is not the mere avoidance of the disvalue. More generally, I will discuss several distinct race-related virtues and vices, attempting to demonstrate the plurality of value in the racial domain, and especially the interpersonal part of that domain.

The plurality of racial value has also been masked by two common approaches to value issues in the racial domain. One is to think that color blindness or race blindness is an adequate overarching norm that should govern all of our actions, and thoughts, in this domain—that we should endeavor to ignore people's race as much as possible. I will reject this claim, in part because it is sometimes appropriate to acknowledge persons' racial identity, and in part because there are several virtues that bear some resemblance to color blindness but are nevertheless distinct from it and from each other.

The second approach is to focus only on 'racism' as the general form of all disvalue in the racial domain. While occasionally the term 'racism' is indeed used as a general term for all racial disvalue (so that focusing on it would not exclude any racial disvalue), more commonly it is used with a narrower scope, to refer to a belief in racial superiority, to racial discrimination or exclusion, or as a catch-all term for the most serious racial wrongs or ills.[1] Some racial value and disvalue would then lie outside the scope of racism, so focusing only on racism will tend to mask that broader domain.

GARCIA'S ACCOUNT

I will find it convenient to approach this topic through a critique of Jorge Garcia's work. Garcia has worked out, with great subtlety, a virtuist or, more precisely, a 'vice-ist' account of racism. Garcia sees racism as most fundamentally an individual vice. His best-known piece in this vein, 'The Heart of Racism', has been reproduced in several canon-defining collections on race and racism, and he has further developed his virtue theoretic approach in three later articles (1996, 1997, 1999, 2001). I will argue that Garcia's analysis does not provide a sufficiently psychologically rich description of the phenomena he encompasses within his own definition of 'racism'. In particular he tends to conflate motivational and emotional dimensions of racism. In addition, his account of racism provides insufficient guidance to the plurality of race-related value. Focusing almost solely on racism, Garcia does not place the racial ills encompassed by 'racism' in the context of the wider set of racial values and disvalues. Finally, Garcia's account fails to capture some of what is distinctive about vice and virtue as they operate in a race-related manner, and this failure points up a more general failure of much work on the virtues. That failure is to confine virtues and vices too much to 'standard issue' virtues and vices, generally designated by single terms such as justice, honesty, benevolence, charity, temperance, perseverance, and the like. Diverse as the standard issue virtues are (and not only moral ones, though I will confine my discussion of race-related vices and virtues largely to moral ones), they still do not encompass or account for the full range of types of virtue-related value and disvalue. Looking at the case of race will help to reveal something of the character of this broader domain.

Let me briefly set the context for Garcia's work. Prior to Garcia, one might say that there were two reigning conceptions of racism. One, with origins in the first uses of that term in the 1930s, views racism as an ideology or set of related, false

---

[1] I discuss different meanings of 'racism' in popular and scholarly discourse in Blum (2002, 2004b).

beliefs about the innate character of large, intergenerational groupings of human beings called 'races'. Charles Taylor expresses this view in his book *Sources of the Self*: 'Racists have to claim that certain of the crucial moral properties of human beings are genetically determined: that some races are less intelligent, less capable of high moral consciousness, and the like' (1989: 7). Anthony Appiah propounded a complex form of this account in his canonical 1990 essay, 'Racisms'. Appiah essentially defined racism as (1) belief in innate differences among 'races' (a view Appiah calls 'racialism'), (2) belief that these differences involve significant inequalities in characteristics of mind and temperament, and (3) a belief that it is justifiable to treat persons of different racial groups differently in light of the latter differences (1990).[2] So Appiah's view linked belief—the original meaning of 'racism' that Taylor's view reflects—with discriminatory action, or at least a belief in its justifiability.

The second conception of 'racism'—generally less theoretically elaborated in the philosophical literature but a dominant conception of racism in much popular anti-racist thought and in some social science literature—is a structure of unjust inequality between racially defined groups. When we speak of racism, or of something's being racist, we must in some way be referring to such structures. (These structures need not be, on this conception, the direct result of acts of racial discrimination. The relation between racial discrimination and racism is generally undertheorized on this 'systemic' account of racism.)

Garcia rejects both the doxastic and the systemic accounts. Both fail to root themselves in what Garcia takes to be the fundamentally moral character of the terms 'racism' and 'racist'. The label 'racist', Garcia says, 'is today thoroughly moralized. To call a person, institution, policy, action, project, or wish "racist" is to present it as vicious and abhorrent' (1997: 7). Although the systemic definition builds in a notion of injustice and thus provides a morally based account of racism, Garcia regards it as omitting or providing an inadequate account of forms of *individual* action and motivation that are standardly referred to as 'racist', such as racial bigotry and race-hatred. Against Appiah's cognitive account, he argues that false belief cannot be a core moral failing, that forms of individual racial wrong do not require racist beliefs, and that mere differential treatment by race is not in its own right morally wrong, and indeed may in some cases be justified.

Garcia sees racism, understood as an individual vice, as taking two distinct but related forms—race-based ill will or hatred, and 'racially based or racially informed disregard' (1997: 13; 1996: 6). Racism is morally bad because it is a type of vice, a vice Garcia often describes in terms of its being the opposite of, or offending against, certain virtues, especially benevolence and justice (1999: 13), but which he also describes as a form of (the vice of) malevolence.

What Garcia calls 'racism' involves both motives and feelings. Ill will or hatred motivates the racist to engage in actions harmful to others (those of a racial group other than her own, or, in the case of internalized racism, toward members of her own

---

[2] Appiah is not entirely consistent in point (3); for he also says that racial favoritism, especially on the part of members of subordinated groups, can be permissible and even admirably supererogatory, if it does not contravene what is owed to all equally.

group). But racial ill will or disregard also manifest themselves in certain feelings or emotions that do not necessarily prompt action. Delighting in the ill fortune of the racial other, anger or dismay at the racial other's successes, aversion to the presence of the racial other, glee when the racial other is humiliated, consternation that one's offspring or friend has befriended a member of a stigmatized race are or can be examples of such emotions.[3] Garcia does not give any attention to these emotions and feelings, and sometimes talks as if his account of virtue and vice concerns only the contents of the will; for example, he refers to his account as 'a volitional account of racism' (1996: 6). But the strength of a virtue account is its capacity to express the range of psychic phenomena involved in forms of goodness and badness. A racist is not someone who only has bad intentions, but someone who has bad and inappropriate feelings as well. Generally, the intentions and the feelings are conceptually linked. We would not attribute ill will to someone who was never motivated to cause harm to the object of his ill will; but nor would we do so if he did not sometime feel delight or pleasure in the ill fortune of that object. Both feeling and motive are integral to what it is to possess various virtues and vices. Nevertheless, it would be appropriate to attribute vicious racial attitudes to someone who never actually engaged in racist actions but who nevertheless thought of another racial group as inferiors, or who wished them ill. Perhaps the non-acting person fears disapproval or getting in some sort of trouble, or is too timid to act on these vicious attitudes, and this is why, after a while, he loses motivation to engage in the sorts of actions that naturally express such attitudes. Not all forms of vice require vicious motivation.

In general, Garcia does not explore the range of psychic phenomena constituting racial vice. For example, he does not look at the characteristic ways that the racist views or perceives the racial other, or the sorts of thoughts the racist might characteristically have. The racist, for example, might fail to notice types of accomplishment in a racial other whose group is seen as inferior; or he might acknowledge the accomplishment but see this is a fairly rare exception, atypical of the group in question.

Thus, although Garcia helpfully and convincingly construes racism as an individual vice, and though he plausibly takes racial ill will to be a form that vice takes, he does not give a psychologically adequate account of the character of the vice in question. He fails to avail himself of the full resources of virtue theory.

A second limitation in Garcia's account is his failure to articulate the plurality of virtues and vices related to race. I have developed this criticism of Garcia elsewhere (2004b), and will summarize those arguments here. The limitation takes two forms. First, Garcia fails to pay adequate heed to the diversity within what he himself takes to be encompassed by the term 'racism'.[4] Secondly, he fails to situate racism within a broader panoply of racial ills and vices.

On the first point, Garcia occasionally describes the vice of racism as involving inadequate concern *or* respect, or an offense against *either* benevolence *or* justice (1996: 10 and elsewhere). Since benevolence and justice are distinct virtues (and

---

[3] Hursthouse (1999: 114) mentions these and other emotions characteristic of a racist.

[4] One part of that diversity is the 'ill will' and the 'disregard' strands of racism. In Blum (2004b) I argue that Garcia nowhere provides a satisfactory account of the relation between these.

malevolence and injustice distinct vices), and since inadequate concern is not the same as inadequate respect, this appears to acknowledge two distinct sub-forms of racism. In '*I'm Not a Racist, But . . .*', I argue that these two forms are best understood as antipathy (toward a racial group), and inferiorization, viewing or treating the racial other as humanly inferior (Blum 2002). But Garcia does not consistently recognize these as two distinct forms of racial disvalue. Indeed, he explicitly argues that the inferiorization type is a mode of the antipathy (ill will) type (1996: 9). This argument is not successful. A racial hater might not see the racial other as inferior; one can hate a racial group seen as superior, or as neither superior nor inferior. Conversely, a racial inferiorizer does not necessarily harbor ill will toward the racial other. Although ill will can accompany inferiorizing, these are two distinct forms of racial wrong, and any account of racial disvalue must distinguish them.

Garcia's account also understates the range and plurality of racial value and disvalue by failing to situate what he designates as 'racism' within a larger domain of race-related vices. On rare occasions, Garcia does mention items that are plausibly seen as falling within that category—engaging in racial stereotyping, giving credence to the false doctrine of racialism (what Taylor means by 'racism'), seeing persons primarily as members of racial groups rather than as individuals (1997: 21). But in general, there is no articulation of wrongs and ills in the racial domain that are other than racism, and no attention to the valuational bases of ills or vices other than race-based ill will or disregard.

Even if Garcia had recognized the plurality of standard-issue virtues and vices bearing on race (justice, malevolence, disrespect, and so on), an important dimension of race-related value and disvalue would have been omitted. Garcia generally implies that the reason *race-based* ill will is bad is simply and solely that it instantiates the vice of malevolence. Malevolence is a vice in its own right, independent of whether race is involved as its basis. Garcia's implication is that if I hate Andres and wish him ill out of jealousy, this is as bad—because equally a form of malevolence—as if I hate him because he is black.

We do not, however, generally look at malevolence in this way. We tend to think that race-based ill will is a *worse* form of ill will than are many other forms. The concept of a 'hate crime' is a legal analogue to this moral intuition. The idea behind a hate crime is that a crime, such as assault, committed out of hatred of someone grounded in certain group-based characteristics, such as race, ethnicity, religion, gender, sexual orientation, and the like, is worse, and deserving of more severe punishment, than the same crime committed for a different reason. (Indeed, the term 'hate crime' is somewhat misleading, since it is not hatred as such that warrants the more severe punishment, but only certain group-targeted forms of hatred.)

Thus, race-based ill will seems to be bad not only because it involves ill will, but because the ill will is based on race. Whatever the explanation for this, it suggests that ill will comes in morally distinct sub-varieties (and perhaps the same can be said for disrespect, disdain, disregard, and so on). One might even say that race-based malevolence is a different vice from jealousy-based malevolence, in having a distinct moral valence and perhaps a somewhat distinct psychic structure. On the other hand, one might not want to call these sub-varieties distinct vices, on the grounds that they are recognized to be sub-varieties of a standard vice; but one would still want a virtue theoretic approach to recognize the form of distinctiveness in question.

The latter concern raises the question what a virtuist account of something consists in. How do we know when a moral phenomenon constitutes a virtue, or vice? A natural way of reading Garcia's account is to say that he sees a virtuist account as one that construes the phenomenon in question as an instance of an already recognized virtue or vice—in his case malevolence (or disregard). Much philosophical literature on the virtues appears to proceed on the assumption that we know what all the virtues and vices are, that they are generally represented by single words—honesty, cruelty, hypocrisy, compassion, and so on—and that what the virtues and vices are recognized to be has not much changed in hundreds, even thousands, of years. James Rachels, for example, in his popular ethical theory textbook, *The Elements of Moral Philosophy* (4th edn.), lists twenty-four virtues in his section 'What Are the Virtues?' —all single-word virtues (2003: 176). Zagzebski articulates this approach to the virtues: 'Those qualities that have appeared on the greatest number of lists of the virtues in different places and in different times in history are, in fact, virtues. These qualities would probably include such traits as wisdom, courage, benevolence, justice, honesty, loyalty, integrity, and generosity' (1996: 89).

True, this is not absolutely inconsistent with there being other virtues. But I think it fair to say that most contemporary writers on the virtues make the at least tacit assumption that all the virtues, or at least the important ones, have already been marked out for us by our current terms designating virtues. When a general point about virtue is being made, these standard issue virtues are always the ones chosen in illustration.

However, if a (moral) virtue is an excellence of character and a vice a deficiency of character, why could there not be many virtues and vices that are not on the standard lists, and that are not designatable by a single term or two ('ill will')? Why, and this is a separate point, couldn't there be virtues (or vices) that have come to be recognized only fairly recently, or, indeed, have come to *be* virtues (or vices) only fairly recently? I want to suggest that we cannot do justice to the variety of value and disvalue in the racial domain unless we are willing to accept a positive answer to these questions.[5] In the remainder of the chapter, I will suggest several distinct virtues and vices related to race, ones which standard virtue/vice terminology does not adequately express. Although some of these virtues/vices may be seen as exemplifications of more general ones, this does not mean they are not in some way importantly distinct as excellences of character.

Let us begin by noting that 'racism' itself appears to be a relatively recent vice. The term itself, in English and other European languages, was not used until the first third of the twentieth century (Blum 2002: 3f; Frederickson 2002: 5). This does not mean, of course, that the phenomenon it denoted had not previously existed; but it does suggest, what historical scholarship appears to support, that racism had not hitherto been generally seen as a vice, or more generally, as a wrong or ill. This does not, of course, mean that it was not actually a vice previously, and certainly some abolitionists in the

---

[5] On virtues other than standard issue ones, see Rosalind Hurtshouse's contribution in Chapter 7 of this volume, in which she suggests virtues related to treatment of the environment.

U.S. and Britain and elsewhere recognized prejudice and oppression based on race to be an important evil.[6] This recency of recognition certainly distinguishes racism from Zagzebski's way of thinking about vices and virtues—that one looks cross-culturally and cross-historically for those most generally cited, as a way to discern what are truly virtues and vices. But in addition the notion of race itself, in the sense in which it is understood as part of 'racism', did not come into being in Europe until the fifteenth and sixteenth centuries, and did not come into full flowering in the sense arguably required for our notion of racism until the nineteenth. In that sense, racism could not have been named a vice prior to the fifteenth century at least, and arguably until the nineteenth.[7]

RECOGNITION OF BLACKS

With the example of racism in the background, let me proceed to my proposed examples of racial virtues and vices. I begin with a racial, or race-related, virtue, that I draw from a vignette from Vivian Paley's book *White Teacher*. Paley (in this book) is a kindergarten teacher in a racially mixed school. The book is an account of her attempt to deepen her understanding of how she, a white teacher, can be a good teacher for a racially and ethnically mixed group of pupils.

Paley describes meeting a black parent of one of her black pupils. The parent, Mrs. Hawkins, relates to Paley that in her child's previous school the teacher, who was white, had said to her, 'There is no color difference in my classroom. All my children look alike to me.' Mrs. Hawkins comments to Paley, 'What rot! My children are black. They do not look like your children. They know they're black and we want it recognized. It's a positive difference, an interesting difference, and a comfortable, natural difference' (Paley 2000: 12).

Mrs. Hawkins is asking something from her child's non-black teachers. She wants them to act and be a certain way with her children, and she implies that she wants the teachers to promote those values in her children's schoolmates. Mrs. Hawkins desires that these non-black children be comfortable with her child's blackness, that they see it as a positive and interesting difference, presumably analogous to other racial, ethnic, cultural, religious, and so forth differences among the children.[8] She desires that Paley recognize and affirm the comfort and positivity that her child already feels about his racial identity.[9]

---

[6] The word 'racism' was coined, in response not to anti-black prejudice, discrimination, and oppression, but to Nazism; and it was in response to the Nazi horrors, especially to their full extent revealed only after the Second World War, that the term came into general use, where it was eventually extended to forms of segregation (including South African 'apartheid'), and colonialism rationalized by racialist ideologies, in which persons of non-European provenance were its victims.

[7] Racism is not simply an in-group prejudice against an out-group, a form of prejudice which has certainly existed since human groups have existed. See Frederickson (2002).

[8] When Mrs. Hawkins speaks of her child's blackness as 'natural', I do not take her to be subscribing to the (largely discredited) theory that races are natural kinds, but rather that phenotypic variation of a sort generally associated with race (for example, skin color) is a natural part of human diversity.

[9] I think we can assume that when Mrs. Hawkins speaks of 'black', she is not necessarily embracing an understanding of what it means to be black that an African or Afro-Caribbean might

I want to draw from Mrs. Hawkins's remarks a suggestion of a more general virtue that can be exemplified by adults toward one another. Part of this virtue is recognition, as Mrs. Hawkins says, which I understand in something like Charles Taylor's sense of acknowledging a group or an individual in light of a group identity that is important to her (Taylor 1994). I want, however, to add an element that Taylor only ambiguously includes in his sense of 'recognition' and that is that the non-black view the black person as a *peer* in the shared enterprise or context that provides the setting of the recognition.[10]

The idea of 'peer recognition' rules out a patronizing form of recognition, in which the proffered recognition carries the message that without the recognizer's publicly conferring her recognition on the recognizee, the latter is without legitimate standing. Peer recognition construes the recognizee as a peer—as someone with, and already possessed of, standing equal to one's own in the context in question—and behavior toward the recognizee expresses that peer regard. (The equal standing, for example as a colleague, does not of course require being seen as an equal in every respect.)

Not every particular context is appropriate for acknowledging blackness, or other comparable groups and group identities; for example, the connection between the two parties may be too tenuous, such as riding on the subway with persons of different races. In general, the idea of peer recognition requires a shared or common enterprise, endeavor, or community of some kind. Recognition is appropriate only when the potential target of the recognition desires it. Mrs. Hawkins's view of this matter may not represent all African Americans. Some may desire to distance themselves from their black identity as they understand it. Nevertheless, it can be said that in general, black Americans do desire *some* acknowledgment of their black identity (in appropriate contexts). Even a black person who wishes to be seen first as a lawyer, a Christian, a world citizen, a Bostonian, and so on, rather than as black, would not characteristically wish her blackness to be entirely overlooked, or rendered invisible.

The recognitional virtue I envision here goes beyond recognition in the sense of a mere acknowledgment of a distinct identity, to involve a positive valuing or appreciation of the identity in question.[11] This is not only (although it includes, as Mrs. Hawkins sees it as well) a recognition of the value of the identity *to black people*. It goes beyond this to involve the non-black agent herself regarding the presence of black people as peers in the enterprises she shares with them as likely to be of positive value to those enterprises and, through doing so, enriching her own experience of those enterprises. What is valued, in this virtue, is inextricably connected with the black people's blackness, their racial identity. Of course, not everything that a peer

---

have, but rather a specifically African-American notion of blackness that may or may not be fully shared by other, non-African-American, blacks.

[10] In the beginning of his essay, Taylor clearly differentiates a form of recognition of the other as an equal from recognition of the other in her distinctness (generally a group form of distinctness) from the recognizer. As his essay proceeds, the equality dimension of recognition drops out of the picture. The notion of equality remains in play, but as a purely political and legal value rather than a recognitional one (Blum 1998).

[11] Susan Wolf, in her comment on Taylor's essay, similarly distinguishes 'recognition of the existence' and 'seeing the value' dimensions of what Taylor calls 'recognition' (Wolf 1994: 75).

contributes to a shared enterprise is connected with her racial identity and, indeed, it would involve the wrong sort of valuing to be unable to see that particular blacks, and particular members of any comparable group, contribute in ways unrelated to their racial identity. Nevertheless, in many contexts and enterprises, what is of value will be related to the racial and ethnic identity of the black people involved (in a manner elaborated below). It is this aspect of what is valued that I mean to highlight in speaking of peer recognition and valuing of blacks as blacks, which I will hereafter refer to simply as 'recognition of blacks'.[12]

CONVEYING RECOGNITION

Recognition of blacks, as here envisioned, involves conveying to one's black peers the appropriate forms of recognition and valuing, so that those peers experience themselves as recognized and valued in appropriate ways, at least by the agent herself. (If Lily recognizes her black colleague but he is not similarly recognized in the larger institution within which he and Lily function, then he will not feel himself to be appropriately recognized in an overall way, but may still feel so by Lily.) Having the appropriate attitude of recognition and valuing does not guarantee conveying that attitude to its target(s) in an appropriate manner. Generally, it would be inappropriate, for example, to greet a new black colleague by saying 'I'm sure glad to have a black person around here; we're so undiverse right now.' New colleagues wish their professional merits rather then their racial identity to be in the forefront of one's regard for them.

By contrast, if a black colleague proffers an insight about racial dynamics among the organization's clientele that one sees to be very likely correct and something one's other colleagues would have been unlikely to notice, noting that fact publicly in the setting in which the insight is proffered might be an appropriate way to convey the appropriate race-related recognition/valuing. In doing this, one recognizes the colleague as an individual and as a colleague contributing to a shared goal, and the black identity is part of and appropriately secondary to that colleagueship.

Thus, appropriately conveying recognition and valuing involves particularistic judgment and knowledge, of the particular black persons in question, and of the particularities of the situation. One gets to know how it is appropriate to express

---

[12] One might attempt to characterize the general social conditions in which a more general version of 'peer recognizing/valuing blacks' is a virtue: (a) The group must be a stigmatized, underappreciated, or marginalized group in the society, community, or institution in question. (b) The group must be involved in or have a perspective on the society, community, enterprise, or institution. (c) The group must desire inclusion in the enterprise, society, community, or institution. (d) The group must have a legitimate claim to inclusion in the enterprise, institution, society, or community. From these conditions, one might derive, for example, 'recognizing handicapped persons', or 'recognizing Muslims' (in various nations) as analogous virtues. But it would rule out 'recognizing Basques' in Spain, if Basques do not wish to be part of the Spanish national community. The more general version might then be something like 'recognizing stigmatized, underappreciated, or marginalized groups in their specificity as those particular groups'. The groups could be defined by any number of characteristics other than race, depending on particular context—religion, other creed/political ideology, handicap, national origin, region, sexual orientation, and so on.

such recognition to one's particular colleagues, although some rough guidelines can no doubt be crafted prior to such extensive contact with particular persons. Indeed, there seems a general epistemological dimension to the virtue of recognition. The recognition and valuing of blacks must be grounded in some knowledge of the group that enables the recognizer to have a personal basis for seeing blackness or black people in a positive light. The epistemological requirement here is not overly stringent. The recognizer need not be an expert on black history or culture. A recognizer could recognize that she knows little about black history, culture, or life, and indeed welcome the opportunity to correct her ignorance (though it would not be virtuous to treat the recognized black person as one's only source of such knowledge). Still, she must have some knowledge both to have a positive view of blackness, as well as to know how appropriately to engage in recognizing.[13]

One might also say that, *ceteris paribus*, the more one knows about black life, history, and culture, the better positioned one will be to engage in the appropriate forms of recognizing behavior. Such knowledge will therefore provide the possibility, and indeed the likelihood, of a more excellent form of the virtue of recognizing blacks.

THE COMFORT FACTOR

One general guideline regarding the appropriate form of verbal behavior involved in recognition of blacks is suggested by Mrs. Hawkins's remark that one should be able to refer to black identity and be comfortable in doing so. For discomfort will suggest that the teacher fails to view blackness, or black identity, as something positive or comfortable.[14] Philippa Foot, in her important early virtuist essay, 'Virtues and Vices', says 'a virtue such as generosity lives as much in someone's attitudes as his actions' (1997: 166). This is by now a commonplace in virtue theory. If I offer money to a friend in need, this does not constitute an instance of generosity if I feel resentful toward the friend but have been shamed into this action by another friend. Similarly, referring to black identity but being uncomfortable doing so will not instantiate the virtue of recognizing/valuing blacks.[15]

Furthermore, it would not be adequate to the virtue in question if the non-black person felt comfortable with black people, but only when they avoid anything that

---

[13] Epistemic virtue is also involved in understanding the racial dynamics of one's society. That is independent of the role race-related knowledge plays in affirming and valuing the particular racial identity of racial others. For instance, many white people do not (at least not explicitly, or even consciously) embrace their white identity and would feel uncomfortable with that identity's being recognized. Nevertheless, it is a civic good to understand how white identity functions in society as part of understanding the role race plays in one's own society.

[14] One caveat here: Some teachers might have adopted such a strong belief in 'color blindness', or, more accurately, 'color muteness' (a commitment to not referring to racial identity) (Pollock 2004), that this by itself is enough to produce discomfort in referring to black identity, independent of any specific feelings the teacher has about blacks.

[15] Discomfort may preclude the virtue with which I am concerned here, but it does not preclude all virtue regarding racial interaction. Certainly one can accord an appropriate kind of identity recognition to an ethnic or racial other without feeling comfortable with that person because of that very feature of her identity.

calls attention to their black identity, for example by never mentioning it, nor mentioning or alluding to cultural markers of blackness such as certain foods, music, film stars known to be black, and so on.[16] Thus, the virtue would characteristically require the *absence* of certain kinds of feelings and emotions, such as a feeling of self-consciousness or anxiety in referring to blackness or black people's black identity. However, the excluded emotions in question are not simply the more distinctly racist ones of race-based contempt, fear, delight at the woe of the racial other, satisfaction at their being bested by members of one's own race, and so on.[17] The virtue I envision does presuppose the absence of such emotions, but also those other emotions just mentioned, less clearly rooted in either racial antipathy or an inferiorized view of the racial other.

'Comfortable peer recognition/valuing' of blacks is a virtue both in the sense that it can come in a trait version but can also be manifested by someone on one occasion, without the person's possessing the trait version. That is, a non-black person could have a standing and deeply rooted disposition to view blackness and black identity as natural and positive, and to accord blacks appropriate peer recognition and valuing. Or she could do this on one occasion without possessing the underlying disposition or state.

Recognition of blacks shares two other features with virtues traditionally understood. First, it refers not simply to the performance of particular discrete acts, nor a bare disposition to do so, but to forms of behavior that are inseparable from an underlying sensibility, characteristic emotions, and moral understandings.[18] Secondly, possession of the characteristic in question is only partly within the direct scope of the will. One cannot just *choose* to recognize/value blacks as peers, if one's attitudes and sentiments are not currently aligned with that value. Exemplifying the virtue requires attempting to change one's characteristic ways of thinking and feeling about, regarding, and responding to black people.

Moreover, the value in question involves a good to the agent—the good involved in the black peers' contribution to their shared enterprise as acknowledged by the agent. (The good could exist, however, without the agent acknowledging it.) For

---

[16] David Shipler cites a good example of a non-black (in this case white) person who exemplifies a certain comfort with blackness as long as it is not being called attention to: 'A white boss who loved *The Cosby Show* "became very irate when the youngest daughter named her twins Winnie and Nelson [after the Mandelas] because then the show became too black"' (1997: 135).

It is an interesting question, bearing on the more general issue whether virtues have a built-in success-tracking quality, whether the cultural markers of blackness in question are in some way 'objective', or subjective to the agent. Suppose that a black employee wears some African attire to work, and her white colleague is entirely comfortable with this, but only because she does not recognize the African provenance of the attire. (I am drawing this example from the character played by Anna Deveare Smith in the film *Philadelphia*.) This would seem not to count as comfort with blackness in the sense required. Or suppose a non-black wrongly takes a certain style of speech developed by Indian-American youth to be black and is uncomfortable with it for that reason (though she remains comfortable with blacks who do not exhibit any cultural behavior that she takes to be black). This would also seem to preclude the comfort with blackness required by the virtue in question.

[17] In Blum (2002: chapter 3), I argue that the sort of racial discomfort referred to in the previous paragraph may be, but often is not, rooted in racist views of the other.

[18] See Crisp and Slote in their introduction to *Virtue Ethics*: 'Another striking feature of virtue ethics is its focus on moral agents and their lives, rather than on discrete actions (telling a lie, having an abortion, giving to a beggar) construed in isolation from the notion of character' (3).

those who see virtues as necessarily contributing to the agent's own good, the value in question shares this feature with virtues.[19]

SOME OBJECTIONS TO THE PROPOSED RACIAL VIRTUE

Yet one element of recognition of blacks may seem troubling, calling into question whether it should be seen as a positive value at all, or at least mitigating that value. Why should blacks or 'blackness' as such be valued? For one thing, many contemporary race theorists and scientists have argued that there are no races in the sense in which 'race' is commonly understood; if so, there seems no blackness to be valued (Zack 1998; Appiah 1996). However, although there may be no races, the groups we designate by racial terms are genuine historical groups—groups with a shared history and social existence arising from their having been viewed and treated as if they were genuine races. They are, in that sense, 'racialized groups' (Blum 2002: chapter 8). Especially in the case of blacks in the United States, becoming a racialized group has meant adopting a self-identity as a distinct group, developing cultural forms and ways of life that express that identity and express the historical experience of being an inferiorized and generally stigmatized group. This response to inferiorization has also involved multiple and complex forms of resistance to that inferiorization. In that sense, blacks have developed a positive self-identity out of the negative experience of racialization and racial discrimination. It is this positive identity that is an appropriate focus for the positive valuing that Mrs. Hawkins suggests. And this positive identity provides an answer both to the objection that races do not exist, so there is no 'blackness' to value; and also to the objection that if 'black' is a historically constructed identity, it is so by virtue of being created as a stigmatized and inferiorized identity, and so is not an appropriate object of positive value.

A different worry about this alleged virtue is that it would seem to require stereotyping. What could the 'blackness' or black identity be that is recognized unless it is a set of stereotypes and stereotypical expectations of black people? I would say that such a stereotypical form of this recognition is a corrupted form of the virtue in question, not an inevitable one. A non-black can expect that her activities that are shared with blacks will be enriched by their presence, and will be so in a manner that is in some way related to the historical experience, cultural forms, and distinctive identity of black people, without necessarily expecting specific opinions or types of behavior from the particular black people engaged in the shared activities. To constitute a distinct and coherent identity, blackness need not be stereotyped or 'essentialized', even if it is an identity that has in fact been prey to powerful stereotyping.[20] Surely most black people possess their own black identity in a non-stereotypic manner, as members of any ethnic or ethnoracial group do. When a non-black is interacting with a black person in a way that expresses the appropriate sense of recognition and

---

[19] I am indebted to the editors of this volume for reminding me of this feature of virtues, according to many theories of virtue. I do not myself subscribe to the view that virtues must always be good for their possessor, although most of them will.

[20] How one cognizes group identities without stereotyping is further explored in Blum (2004a).

appreciation, she acknowledges the black person's individual way of understanding her black identity; the non-black should not impose, or expect, the individual black person to have a particular understanding of that identity. So, although recognition of blacks necessarily has a group-focused dimension, it need not involve stereotyping and can be applied to individuals in a way that allows for individuality, for individual forms of appropriation and understanding of that group identity.[21]

A final point of clarification: As I am construing recognition of blacks, in the spirit of Mrs. Hawkins's remark, it necessarily involves a person focus. Merely enjoying cultural products of blacks will not count; it will not count as valuing blackness if someone loves movies with Denzel Washington, Angela Bassett, and Mos Def, but does not wish to be in the presence of black people.[22] It is black *persons* (specifically, peers) who are to be recognized and valued in the appropriate manner.

RECOGNIZING/VALUING BLACKNESS AND THE DIVERSITY RATIONALE FOR AFFIRMATIVE ACTION

Some doubts about recognizing blacks as a virtue may perhaps be dispelled by relating it to the so-called 'diversity rationale' for affirmative action, which was given expression by the majority opinion in the U.S. Supreme Court's 2003 *Grutter v. Bollinger* case. The opinion (written by Justice O'Connor) said that having a critical mass of the major racial groups present in each class in a selective law school was 'a compelling state interest that can justify the use of race in university admissions' (*New York Times* 2003: 2). Several benefits of this policy were cited by the Court—improved understanding of persons of races other than one's own; breaking down racial stereotypes; preparing students for a diverse, multiracial world; more stimulating and enlightening classroom exchanges. The critical mass was justified on the grounds that it made members of the racial minorities in question feel sufficiently comfortable in the institution; that goal, in turn, was regarded as necessary for the others. Without it, the minorities would not participate in the intellectual and social life of the institution in a way that would contribute to the enhanced learning of all.

Justice O'Connor assumed that because 'of our nation's struggle with racial inequality' in a society in which 'race still matters', racial identity is likely to affect the views of members of a given racial group (*New York Times* 2003: 3, 5). At the same time, she rejected the view that this truth entails that 'minority students always (or even consistently) express some characteristic minority viewpoint on any issue' (3). Indeed, undermining the latter belief is one of the purposes of attracting a mix of students of different racial groups in sufficient numbers, so that the actual diversity of viewpoints within each group is made manifest to the larger community.

---

[21] Although persons can put an individual stamp on the meaning of their racial identity, there are obviously limits to these meanings. There is no getting around the way that racial identity is an entirely involuntary identity, yet one fraught with great social significance.

[22] On liking black culture while remaining prejudiced toward blacks, see Ralph Ellison's vignette of a white youngster enjoying a Stevie Wonder song while spouting racist epithets at blacks swimming at a public beach (1986 (essay originally 1977): 21).

In a way, the Court could be taken to be affirming the value of recognizing blacks, or at least a part of that value. (I will now refocus the discussion on blacks specifically, rather than racial minorities more generally.) The University of Michigan Law School's policy aims to make black students feel comfortable and recognized in the institution. But what is being implied about individual non-black students with respect to this virtue or value? Certainly the University is saying that it is good for the non-black students that black students are present in sufficient numbers—good for them educationally, personally, and perhaps as citizens as well. And this benefit depends on the black students' blackness. Presumably, also, the non-black students recognize that they are benefiting in these ways from the presence in sufficient numbers of the black students, and to that extent they are pleased that the black students are present.[23]

At the same time, Justice O'Connor's argument does not go as far as saying that the non-black students should exemplify or cultivate the virtue of recognizing blacks (or other groups), or, more generally, that each group should extend a comparable recognition and valuing to the others. For it is not implied that the non-black students are to do anything to make the black students know that they are appreciative of their presence, in contributing to the non-blacks' opportunity to learn and grow educationally and personally. It is not a deficiency in the argument about affirmative action that it fails to engage with this level of individual virtue. But it does suggest a way that a virtue approach illuminates something about the terrain in which affirmative action operates that the standard social, legal, and moral philosophical arguments about affirmative action characteristically do not.

I cite the affirmative action diversity rationale in part to lend credence to recognizing blacks as a virtue; but also to bring out how the social, legal, and moral arguments involved in this rationale are enriched by the virtue perspective that highlights the attitudes, values, and qualities of character that are desirable in a community that has been created according to that rationale.

CIVIC RACIAL EGALITARIANISM AS A VIRTUE

Peer recognizing of blacks—and specifically the dimension of that virtue involving the positive valuing of blacks in shared enterprises and contexts—is not equivalent to seeing and treating members of racial groups other than one's own (in particular, non-blacks seeing blacks) as civic *equals*. The differences between these two virtues are instructive. Civic equality is particularly pertinent to the case of blacks in the U.S. because for so long blacks were legally 'second class citizens', and the civic standing of blacks is still problematic in some respects. Blacks are stereotyped and stigmatized as welfare dependents, as complainers, as not adhering to the American work ethic—all markers of civic deficiency in the minds of many white Americans.[24]

---

[23] Richard Light found that students at selective universities were virtually unanimous in being pleased at the racial diversity on their campuses, and in feeling that their academic and personal development was enhanced by that diversity (Light 2001: chapters 7 and 8).

[24] See Sears, Sidanius, and Bobo (2000); Roberts (1997).

Let us see 'civic egalitarianism' (here, a virtue, rather than a set of beliefs) as involving regarding the other as deserving of all the rights and privileges of a citizen of one's polity, such as political expression, political participation, having one's voice heard and taken seriously in appropriate civic venues, the right not to be discriminated against in education, housing, and other basic domains of social existence, and so on. To see someone as an equal is not simply to lack certain objectionable attitudes toward that person. It is to have a positive take on that person as someone whom one has reason to respect and to take seriously in civic venues. For example, it involves not only recognizing that it is illegal to engage in racial discrimination in housing, but recognizing why and how it wrongs the discriminated-against individual for her to undergo that discrimination. It means not only countenancing persons giving voice to political positions one disapproves of, but recognizing why such political expression is or could be important to that individual, and appreciating why she has as much right to that expression as one does to one's own political expression. Thus it also requires that one be disposed to protest against injustices committed against one's civic equals, to sympathize with their plight, to feel indignation and anger toward the perpetrators of discrimination, and the like.

I am interested in a sub-variety of civic egalitarianism related to race—'civic racial egalitarianism'—and will again use blacks as my primary example, although other racial and ethnic groups have historically presented comparable concerns. This virtue has both an individual and a group dimension. It involves recognizing that blacks are a distinct socially and civically significant group, whose history of being treated unequally raises particular concerns about their being treated equally. So the virtue will involve being concerned that blacks as a group come to have equal civic standing. One's response to individual instances of, for example, discrimination in housing, will involve recognizing the larger group context; one will, for example, be inclined to regret, protest, and support redress of discrimination not only because it wrongs the discriminated-against individual, but also because it bears on the group's civic standing. The civic racial egalitarian is not merely someone who lacks racism (in the form of racial inferiorizing attitudes) toward certain racial groups. This is part of the complexity and variety of racial value and disvalue. Merely lacking racism does not guarantee the appreciation of the importance of the civic domain and of the wrongness of discrimination in public or public-related venues, nor the range of attitudes and reactions that express that appreciation, involved in civic racial egalitarianism.

Viewing blacks as civic equals involves certain considerations not necessarily present with respect to every ethnic, racial, or other socially distinct group. 'White cultural values fundamentally disvalue African Americans', Mary Waters writes in her study of West Indian immigrants to the U.S. (Waters 1999: 148). Although African Americans have formal rights equal to those of other Americans, they are often both stigmatized and discriminated against in major life activities and domains.[25] Waters's study is instructive in this regard. Her respondents—mostly blacks from the English-speaking Caribbean—are shocked by the stigmatization of African Americans, and of

---

[25] See Loury (2002) for a sustained argument that 'blackness' remains a stigmatized identity in the U.S. See also M. R. Banaji (2001).

blackness more generally, that they find when they arrive in the U.S.; they have not experienced anything like this in their countries of origin, which are nevertheless in no way racially egalitarian societies. Many, Waters finds, attempt to distinguish and often distance themselves from African Americans in hopes of exempting themselves from this stigma, though they share 'blackness' with African Americans.

If there is a pervasive devaluing of blacks and blackness, then seeing and treating blacks as civic equals poses a challenge not necessarily present in the case of other groups.[26] For most non-blacks, seeing blacks as civic equals will mean becoming aware of the cultural influences on themselves that foster the devaluing of blacks, acknowledging their own subjection to those influences, and finding ways to counter them. It is not necessary to claim that all non-blacks will need to engage in such forms of struggle (and certainly not to the same degree) in order to see blacks as civic equals. Perhaps some persons are brought up with such strong egalitarian beliefs, and a set of natural or learned predispositions to see their fellow citizens as equals independent of race, that civic racial egalitarianism comes relatively easy to them. This is a dimension of moral luck comparable to that present in all virtues. What for most people stand as obstacles to compassion, courage, honesty, and the like are, for various reasons, barely operative with respect to other persons.

Philippa Foot says, 'As Aristotle put it, virtues are about what is difficult for men' (1997: 169). She understands this difficulty in terms of temptation to be overcome, or a deficiency (e.g. of motivation) to be made good.[27] This is a plausible view about virtues; the patterns of action, feeling, and understandings constituting virtue must be developed by human beings against a background of difficulty of some sort. At the same time, although this is true of human beings in general, it can well be more true of some than others. Courage comes easier to some than to others; the latter must work hard to achieve the level of courage that comes easier to the former.

The race-related virtues I discuss here follow the same pattern. They come more easily to some than others, but in general they involve a kind of difficulty, an over-coming of deficiency, or moral effort. Yet there is an important difference here from the way Foot sees the difficulty or deficiency involved in virtue. For her this is always purely individual; a particular agent lacks natural empathy, or feels pulled by fear not to want to stand up to the bully. But in the race case, the deficiency is in the larger culture and in that sense affects individuals in light of their particular social location. The difficulty involved in seeing blacks as civic equals is socially produced rather than a purely individual psychic deficiency.

Treating blacks as (civic) equals and recognizing blackness are not the same virtue. Someone who sees blacks as equals need not also value blackness. She may entirely avoid sharing in the larger society's stigmatizing of blackness and entirely respect

---

[26] Arguably, some other ethnoracial groups besides blacks—for example, Native Americans, Mexican Americans, Puerto Ricans—suffer some form of stigmatization.

[27] Von Wright (1963: chapter 7) takes a similar, slightly narrower view, that the virtues are all forms of self-control. Zagzebski proposes a more plausible, weaker criterion—that there be at least some chance that the person develop the corresponding vice rather than the virtue—that is still consistent with the idea that virtues are not merely natural dispositions but require moral effort of some kind (1996: 105).

blacks as fellow civic participants, without herself having a positive take on blackness as a distinct cultural/communal entity. This does not mean that the civic egalitarian must also be an assimilationist—someone, described earlier, who accepts blacks in shared enterprises only insofar as they do not call attention to their blackness. Such a person would not be a civic (racial) egalitarian in my sense. The egalitarian cannot be put off by the appropriate and reasonable invoking of blackness and black identity; but she need not attach any distinctive positive value to it either. The civic racial egalitarian need not feel that her shared civic activities are enhanced by the presence of black people; she need only feel that they are not diminished.

I am not certain, however, if the implication goes in the other direction. That is, could a valuer of blackness fail to be a civic racial egalitarian? It might seem not, since a valuer of blackness would also have to have entirely rejected any stigmatizing of black people or blackness, and would in that way have to see blacks as equals. But perhaps a civic egalitarian must have a deeper appreciation than is required by recognizing/valuing blackness, of the importance of the civic domain, and of how equality operates in that domain. A civic racial egalitarian would perhaps be more likely to be angry and indignant about a serious case of racial discrimination against blacks than would a valuer of blackness.

Note that even though recognizing/valuing blacks is not the same as egalitarianism, this does not mean that the valuer of blackness thinks *more highly of* blacks than of other ethnoracial groups regarded as equals. It is not a matter of comparing the value of different groups. The blackness valuer could also value Chinese-ness, Asian American-ness, Mexican American-ness, and so on. She need only see a distinctive value in different groups; she need not see that value comparatively.

Racial egalitarianism with regard to blacks also involves an epistemic dimension, but it is different from that in recognizing blacks. The non-black civic egalitarian (with respect to blacks) will characteristically know that blacks are stigmatized in her society and that she herself to some degree participates, even if unwittingly, in that stigmatizing. She will characteristically recognize that racial ideologies and existing and persistent socio-economic inequalities encourage us to view racially disadvantaged groups not as equals but as inferiors, and that these inferiorizing tendencies can be difficult to acknowledge because they run embarrassingly contrary to the ideal of equality in which we are meant to believe. For most non-blacks, such knowledge is required for them to work themselves toward an attitude of genuine civic equality with blacks, though I have allowed that a rare few non-black persons might be able to attain the civic equality stance without having been touched by the stigmatizing of blacks.

The difference in the epistemic dimension of the two virtues is this. With regard to valuing, one must particularistically value blacks and blackness and thus know particulars about black history, culture, and life as a basis for doing so. With regard to civic egalitarianism, this sort of particularistic knowledge is not necessary; all that is required is that one recognize that blacks have been subject to stigmatizing and inferiorizing assumptions and treatment that have prevented them from attaining full civic equality, and that continue to pose psychic obstacles to blacks' struggle to achieve civic equality.

SEEING OTHERS AS INDIVIDUALS

I have delineated two distinct race-related virtues—racial civic egalitarianism, and recognizing blacks—as part of attempting to show that the domain of race-related value is multifarious, and that a virtue approach can help us to access this complex domain. I will now discuss a third virtue, that exists in moral complementarity with recognizing blacks. This is the virtue that might be called 'seeing others as individuals and not solely or predominantly as members of racial groups'. Although there may be many particular contexts in which one is perfectly happy to be regarded simply as a representative of one's racial group, overall most persons wish others with whom they come in contact in more than a cursory fashion to treat them as individuals and not simply as a member of (racial) groups. But being so treated is not something one can take for granted. It requires the sort of moral effort, sensibility, and attentiveness involved in virtue. Both cognitive and emotional forces incline us to see other persons through the lens of group identity rather than saliently perceiving their individuality.[28] Race shares with other group identities this homogenizing feature, but it is intensified in the case of race (or at least it can be so argued). Seeing others racially inclines us to see them, wrongly, as fundamentally the same. In the United States, this homogenization has been particularly strong in relation to Asians and blacks; members of these groups tend to be seen by whites (and, often, by the other group) as members of homogeneous groups. (Because people tend not to homogenize their own group, and because whites are the dominant group in American society, whites are less subject to this homogenizing force.) Getting past these social and psychological barriers so as to see racial others as individuals therefore involves moral understanding and effort.

The virtue of 'seeing others as individuals . . .' (I use the ellipsis to indicate that the virtue in question is set specifically against the background of racial group identity) comprises a complex of dispositions of behavior, feeling, thought, forms of awareness, and perception. It involves, for example, one's mental and emotional reactions to a particular member of the group in question not merely being the same as those triggered by the group itself. It means being vividly aware of particularities about the person in question not shared by other members of the group. It means not making unwarranted assumptions about that individual based on her group membership.

Seeing others as individuals rather than predominantly as members of (racial) groups is a race-related virtue like the other two virtues so far discussed. It is a *different* virtue from recognizing blacks, and the two pull in somewhat different directions. Recognizing blacks requires giving someone's racial identity its due in one's interactions with another person. 'Seeing others as individuals . . .' involves not allowing that group racial identity to loom too large in one's response to the other person.

---

[28] Examples of cognitive and emotional factors inclining us to see others in terms of group membership rather than as individuals are that it is mentally easier to think in terms of groups than to make the effort to see the particularity of individuals, and that social distance between groups reinforces the perception of groupness over individuality. The large literature on stereotyping explores these matters. See, for example, Oakes et al. (1994).

It might seem that the particularistic dimension of recognizing blacks already encompasses the virtue of seeing others as individuals, since one needs to be aware of individual particularity in order to see how appropriately to give recognition to a particular black person. But how the recognizee relates to her black identity and how she would be likely to experience various expressions of recognition is only a part of her individuality. To oversimplify a bit, recognizing blackness takes account of someone's individuality in relation to her black identity, while seeing others as individuals in light of their racial identity takes account of her individuality as going beyond her black identity.

Our various group memberships are partially *constitutive* of our individuality; they do not only threaten to mask it. In addition, our individuality is expressed in the particular meanings we give to our particular group identities, the extent to which we embrace our group identity or distance ourselves from it, and the like. That is why an individual black person at a particular period in her life might wish to distance herself from black identity as she understands it, or as she recognizes others to understand it. Still, to be seen as an individual involves not being seen too exclusively in terms of a specific one of those memberships, however construed by the individual.

Combining the two virtues requires sensitivity and judgment; yet clearly it is a manageable goal. In our initial example, Mrs. Hawkins surely wanted her child to be seen and valued both as an individual *and* as black. She did not think the two incompatible, nor did Paley in commenting on the exchange with Mrs. Hawkins.[29] (Moreover, though the two virtues are distinct, it is quite possible to exemplify neither one—neither to see members of a racial group as individuals nor to give their group membership proper recognition. A racist in Garcia's sense, for example, does neither.)

Note that seeing others as individuals is not the same as the virtue of civic racial egalitarianism, or even of egalitarianism of any kind. Seeing someone as an individual is compatible with not seeing her as a civic equal; and seeing her as a civic equal is compatible with privileging her group identity in a way that is not consistent with seeing her as an individual. The lived sense of a racial other as *equal* is different from the lived sense of the racial other as an *individual*. The two virtues are not, of course, inconsistent with one another, and they do naturally go together; but they are distinct.

'COLOR BLINDNESS' AS A RACE-RELATED VIRTUE

I mentioned earlier that one reason many people fail to see the diversity of race-related value and disvalue is that they think that color blindness should be the overarching principle governing all racial matters including interracial interactions. We are now in a position to assess this idea. 'Color blindness' does not really refer to a single principle or value. In public policy contexts, it is taken to mean that social policies should not mention race, and thus should not explicitly call for the disparate treatment of

---

29 Paley's book and a later companion volume, *Kwanzaa and Me*, are particularly good resources for seeing the operation of these two complementary virtues. These books can be read as a record of Paley's journey toward attempting to give appropriate recognition (and valuing) to her pupils' racial identities, while continuing to see them as individuals.

different racial groups. Several commentators have noted that some public policies which do not mention race are nevertheless intended to have race-differentiated effects (Blum 2002: chapter 4; Loury 2002). It is not clear, then, if it is the absence of intended effect or the lack of explicit mention of race that should count as color blindness.

The policy debate is not necessarily pertinent to our concerns with personal virtues. Yet here too there is no clear agreement as to what color blindness entails. Should it be equated with 'colormuteness', that is, not making explicit (or implicit?) reference to persons' racial identities in personal interaction (Pollock 2004)? Or should it be understood as a principle governing behavior toward other persons—that one should never treat persons differently because of their racial identity? Finally, it could also be taken to mean that one should strive to be blind to—actually not to notice—the physical characteristics taken as markers of racial identity, as the teacher cited by Mrs. Hawkins could be taken to have claimed, when she said: 'All my children look alike to me'. Finally, color blindness could be something about not what one notices, but what one attaches importance to; the principle could be that one should not attach any importance to racial identity. (This in turn could lead to the 'no differential treatment' form.)

The 'colormuteness' form seems normatively superficial, so let us take the other three as plausible candidates.[30] There are certainly contexts in which color blindness in any of these three senses is entirely appropriate, or even morally required. I will not attempt to characterize such contexts. But of the three race-related virtues I have discussed, recognizing/valuing blacks obviously requires attention to racial identity in thought, feeling, and behavior. An all-encompassing color-blind stance would make it impossible to realize this virtue. Seeing others as individuals and not only as members of racial groups seems closer to a form of color blindness, since it does not make specific positive reference to racial identities. Still, this virtue is not color-blind. It does not prescribe *ignoring* racial identity in how one sees or treats persons; it says only that persons should be seen as individuals and not *only* as members of racial groups. Insofar as one's racial identity is a part of one's individuality, color blindness would be at odds with this virtue. If I am Mexican American and think that a colleague, Revan, attaches no significance to this identity and tries to ignore it, I may well feel that Revan is unable to see me for the individual I am. So treating others as individuals, not only as members of racial groups, is distinct from color blindness (in some of its plausible forms), and can be at odds with it.

Of the three, only civic racial egalitarianism involves (one type of) color blindness. For it says that racial identity should not affect one's seeing and treating fellow citizens as civic equals; they should be treated as equals, no matter of what racial group. It must be noted, however, that this does not entail that persons' racial identities should be ignored, nor that they should never be grounds for differential treatment. For, I have argued, to acquire the virtue of civic racial egalitarianism, a non-black must

---

[30] Although colormuteness does not seem a plausible normative principle, its implementation can be harmful, in not allowing people to pay the appropriate attention to racial differences, for example, with respect to racial inequalities (Pollock 2004).

characteristically be aware of the role anti-black racism has played in relegating blacks to less than civic equality. This will, then, often mean paying a certain kind of attention to blacks' racial identity, and possibly engaging in race-sensitive behavior (or supporting race-sensitive policies) intended to support blacks' efforts to secure civic equality.

In sum, color blindness in its several forms cannot serve as an overarching virtue governing race relations in interpersonal and civic settings. It may, in some form, survive scrutiny, and take its place among the panoply of race-related virtues (Blum 2002: chapter 4). But at most it will be one among several such virtues.

ARE RACE-RELATED VIRTUES TOO LOCAL TO COUNT AS VIRTUES?

Two objections can be raised to calling the race-related qualities of character that I have discussed virtues. First, it might be felt that they are too local in character, and thus of insufficient significance, to count as virtues. They pertain only to the racial domain of life, while standard issue virtues such as justice, honesty, integrity, and compassion are not so limited but apply across multiple domains.

Three replies can be made to this objection. First, standard issue virtues themselves vary quite a bit in the extent to which they apply in daily life. Honesty is arguably a virtue that is pervasively relevant. But courage seems a virtue that may not be pertinent to the lives of many persons for long stretches of time. Moreover, in particular societies and contexts within those societies, all three of the race-related virtues so far mentioned seem applicable across a broad range of contexts. If a non-black interacts with blacks on a daily basis, all three virtues will frequently be appropriate (especially if racial egalitarianism is construed not only as civic egalitarianism but as human, social, and political racial egalitarianism as well). So, depending on the social world involved, frequency of contexts of appropriateness will not necessarily favor all standard issue virtues over these race-related ones.

Furthermore, race-related virtues are arguably of vital importance in the United States, plagued as it is by a continuing legacy of troubling racial inequities in many domains of life, as well as segregative processes and other factors making interactions between those of different ethnoracial groups less than ideal.[31] So, for example, rejecting the negative value often attached to blackness and attaching positive value to blackness (valuings involved in civic egalitarianism and recognizing blacks, respectively) in one's interactions with black people and in one's life more generally are arguably important civic or civic-like virtues. These two virtues are somewhat analogous to but are more demanding than a general courteous respectfulness in dealing with those of ethnic, religious, political, racial, and linguistic groups other than one's own. This civic courtesy requires a lower level of engagement with the structures and processes of social value attached to different racial groups than do the two race-related virtues discussed.

---

[31] On racial inequities in important life domains, see Loury (2002: appendix).

Moreover, both these virtues arguably bear some empirical relationship to social justice. This is true of the racial civic egalitarian by definition; she must care that blacks and other racial groups not suffer from race-based injustices. Recognizing blacks is less directly civic in import; but it seems plausible that a recognizer of blackness will care about blacks and therefore about social injustices from which they suffer.

Secondly, I would note John Doris's argument that local virtues have an empirical reality that standard issue virtues generally lack (Doris 2002). Some people are 'honest in the context of family life' but not 'honest at work'; but only a very very few are 'honest' overall, in the way generally understood in attribution of traits. Although Doris does not attempt to characterize the form of localism in question, it seems plausible to see the race-related virtues I have delineated as, on Doris's account, more likely to have psychic reality than standard issue virtues. (How pertinent this point is to the normative adequacy of a proposed virtue is another matter.)

A third response to the 'too local' objection would be to question why more local worthy traits of character should not be thought of as virtues even if they lack the scope of some of the most important and pervasive standard issue virtues. They would still involve the psychic complexity of virtues, encompassing behavior, forms of perception, feelings, modes of moral understanding, and the like. They would still be traits of character that would enable persons to live well. One would have to give up the idea that a virtue must be for human beings as such, rather than applying much more to some societies (or other all-encompassing social contexts) than others. (The race-related virtues would be much less pertinent in racially homogeneous societies.) But jettisoning that view seems to me a gain for virtue theory. We seem already to accept some departure from this universalist ideal in the notion of role-related virtues, such as virtues attached to particular professions.

A second objection to calling the race-related traits virtues might be that they are no more than subspecies of more general, standard issue, virtues—or the same virtues applied in distinct contexts. Civic racial egalitarianism would be a subspecies of civic egalitarianism, which can perhaps be seen as a form of justice. With regard to treating the racial other as an individual and recognizing blacks, it is less clear of what standard issue virtue these would be subspecies. It is not justice, for example, since justice does not require the positive valuing of blackness. One possible candidate is respect. Indeed, Taylor's argument in 'The Politics of Recognition' can be read as suggesting that both regarding others as equals and appreciating others' individuality are forms of a common respect (Taylor 1994).[32] In turn, the latter form of respect can be seen as one variety of an intermediate subtype of respect, namely respect for distinctness, which also comes in the form of appreciating persons' *group* distinctness.[33] The latter, in turn,

[32] For Taylor, respect is not distinctly construed as a virtue, but only as a value. However, it can be construed as a virtue, and so can the sub-forms that Taylor derives from it. That is, respect can come in a trait form (perhaps 'respectfulness') and in a non-trait form that still refers to a complex of behavior, attitude, emotion, perception, and so on.

[33] I criticize Taylor for not fully appreciating that recognition of someone as an equal is not the same as recognition of her as a distinct individual (Blum 1998). Appiah criticizes Taylor for failing to appreciate that the group and the individual forms of 'respect for distinctness' can be at odds with one another (1994).

can be seen as a more general form of (at least a part of) the virtue of recognizing blacks. So Taylor can perhaps be read as suggesting a more general version of all three of our race-related virtues, as well as suggesting that all are forms of respect.

However, Taylor's 'recognizing group difference' would not actually be the more general form of the recognizing of blackness virtue, since Taylor's virtue does not require the morally significant element of marginalization, underappreciation, or stigmatizing of the group. This condition brings out that 'recognizing blacks' could conceivably disappear as a virtue in a particular society, if blacks became fully integrated and accepted, and the stigma of blackness entirely disappeared. Similarly, if blacks no longer came to constitute a group with a distinct group identity, or, in another direction, if certain cultural nationalist strands of thought became pervasive in the black community, so that blacks no longer wished to be included in major institutions and venues, it would also cease to be a virtue. That the virtues in question are not timeless but socially and historically context-dependent in no way impugns their moral significance in the contexts in which they do apply.

Even if the three virtues were all forms of some kind of respect, this would simply suggest that respect comes in importantly morally distinct sub-varieties that need to be distinguished from one another. The respect involved in civic equality differs from the respect involved in recognizing blacks, and both differ from the respect involved in seeing others as individuals not only as members of (racial) groups. Whether they are seen as fully distinct virtues seems less significant, once one recognizes that they involve both distinct values and distinct psychic structures, as I have argued above.

Moreover, there are certainly forms of the virtue of 'respect' that do not require the kind of positive group identity affirmation involved in recognizing blacks. I can respect someone with whose political views I deeply disagree. I do not value his views, but I respect him, and, let us say, I recognize that his, to me regrettable, views are honestly and conscientiously arrived at. I respect him and I respect his holding those views; but I do not confer value on the political identity he has adopted. We have reason to confer value on black identity, and perhaps other ethnoracial identities, that we do not have for some other sorts of identities. In this sense, there are certainly morally distinct forms of respect.

Not only are the three more general forms of the virtues I have discussed—recognizing groups, civic egalitarianism, and seeing as an individual . . .—distinct from one another, but, I have argued, the specifically racial form of each of the virtues is psychologically and morally distinct (at least in respect of involving distinct moral capacities and understandings) from other forms. Someone might exemplify the racial form but not some other form. For example, he might be a civic racial egalitarian but not a civic gender egalitarian, seeing blacks as civic equals, but not women. Someone might be a recognizer of blacks, but not a recognizer of Muslims, or of Mexican Americans. Though I would not advocate that each of these sub-forms differentiated by group be thought of as a fully distinct virtue, their distinctness does require recognition in a fully adequate account of them as morally valuable traits of character.

I have argued that the domain of race is a rich venue of value and disvalue. Drawing on Jorge Garcia's work, I have attempted to show that the virtue tradition provides important resources to articulate the values in question. Amplifying Jorge Garcia's account of 'racism', I have mentioned several distinct vices (racial ill will, racial inferiorizing, racial disregard). I have also suggested several distinct race-related virtues, which are more than the mere absence of these forms of vice—peer recognition/valuing of blacks, civic racial egalitarianism, and treating persons as individuals rather than solely as members of racial groups. I argued that these virtues are distinct from one another, and have suggested thereby that there are likely to be other virtues and vices of a race-related character.

REFERENCES

Appiah, K. A. (1990). 'Racisms,' in David Theo Goldberg (ed.), *Anatomy of Racism*. Minneapolis: University of Minnesota Press, 3–17.

——(1994). 'Identity, Authenticity, Survival: Multicultural Societies and Social Reproduction,' in A. Gutmann (ed.), *Multiculturalism*. Princeton Princeton University Press.

——(1996). 'Race, Culture, Identity: Misunderstood Connections,' in K. A. Appiah and Amy Gutmann, *Color Conscious: The Political Morality of Race*. Princeton Princeton University Press.

Banaji, M. R. (2001). 'Ordinary Prejudice.' *Psychological Science Agenda*, 14 (Jan–Feb): 8–11

Blum, L. (1998). 'Recognition, Value, and Equality: A Critique of Charles Taylor's and Nancy Fraser's Accounts of Multiculturalism,' in C. Willett (ed.), *Theorizing Multiculturalism: A Guide to the Current Debate*. Malden, MA: Blackwell's.

——(2002). *'I'm Not a Racist, But...': The Moral Quandary of Race*. Ithaca, NY: Cornell University Press.

——(2004a). 'Stereotypes and Stereotyping: A Moral Analysis.' *Philosophical Papers*, 33/3: 251–89.

——(2004b). 'What Do Accounts of "Racism" Do?', in M. Levine and T. Pataki (eds.), *Racism in Mind: Philosophical Accounts of Racism and Their Implications*. Ithaca, NY: Cornell University Press.

Boxill, B. (ed.) (2001). *Race and Racism*. New York: Oxford University Press.

Crisp, R., and Slote, M. (1997). 'Introduction,' in R. Crisp and M. Slote (eds.), *Virtue Ethics*. New York: Oxford University Press.

Doris, J. M. (2002). *Lack of Character: Personality and Moral Behavior*. New York: Cambridge University Press.

Ellison, R. (1986). 'Little Man at Chehaw Station,' in *Going to the Territory*. New York: Random House.

Foot, P. (1997). 'Virtues and Vices,' in Roger Crisp and Michael Slote (eds.), *Virtue Ethics*. Oxford: Oxford University Press, 163–77.

Frederickson, G. (2002). *Racism: A Short History*. Princeton Princeton University Press.

Garcia, J. L. A. (1996). 'The Heart of Racism.' *Journal of Social Philosophy*, 2: 5–45 (reprinted in Boxill (2001) and Harris (1999)).

——(1997). 'Current Conceptions of Racism: A Critical Examination of Some Recent Social Philosophy.' *Journal of Social Philosophy*, 28 (2): 5–42.

——(1999). 'Philosophical Analysis and the Moral Concept of Racism.' *Philosophy and Social Criticism*, 25 (5): 1–32.

——(2001). 'Racism and Racial Discourse.' *Philosophical Forum*, 32 (2): 125–45.

Harris, L. (ed.) (1999). *Racism*. Amherst, NY: Humanity Books.

Hursthouse, R. (1999). *On Virtue Ethics*. Oxford: Oxford University Press.

Light, R. J. (2001). *Making the Most of College: Students Speak Their Minds.* Cambridge, MA: Harvard University Press.

Loury, G. (2002). *The Anatomy of Racial Inequality.* Cambridge, MA: Harvard University Press.

New York Times, 'Excerpts From Justices' Opinions on Michigan Affirmative Action Cases,' June 24 (2003). 1–9 <http://www.nytimes.com/2003/06/24ATEX.html?pagaewanted= print&position=>.

Oakes, P., Haslam, S. A., and Turner, J. C. (1994). *Stereotyping and Social Reality.* Oxford: Blackwell's.

Paley, V. G. (1995). *Kwanzaa and Me: A Teacher's Story.* Cambridge, MA: Harvard University Press.

_____ (2000 [1979]). *White Teacher*, with a new preface. Cambridge, MA: Harvard University Press.

Pollock, M. (2004). *Colormute: Race Talk Dilemmas in an American School.* Princeton: Princeton University Press.

Rachels, J. (2003). *The Elements of Moral Philosophy* (4th edition). New York: McGraw-Hill.

Roberts, D. (1997). *Killing the Black Body: Race, Reproduction, and the Meaning of Liberty.* New York: Vintage.

Sears, D. O., Sidanius, J., and Bobo L. (eds.) (2000). *Racialized Politics: The Debate About Racism in America.* Chicago: University of Chicago Press.

Shipler, D. K. (1997). A *Country of Strangers: Blacks and Whites in America.* New York: Vintage.

Taylor, C. (1989). *Sources of the Self. The Making of Modern Identity.* Cambridge, MA: Harvard University Press.

_____ (1994), 'The Politics of Recognition,' in A. Gutmann (ed.), *Multiculturalism.* Princeton: Princeton University Press.

Von Wright, G. H. (1963). *The Varieties of Goodness.* London: Routledge and Kegan Paul.

Waters, M. (1999). *Black Identities: West Indian Immigrant Dreams and American Realities.* Cambridge, MA: Harvard University Press.

Wolf, S. (1994). 'Comment,' in A. Gutmann (ed.), *Multiculturalism.* Princeton; Princeton University Press.

Zack, N. (1998). *Thinking About Race.* Belmont, CA: Wadsworth.

Zagzebski, L. T. (1996). *Virtues of the Mind: An Inquiry into the Nature of Virtue and the Ethical Foundations of Knowledge.* New York: Cambridge University Press.

12

Virtue and a Warrior's Anger

Nancy Sherman

And what about when your warrior's anger goes home? What is it like with his wife and children? Is it useful then, too? (Cicero, *Tusculan Disputations*, 4.54 (Graver 2002))

Marvin served as a marine in Okinawa during the Second World War. The fighting during April and May, 1945 was ferocious, with men typically spending fifteen days at the line, armed with bayonets and knives, living on three to four hours sleep, pumped with Benzedrine (speed) for those campaigns in which they had to fight for forty-eight hours straight. Battle rage still visits Martin, in anger at employers whose voice and attitude bring back the feel of being given military orders, in mini-flashbacks that transform a car that cuts him off on the road into an enemy with a one and a half ton weapon out to hurt him. Recently, Marvin was taking a walk in a neighborhood park when young boys on mountain bikes crossed his path. They weren't supposed to be riding in the park, and he bellowed out a threat to them: 'Tomorrow I start target practice.' When they left, he about faced and marched through the woods as if he were in the front again. At that point another cyclist came into view, and his fury surged. His body started to tremble and he imagined his hand coming down on the boy's collarbone and breaking it. 'That would immobilize him. Then he would be at my mercy.' Battle rage had exploded a half-century after the campaign (from personal conversations with Marvin Brenner).

Hugh Thompson, the American helicopter pilot who ordered his side gunner to open fire on the GIs if they blocked his attempts to stop the My Lai massacre, returned to Vietnam some thirty years later. A frail, aging woman who survived the massacre rushed up to meet him. She implored, 'Why didn't the people who committed the murder come back with you . . .' She finished her thought without pause but the interpreter's translation lagged behind. '. . . so that we could forgive them.' This was not how Thompson thought the sentence would end. At that point, he recalls, 'I totally lost it. How could this woman have compassion in her heart for someone who was so evil? She's a better person that I am' (from personal conversations with Hugh Thompson).

1. INTRODUCTION

Anger is as much a part of war as weapons and armour. The greatest of war epics, Homer's *Iliad*, is arguably about warrior anger—about the fury of a warrior like Achilles and the injuries to honor that can lead to that fury. Anger 'whets the mind for the deeds of war', says Seneca, reporting the conventional ancient view.[1] In modern terms, it is linked with the adrenaline rush that allows non-killers in civilian life to become killers in war. But unlike weapons and armour, anger, warns Seneca, is not easily thrown off after the battle.[2] It is a 'runaway emotion', easy to turn on but hard to turn off. Combat veterans, like Marvin, described above, all too often live out that truth. They bring home a rage that has lost its targets and finds new ones that are far less appropriate. In recent news, the point was brought home in an all too ugly incident in Fort Bragg, North Carolina. Four Army men in the elite special operation forces returned from Afghanistan, each to kill their wives in brutal fashion. However complicated the motives, on the surface, at least, the combat anger button couldn't be turned off.[3] Anger that might have been adaptive in combat became sorely maladaptive at home.

Issues of warrior conduct have, in some ways, always been central to virtue ethics. Courage, after all, on Plato and Aristotle's view, is pre-eminently a warrior virtue that only derivatively finds a home off the battlefield. And pivotal to the discussion of courage is anger. Thus, in the *Republic*, Plato regards anger as the special province of the warrior class. It is the fire in a warrior's belly, or more precisely, in the *thumos*, or spirited part of the soul. While Aristotle explicitly denies that courage is itself animal-like rage, he nonetheless leaves room within his account of virtue for a kind of moral outrage that might motivate many a warrior to combat. The Stoics, however, deny any such role for anger. The renunciation becomes most explicit in Seneca's *On Anger*. Anger, like other emotions, Seneca argues, is the expression of vulnerability; it is a sign not of might or strength, but of defensiveness. It is an exaggerated response to injury and loss, from which the self-sufficient person should be able to detach. The rage of an Achilles is a 'bite-back' impulse of revenge, a vindictiveness that is misplaced on the battlefield and off.

In this essay, I examine this Stoic position in greater depth. The discussion is informed by my own experience as Distinguished Chair in Ethics at the United States Naval Academy (1997–9) and by extensive interviews and conversations I have had over the years with military personnel in the United States and Great Britain.[4] With Seneca, we might feel uncomfortable about commanders exploiting their subordinates' feelings of revenge as part of combat motivation. Apparently, this is just what Captain Medina of the Charlie Unit did the night before his unit carried

---

[1] *On Anger* 1.9 using throughout Cooper and Procopé (1995). For the Latin text, Seneca (1989).
[2] *On Anger* 2.35.1.
[3] For this terminology regarding combat anger, see Shay (2002); also Shay (1994).
[4] The interviews are background for my book, *Stoic Warriors* (OUP, 2005). This essay is an abbreviated version of one of the chapters.

out the My Lai massacre in March 1968. Sergeant Kenneth Hodge later recalled Medina's pep talk: He made it clear to us that 'this was a time for us to get even. A time for us to settle score. A time for revenge—when we can get revenge for our fallen comrades' (Bilton and Sim 1992: 98–9). But is retaliative anger itself a bad thing for a soldier to feel? Consider anger in response to terrorism or violations of just conduct in war (such as the use of human shields, or feigned surrenders, or combatants disguised in civilian garb). Presumably, resentment and indignation are here justified, and I would add (though not all would agree) some impulse to retaliative punishment. But how does that impulse then translate into battlefield action and attitude, given the constraints of just conduct in war that guide the honorable soldier's actions? And, moreover, how does one respond to the objector who argues retaliative anger, even in a soldier trained to kill an enemy, is an ignoble thing? In exploring these questions, I turn to Aristotle for guidance, but also to Seneca, who raises the challenges any defender of anger within virtue must meet.

The plan of the chapter is as follows: I set the scene (in Section 2) by taking a brief glimpse at the *Iliad* and its traditional view of warrior anger. I then move (in Section 3) to an Aristotelian analysis of anger and to the claim that anger plays a normative role in both military and civic virtue. I next turn (in Sections 4 and 5) to the Stoic critique of anger as limned by Seneca in *On Anger*. I focus on the Stoic claim that emotions, like anger, are irrational and require elimination. I raise objections to this view (in Section 6), in part, by turning to concrete, contemporary examples of what we might call rational warrior anger. Finally, I conclude the discussion in (Section 7) with Stoic recommendations for treating anger. Here, I take as background the Stoics' self-description as doctors of the soul who advocate psychic *therapeia*, or what we would call, psychotherapy.

2. INSULT, INJURY, AND REVENGE

In locating anger or *thumos* in a special function and seat of the soul (*psychē*), Plato paints a psychological portrait of the notion of a warrior's rage familiar to every Greek through Homer's Achilles. Achilles is the angriest, 'most violent man alive', proclaims Agamemnon (*Iliad* 1.170). But Achilles has much angry company in the *Iliad*—both divine and human. Famously, it is Agamemnon's own vindictiveness that sets the epic in motion. Apollo and his priest demand that Agamemnon, chief of the Achaeans, surrender to them his war bride, Chryseis, daughter of the priest, in return for a handsome ransom. Agamemnon will not have it. Chryseis is his war prize (his *timē*), a sign of his honor and status; to snatch the prize is tantamount to stripping him of his medals before his troops. He dismisses the priest, only to face Apollo's wrath in nine days of relentless arrows that cut down his men 'in droves'. Finally, Agamemnon relents, but he won't tolerate a full dressdown before his men. He'll give up the girl, but not without a proper replacement. 'Fetch me another prize,' he orders, 'else I alone of the Argives go without my honor' (1.138–40).

(The pressures to surrender the symbols of military honor bring to mind more recent examples. In the spring of 1996, it was alleged that the 'v' device that ADM

Michael Boorda, Chief of Naval Operations wore (for valor in engaging the enemy in face to face combat) misrepresented his actual combat record in Vietnam. The facts surrounding the allegation are complex, but not insignificant was that Boorda had been appointed CNO in the wake of the Tailhook sexual abuse scandal in 1991 within the naval aviation community and many of the old guard in the Navy believed that the new leadership, including the new CNO, had become overly supportive of women's causes (Philpott 1995). On 16 May 1996 Boorda committed suicide by shooting himself in the chest, in the very place where he once wore his medals.)[5]

For Agamemnon, restoration of honor is a matter of a transfer of fungible goods— he'll replace his lost war bride with Achilles' (*Iliad* 1.217–21). This is the insult that unleashes Achilles' unrelenting fury. He digs his heels in and refuses to fight under Agamemnon's command. The plot that ensues is well known: While the hero stays home, Patroclus, Achilles' beloved comrade-in-arms, disguises himself in Achilles' famous arms only to meet his death at Hector's hand. With this fresh and inconsolable loss, Achilles' wrath turns from Agamemnon to Hector. If Achilles' anger towards Agamemnon is a response to jealousy and competition, then his second anger toward Hector is a response to both loss and survivor guilt—for Achilles, after all, yielded to Patroclus' entreaty to let Patroclus impersonate him by wearing his armour. The friendship of Achilles and Patroclus has become the archetype of war buddies. We can speculate, as many have, whether this friendship was, in addition, a homosexual relationship of the sort the U.S. military demands be kept under wraps and that the Greeks welcomed as a fitting part of an aristocratic boy's development. But the more pressing point is that Achilles has, in some real sense, died with Patroclus. 'My spirit rebels—I've lost the will to live.' 'The man I loved beyond all other comrades, loved as my own life—I've lost him' (18.105; 94–6). Achilles experiences what many soldiers feel in losing their 'brothers'—that it should have been themselves, that they would give anything to switch places. In Achilles' case, he would give anything to undo the original switch. His may be the archetypal case of survivor guilt.[6]

Revenge once again consumes Achilles, but this time it launches him into the war effort—to 'fight in the front ranks' with a 'soldier's strength and nerve' (9.857–61; 65). We might argue that Achilles' revenge has finally found an appropriate object: for a warrior is entitled to some sense of restitution, even if we moderns bristle at the idea of a *private* vendetta, on the battlefield or off. But the revenge turns ugly quickly with Achilles' desecration of Hector's corpse by dragging it facedown around Patroclus' tomb. The poet's voice finally becomes decisive: Achilles' rage transgresses the decorum of war: 'That man without a shred of decency in his heart . . .'. He outrages even 'the senseless clay in all his fury' (22.398–405; 24.64–5). Priam's tragedy, however, will be softened by the gods' intervention that keeps Hector's body intact, despite Achilles' brutality.

---

[5] I have been told that the Commandant of the Marines, Mike Hagee, removed three medals before being sworn in, because he lacked properly documented citations. In this regard, several officers have told me that medals are often awarded in haste without proper documentation.

[6] For a moving discussion of survivor guilt in the context of a study of Vietnam veterans, PTSD, and Homeric values, see Shay (1994, 2002).

But not all soldiers' families are so lucky. I am reminded of a conversation I once had with Sybil Stockdale, the wife of ADM James Stockdale, the senior POW in Vietnam.[7] The husband of a close friend of hers had served in Laos and was listed as missing in action. But many years after the war, her friend received confirmation that her husband had been killed shortly after his capture. The news came from an officer who had served beside her husband, and who had seen his severed head used by the enemy in a gruesome game of soccer.

Homeric Achilles is the archetype of warrior anger gone amok. Still, Homer never gives up on the conviction that anger, and in particular revenge, has military utility. Properly restrained, it can be a reasonable combat motivator. The Stoics, as we have anticipated, deny the claim. A soldier who relies on anger is a soldier who has surrendered control. We shall turn to Stoic arguments momentarily. But first we must turn briefly to Aristotle. For it is against his claims about the role of emotions in the virtuous life that the Stoics propose an alternative.[8]

3. ARISTOTLE ON ANGER

If Plato is the first to construct formally a psyche with *thumos*, or an angry part, Aristotle is the first to analyze anger (*orgē*, as he tends to call it) as part of a systematic study of the emotions, or *pathē*. The account appears in the *Rhetoric* and is intended for orators in the business of manipulating the emotions of a jury or assembly. But despite its practical aim, Aristotle's study is both deep and broad, offering a unified account of emotions unparalleled in the history of philosophy.

Roughly speaking, Aristotle proposes what psychologists (and many philosophers) today call an appraisal theory.[9] As we shall see, the Stoics put forth the view in radical form. On such a view, emotions are constituted by judgments or appraisals about one's situation. To be more precise, an appraisal is an evaluation about the goodness or badness of some perceived or imagined event. Thus, anger requires an evaluation that one has been unjustly slighted by another, fear that there is present harm or danger, grief that something valuable has been lost. In this sense, emotions are more like thoughts than brute feelings or sensations, or as William James once held, the awareness of physiological changes in the viscera and musculature, such as knots in our stomach or tension in our hands. Aristotle never denies that most emotions will have a certain kind of 'feel'. As he puts it, they are 'accompanied' by pleasure and pain, but those 'feels' cannot constitute the emotion independent of the thought content to which they attach. Moreover, it is the thoughts and not the 'feels' that allow us to identify specific emotions. Thus, although emotions may sometimes announce

---

[7] From an interview, October 2001.

[8] For a more thorough review of Aristotle on the emotions, see Sherman (1989), Sherman (1997).

[9] The theory is the reigning view of emotions in cognitive psychology—e.g. Lazarus (1984), Scherer (1993), Frijda (1986), and Oatley (1992). See Zajonc (1984) for an important criticism. Among philosophers, see DeSousa (1987), Stocker (1996), Goldie (2000), and Nussbaum (2002) for a sampling.

themselves to us through a physiological or psychic feeling (i.e. a racing heart or an uplifted mood), those feels on their own are not determinate enough to convey just what emotions we are experiencing (Schacter and Singer 1962; Cannon 1927). The same sort of knotted stomach can be part of fear or indignation, just as a feeling of uplift can be part of excitement or hope. In addition, Aristotle claims, emotions often include a reactive desire, an 'action tendency', as contemporary psychologists call it, that motivates us to action or reactive behavior. Combining the elements, Aristotle says, anger involves an 'apparent' (i.e. perceived, judged, or imagined) 'wrongful slight to self or those near to one' 'accompanied by pain' and issuing typically in a 'desire for revenge' which can bring its own pleasure (*Rhetoric* (*Rh.*) 1378a30–2, my trans.). Aristotle doesn't formally distinguish between emotions as dispositions and as episodes (e.g. anger as irascibility vs. anger as a discrete outburst), in the way contemporary theorists do, but something like the distinction is often implicit in his remarks.

As part of a handbook for orators, the account relies on conventional views about the objects of anger—that it is directed at those who belittle us or hold us in contempt, and that the angry person seeks some form of revenge. As such, the remarks fit, more or less, the Homeric world of hubristic insult and revenge, and indeed, the few quotes Aristotle approvingly cites are from the *Iliad*. But Aristotle is keen to show that the warrior has no exclusive hold on anger, and that the non-battlefield world is ripe with its own kinds of rage and provocation. So, Aristotle suggests anger is appropriately directed at the person who insults us by forgetting our name one time too many, or who regularly makes a joke of what we wish to be taken seriously, or who is eager to listen to gossip about us or dwell on our weaknesses (*Rh.* 2.2). The substantive point is that anger is a response to disrespect, to 'being dissed', to use the street lingo, however local or shared the forms by which we show respect and its opposite.[10]

Significantly, Aristotle has little to say about anger that is objectless (such as *angst* or generalized irritability), and he does not dwell for long on the kind of anger whose object is apparent failure or frustration or helplessness (*Rh.* 1379a22–4). Also, he typically thinks of anger as including some pressure for aggressive behavior, whether or not that behavior is, in the end, acted out or inhibited. Furthermore, he thinks of anger as a state directed against a particular individual—'not humankind in general' (1378a35). We might wonder if this excludes anger against a group or nation, such as the Al Qaeda or the Japanese in the Second World War. We might speculate that Aristotle would answer 'no,' to the extent that any collective group is a determinate enough entity to be held accountable.

Equally, *things* are not the proper objects of Aristotelian anger. My car doesn't deliberately wrong me, so pounding it when it breaks down is misplaced anger. In many such cases, I am really angry with myself for negligence or my mechanic for incompetence. But, of course, not all frustration of this sort is implicitly directed at someone who can be held accountable. In the soldier's life, due diligence, endless training, drilling in conditions of deprivation and stress cannot themselves ensure for

---

[10] Note, Aristotle tends to focus on variants of *moral* anger (i.e. responses to being wronged or slighted); the anger (and hate) that is part of ill will is implicit in the attitude of slighting and its subspecies, contempt, spite, and insolence—*NE* 1378a14.

the perfect execution of missions. There will always be the fog of war, an unexpected mine, inhospitable weather, terror at things more gruesome than any simulation can represent. Some degree of frustration at the unexpected seems an unavoidable part of a combat soldier's lot. And we tend to think of that frustration as either a species of anger or, at least, a distant cousin of it.[11]

Aristotle's appraisal view entails that emotions 'share in some way', as he puts it, in rational capacities (*Nicomachean Ethics* (*NE*) 1103b30). Up to this point, we have been exploring this as a descriptive claim—that emotions are, in part, cognitive constructs. But when Aristotle uses the phrase in the *Nicomachean Ethics*, he means principally that emotions can be made rational. They can respond to reason, 'as a child listens to a parent' (1103b31–2). Thus, that emotions share in reason has both a descriptive and a normative sense. Talk of virtue emphasizes the normative sense— the virtuous persons stands well with respect to her emotions in so far as they are *properly* informed and guided by reason. Aristotle often puts the point by saying that emotions, like actions, must hit the mean. This does not require, as many interpreters from the Stoic period onward have insisted, that appropriate Aristotelian emotions must always be moderate, with no sign of either vehemence or mildness. In his more careful formulation, Aristotle's meaning is clearer: 'The person who is angry at the right things and with the right people, and further, as he ought, when he ought, and as long as he ought, is praised' (1125b32–3). Extreme anger may be exactly the right response in certain circumstances.

So it seemed for some peacekeepers in Bosnia constrained by rules of engagement that left innocents to perish in areas scheduled by the Serbians for ethnic cleansing. The hands-off approach made them feel complicit in the cleansing, though some of their commanders insisted that to remove Bosnians from their homes would itself amount to complicity in the cleansing. When the young officers returned home, they brought with them anger and guilt that would not abate. This is captured well in a BBC dramatized documentary, 'Peacekeepers'. In one scene, a returning reservist lashes out at a whining child in a supermarket for making a scene: Doesn't she know that children in war zones have something *real* to cry about? The mother of the child scoops her away from the raving man. Another newly returned veteran flies into automatic rage when the whirring motor of an earth tiller suddenly becomes enemy artillery. He attacks the person standing nearest to him—his girlfriend, eight-months pregnant.

Aristotle holds that to fail to be angry at the things one ought is the mark of either foolishness or servility (*NE* 1126a2–8). But if one can't turn off anger, however legitimate its initial object, is it still servility to abstain? Might not abstinence, as the Stoics suggest, be a better kind wisdom?

Still, Aristotle has high hopes for the kind of psychic harmony that tames emotions under reason's rule. He insists that the cognitive grounding of emotions makes even anger, in principle, responsive to reason in a way that brute appetites or cravings can never be. Anger, he says at one point, 'seems to listen to argument' even

---

[11] See *Rh.* 1379a22–7 where Aristotle seems to include frustration as a kind of anger.

though it can often 'mishear' it, like a hasty servant who 'muddle[s] the order' (*NE* 1149a25ff.). The Stoics question Aristotle's optimism. Isn't anger more like a disease that needs a doctor than a servant that needs a good talking to? Moreover, they will demand, even if emotions are purely cognitive states (as they themselves hold), why should we assume they are states that use reason *well*. Why should we assume that the intense anger, often felt by combatants in a war zone, knows proper limits? With these anticipations, it is time to turn to the Stoics.

4. STOIC ABSTENTION

In a lesser known dialogue by Plutarch, 'On the Control of Anger', Fundanus, the principal speaker, compares withholding anger to learning sobriety. Anger, like drink, is hard to control once indulged. It is best to give it up entirely and practice full abstention. Fundanus speaks from first hand experience of this AA (Alcoholics Anonymous) method. He, himself, first passed 'a few days without anger, sober and wineless days, as it were', and then a 'month or two', pure of the taint. Though he knows anger is the kind of disease that requires lifelong therapy, the cure seems for now, at least, to be sticking: he is no longer angry towards his household slaves, and in general, is more 'courteous in speech'. Those he interacts with benefit from his new humane (*philanthropon*) spirit, but he himself is the greatest beneficiary.[12]

Plutarch, here, in Stoic voice, rehearses the Roman and Hellenistic preoccupation with anger and its eradication. The wrath of an Achilles is fixed in all minds. But so too are the atrocities of political and military leaders, like Caligula or Nero, and too, the abuses of lesser men—heads of household, like Fundanus, who given the status system of Rome, exercise near monarchical powers over their slaves and dependants.[13] The havoc anger wreaks on others is a constant theme, but even more so, the havoc it wreaks on one's own soul.

The concern strikes a chord with the American military. Stanley Kubrick's notorious drill sergeant in *Full Metal Jacket* paints a picture of sadism with which few professional soldiers would wish to be identified. 'You will be a weapon,' he bellows at his marine inductees at Parris Island. 'But until that day, you are not even a thing.' He screams louder with eyes filled with fury, 'I am hard, but the more you hate me, the more you will learn. Here you are totally worthless. Do you Maggots understand that?' 'Goodnight, Ladies,' he barks, with a sexism woven deep into his anger.

The portrait is a caricature. But that is not to say there aren't caricatures of the drill sergeant in the military itself. In fact, many enlisted military men and women with whom I have spoken would argue that the caricature is the norm. But they also argue that even if drill sergeants typically abuse their power, the role of drill sergeant is itself

---

[12] Plutarch's *Moralia: On the Control of Anger*, 464c–d; 453D (Plutarch 2000). For abstaining from anger on the AA model, see also Seneca, *On Anger*, 2.12.3.

[13] See Cooper and Procopé (1995), for helpful remarks to this effect, in their introduction to Seneca's *On Anger*.

legitimate. By definition, his or her job is to be relentless and 'in your face'. The very point of boot camp is to break down a self in order to build it up again. This, they insist, is what they signed up for. And it is what, at most moments, they are willing to take.

But what is it to break down a self and build it up again? Presumably, part of what is meant is that boot camp experiences crush cockiness and selfish independence. And they teach the sacrifices of service that come to be motivated through horizontal bonding, even when ordered top down. In a deeper sense, boot camp remolds identity so that one becomes a member of a larger cause that binds one to another and to a mission. Most military instructors I have spoken to at the service academies—be it the Naval Academy, West Point, the Air Force Academy, or Coast Guard Academy—insist that the process of breaking down a self ought not, in the ideal case, depend upon either sadism or a response of brute fear. A subordinate must trust that a superior is stripping neither himself nor his subordinates of dignity. We might flesh out the idea by arguing that guilt or moral anxiety comes to replace the fear of a coercer when subordinates can respond to demands and punishments as having legitimate authority, and to a commander as setting reasonable norms (Velleman 1999). The commanding officer who is admired and emulated by his subordinates as a role model can still 'break down' his subordinates, but through a process that involves respect for their capacity to assess the legitimacy of his norms.

While the Stoics would concur that proper disciplining cannot rely on anger, they nonetheless insist that *mock* bullying that makes use of *mock* anger can have a critical role. Indeed, they inveigh against the Peripatetics that 'faking it' can work just as well as showing real anger, with the added benefit, that fake anger, unlike the real thing, remains within an agent's control. Seneca and Cicero make the point in the context of oratorical technique. The orator may need to show the 'guise of doing harm', says Seneca, without actually feeling anger. And Cicero says, in a similar tone, 'even if the orator is not angry himself, he should still make a show of anger in his words and gestures, so that his delivery may kindle anger in the hearer.'[14]

The implication is that the drill sergeant may need to do the same. His subordinates may need to feel the palpable pressure of a cruel punisher whom they can fear during a training session, even though they know in the back of their minds that the commander is no sadist. They play his game for their own advantage. They feel real fear—they are not play-acting that—but it is real fear in the context of a staged drill. Still, there is a crucial structural factor at work that is disanalogous to the oratory case. In the soldier's case, opting out of the play-acting brings 'real' terrible consequences that are simply not there for the orator's audience. Failing in the military drill *is* frightening and humiliating. Thus, the fear is not only a response to the mock bullying anger of a drill sergeant, but also to the real consequences that would ensue were one to fail. The drill sergeant's role is just to 'play' on those fears. And his anger is 'mock' precisely in the sense that it is less a 'read out' of what he is really

---

[14] Seneca, *On Anger* l.6.l, 2.11; 2.14; 2.17. Cicero, *Tusculan Disputations = TD* 4.43.

feeling than a social signal designed to communicate the costs of failure and whin-ing.[15] His job is to make you buy into the system and be frightened of 'screwing up'.[16]

Still, few military educators underestimate the temptation to engage in *real* bul-lying and scapegoating. At the Naval Academy, a handful of entering second-year students, or 'youngsters', as they are called, are selected each spring to become squad-ron leaders for the incoming freshmen or 'plebes' during 'plebe summer'. They will be junior drill sergeants, in effect, marching their troops in formation around the base, toughening them with grueling physical fitness regimens, and in general, overseeing their initial indoctrination into military life. It is easy to overstep the boundaries of this job, especially when the indignities of one's own suffering during plebe sum-mer are still fresh. Annapolis summers can be blistering hot with humidity that often brings the heat index well over 110 degrees Fahrenheit. In the old days, punishment for a slacker in the unit might have consisted in the entire squad doing remedial push-ups into the high double digits, without any break for water afterwards. These days, this is on the banned list as a clear form of bullying.

Yet when training that toughens physical and moral fiber is the explicit goal, the line between sternness and abusiveness can be hard to draw. Marine colonels and Navy captains with whom I taught often took it as their mission to knock the 'Rambo' out of their young cadets. 'They have simply watched too many Rambo movies,' one officer lamented to me. They are too ready to flare up, he complained, in the name of warrior glory. Others worry that some of their students, like Einstein, the brainy RIO (Radar Intercept Officer) in Ward Carroll's naval aviation novel, *Punk's War* (2001), may not themselves be a Rambo, but will end up in the cockpit next to one who is all too eager to use his trigger finger. The worry is about sadistic anger, whether used against subordinates or the enemy.

Indeed, in the back of some officers' minds at service academies and ROTC pro-grams are the careers of a Lt. Calley or Capt. Medina and the atrocities to which warrior rage can lead. Many of the midshipmen I taught had, initially, only a shad-owy grasp of the events that unraveled in My Lai. But on the base were a handful of Vietnam veterans, in particular Marines who struggled hard in Vietnam, often at great cost to their own troops, to make the distinctions that Calley and Medina failed to make between combatant and non-combatant in an enemy that often deliberately blurred that line. In their minds, as military educators, Stoic abstention from warrior anger was a way to avoid another My Lai.

5. THE IRRATIONALITY OF ANGER

Seneca dedicates *On Anger* (*De Ira*) to his elder brother, Novatus, who served as Gov-ernor of Achaea in 51–2. Although Novatus, himself, apparently did not need lec-tures on irascibility (indeed he is remembered by some for his 'sweetness'),[17] the essay

---

[15] For a relevant debate within the social psychology of emotions on emotions as 'read out' vs. emotions as social signals, see Jakobs, Manstead, and Fischer 1999.

[16] I owe thanks to Alisa Carse for helping me to see this point.

[17] See Griffin (1992), 319, n.5, 84, n.5; also Cooper and Procopē (1995), 15–16.

which is addressed to him stands as a bold teaching to those who *do* need exhortation. Seneca opens the essay with a voyeuristic glimpse at the face (and body) of anger:

Eyes ablaze and glittering, a deep flush over all the face as blood boils up from the vitals, quivering lips, teeth pressed together, bristling hair standing on end, breath drawn in and hissing, the crackle of writhing limbs, groans and bellowing, speech broken off with the words barely uttered, hands struck together too often, feet stamping the ground, the whole body in violent motion . . . the hideous horrifying face of swollen self-degradation. (*On Anger* 1.1.3–4)

Like theatergoers watching at a safe distance, we often find fascination in the gruesome. And Seneca's portrait may be intended, in part, to feed our appetites. But however titillated we may be, few among us would wish to be at the receiving end of such a hideous face or themselves wearing one. 'What can the mind be within if the image is so foul?' What is reflected on the face is only 'a tiny fraction of its true ugliness' (2.36.1).

The look of anger, Seneca says, can terrorize in the way a hideous mask strikes fear in a child (2.11.2). Indeed, the face is a mask we read all too well. Research confirms the point. We are exquisite readers of faces and anger is one of the faces we read instantly, from early childhood onward.[18] But it is what we *do* in anger, and not just what we communicate through our eyes or mouths that Seneca worries about most. Anger, Seneca declares, is responsible for far too many of the atrocities to which Romans have grown accustomed:

No plague has cost the human race more. You will see slaughter, poisoning, charge and sordid counter-charge in the law-courts, devastation of cities, the ruin of whole nations, persons of princely rank for sale at public auction, buildings set alight and the fire spreading beyond the city walls, huge tracts of territory glowing in flames that the enemy kindled. Look and you will see cities of greatest renown, their very foundations now scarcely discernible—anger cast them down; deserts, mile after mile without inhabitant—anger emptied them . . . look upon gathered throngs put to the sword, on the military sent in to butcher the populace *en masse*, on whole peoples condemned to death in an indiscriminate devastation. (1.2.1–3)

Seneca could just as well be describing the anger that underwrites many of the atrocities of our own time—the butchery *en masse* in Rwanda, the desolation of Kosovo, the fiery inferno at the World Trade Center. The horrors of war, just and unjust, Seneca suggests, are the work of unrestrained rage. Seneca's style, here and elsewhere, is hyperbolic. But more than any author, he outlines for us the disutility of anger and the inherent difficulties of keeping a lid on its excesses. And with a 'can-do' attitude, familiar to the military, he insists that eliminating it is a practical possibility. We shall have to ask whether, indeed, vice lurks in all or even most species of anger and whether trying to root it out, is, as Seneca insists, the best way to 'cultivate our humanity'.[19] But in order to assess Seneca's specific claims about anger, we need to understand the Stoic conception of emotions more generally.

---

[18] For a lively piece on Paul Ekman's studies of the facial expression of emotion and its implications for law enforcement, see Gladwell (2002).

[19] *On Anger* 3.43.5; see Plutarch, *On the Control of Anger*, 464d for an anger-free soul as a humane (*philanthropon*) soul. Also, see Nussbaum (1994) for an important discussion of this.

Anger, Seneca tells us, is a 'departure from sanity' (3.1.4). But all ordinary emotions, on the Stoic view, are such departures. More specifically, they are perverted cognitive or rational constructs.[20] So, Seneca claims, anger, like emotion in general, 'cannot . . . come into being except where there is a place for reason'. But 'all the same, it is the enemy of reason'.

In viewing emotions as cognitively constituted, the Stoics follow Aristotle. But they take their leave from him in holding that emotions are completely determined by their cognitive nature. They are uncompromisingly judgments or beliefs in a psyche that is itself undivided and homogenously cognitive. In this way, a unitary, rational mind comes to replace the bipartite and tripartite psyches of Aristotle and Plato. As perverted cognitive constructs, emotions are judgments that are, in principle, mistaken or false. The task of Stoic enlightenment is to recognize this and submit to a radical therapy (*therapeia*) that will cure one of ordinary emotions and their habits. The underlying assumption is that it is possible to have dominion over our emotional lives.

The Stoics elaborate in more detail. Emotions are judgments or beliefs in so far as they are voluntary assents to appearances or impressions regarding goods and evils. As Seneca explains, 'anger is . . . set in motion by an impression received of a wrong. But does it follow immediately in the impression itself and break out without any involvement of the mind? . . . Our view is that it undertakes nothing on its own, but only with the mind's approval' (2.1.3–4). Thus, emotions, however spontaneously experienced, are mediated by an appraisal, conscious or unconscious, which is voluntary. They are voluntary in the sense that while we may be 'struck' by impressions, we nonetheless accept or 'assent' to those impressions—for example, in the case of fear, that something in our midst is threatening. In addition, they involve an assent to a second judgment that certain reactions or affective responses (e.g. fleeing or trembling) are appropriate.[21] The overall claim is that emotional experience is, in a substantive way, voluntary.

The view runs counter to much ordinary thinking about emotions. Emotional language is filled with passivity. We are 'bowled over' by love, 'overcome' with grief, 'paralyzed' by fear. And while emotional experience doesn't always leave us helpless victims, there is often lag time before we are able to take charge. We are seduced by impressions, the Stoics will suggest, and give them our assent improperly. The Greek word for emotion, *pathos*, underscores the point. It derives from the verb *pathein*, to suffer or endure, and our Latinate term, 'passion', preserves some of that gloss. The Stoics, however, demand that we cease to view emotions as events that merely happen to us. However possessed we may feel by emotions, we are the possessors, ultimately 'in charge' of our experience. Undoubtedly, the Stoics, once again, push their claim too far. But their views, nonetheless, give us insight into ways in which we *can* take responsibility for our emotions.[22]

---

[20] *Tou logou diastrophos*, Von Armin (1924) (*SVF* I 208).

[21] On the two-judgment view, see *TD* (Cicero 2002) 3.24, 4.14, and Graver's commentary. For further discussion, see Sorabji (2000), 29, Brennan (1998), 335, White (1995), 230–2.

[22] For further related discussion, see Sherman (1999a, 1999b, 2000).

The ancient Greek Stoics classify all emotions into four basic types that divide along two major axes: they are about either goods or evils, and focused on either the future or the present/past. So desire (*epithumia*) is directed at the appearance of a future good in the offing, fear (*phobos*) at the appearance of a future evil. Pleasure (*hēdonē*) is a judgment of a good in the present or past and distress (*lupē*) a judgment of evil in the present or past. All other emotions are conceived as subspecies of these four generic ones.[23] So, for example, the Stoics, fixing on the revenge motive often linked with anger, classify anger as a desire, alongside sexual appetite and love of wealth and honor.[24]

Although the Stoics take emotions to be fully cognitive, this does not entail, on their view, that emotions are flat or affectless. Emotions are accompanied by a kind of mental tension or arousal—'shrinkings' and 'swellings', 'stretchings', 'contractions', and 'tearings'. In Zeno's novel metaphor, emotion is a 'flutter'. Thus, locating emotion in a unitary, rational soul need not detract from emotion's characteristic feel. Zeno underscores the point by adding that the belief must be fresh (*prosphatos*), again, a striking metaphor meant to call up associations with freshly cut meat or corpses that haven't yet decomposed.[25] Cicero, in the *Tusculan Disputations*, gives a temporal gloss to the term, translating with the Latin *recens*. But, of course, emotions like anger can linger and bite (*TD* 3.83)[26] long after a perceived offense. So 'recens' cannot be restricted to a temporal meaning. Cicero himself adds that a judgment remains fresh 'so long as it retains some force (*vis*), some liveliness (*vigeat*) or, as it were, some greenness (*viriditatem*)' (3.75).

At the heart of the Stoic doctrine, as we have said, is the view that emotions are false beliefs, mistaken judgments. They are assents to a mistaken conception of what is good and evil. Reviewing the Stoic conception of happiness or *eudaimonia* is important here. The Stoics regard virtue alone as sufficient for *eudaimonia*. It is the only proper object of choice, the only real good constitutive of happiness. Everything else, as Diogenes Laertius reports—'life, health, pleasure, beauty, strength, wealth, reputation, noble birth and their opposites, death, disease, pain, ugliness, weakness, poverty, low repute, ignoble birth and the like'—(essentially, the Aristotelian list of external goods in *NE* I.10–12) are 'indifferents' (*DL* 7.101–3). Among the indifferents, some will be 'preferred' (*adiaphora kat'eidos proēgmena*)—'things that are in accordance with nature', natural advantages better to have than not to have.[27] But even preferred indifferents are not the sort of things that can make a life happier or more self-sufficient. They are not genuine goods that can make a difference to happiness, in the sense of doing real benefit or harm. As Cicero puts it in *De Finnibus*,

---

[23] *Arius Didymus* 2.90, 19–91, 9 in Stobaeus (1884)=Long (1987a) 65E.

[24] We may think it better classified as a kind of distress at present evil, and close cousins with some emotions that fall under that genus. (The list includes malice, envy, jealousy, pity, grief, worry, sorrow, annoyance, mental pain, and vexation.) But note, in the conversion of ordinary emotions to more rational ones (*eupatheiai*), nothing corresponding to distress will survive—for the only genuine evil that could arouse rational distress is wrongdoing, and the sage is not capable of that. In contrast, emotions corresponding to appetites do survive as rational wishes (*boulēseis*).

[25] For insightful discussion, see White (1995), 230.

[26] Using Margaret Graver's trans. (2002).   [27] See Stobaeus (1884), 2.79,1–80.

they contribute no more to happiness than stretching or contracting a finger or having an odd or even number of hairs on one's head (3.51–2). The Stoics flag the difference between the genuine goods constitutive of happiness and the indifferents by labeling the first as 'chosen' (*haireta*) while the second are 'preferred' (*proēgmenon*) (*De Finn.* 3.51–2). And it will turn out that fine or rational emotions (*eupatheiai*—the only legitimate form of emotion for a sage) will be true judgments about these real goods and evils.

The doctrine of genuine goods and indifferents has important implications for the emotions. For, ordinary emotions are, as the Stoics stipulate, typically ways of taking interest in the sorts of goods that constitute externals or indifferents. To feel anger at an unwarranted insult is to be attached to certain views of oneself that can be lost or tampered with, in the way reputation or honor can be; to fear is to care about threats to such things as health, life, or the health or life of one's children or spouse; to love is to invest in someone outside oneself whom one cannot control or fully protect from the evils of the world; to pity is to view undeserved loss and tragedy as evils that diminish a person's well being. In short, many emotions express attachments and losses to things we cannot control. They express an interest in things, the Stoics would say, that lie beyond inner virtue—the one good over which we have full dominion. In so far as we experience emotions of the above sort, we don't fully grasp the real values of things. We misjudge or make mistaken appraisals. We are taken in by the attractiveness of vivid appearances when we should withhold assent. Given these tendencies, it is clear why a Stoic like Chrysippus demands a therapy to cure the soul of its emotional ills. To tolerate and cultivate ordinary emotions is to encourage false appraisals of good and evil. And so the Stoics advocate *apatheia*, freedom from emotions as a way of securing our rationality.

Emotions are irrational, the Stoics claim, in an additional, perhaps more intuitive sense. By stipulation, they are false judgments of goods and evils. But, also, they are simply excessive. They are heady, impulsive, and magnify the good and evil assessed. They are 'excessive impulses', in Zeno's original formulation. Angry feelings are especially excessive, on Seneca's view. They are like 'bodies in free fall' that 'have no control over themselves'.[28] They drive the mind 'headlong'. Chrysippus' metaphor is apt here. Imagine a runner whose pace doesn't allow him to stop suddenly. In a similar way, emotions rarely proceed at a walking pace; they exceed the measure of natural reason.[29] Excess leads to other evils of irrationality: so anger, Seneca insists, can be unreliable in its judgments, like a serpent whose fangs become innocuous once the venom is dried out. And it can be capricious, leading us to treat individuals in arbitrary ways (*On Anger* 1.17.5–7).

The goal of moral education is to make more accurate calibrations of the place of externals in one's life. And it is the sage who perfectly realizes the goal, and thus comes to release himself from the neurosis of ordinary emotional experience. But significantly, the end result is not that he becomes emotionless. Rather, he now

---

[28] *On Anger* 1.7.4; 3.1.4; also 3.16.2.
[29] Galen, *On Hippocrates' and Plato's Doctrines* in DeLacy (1984), 4.2.10–18 on Long and Sedley (1987a) 65J; also the latter's comments, 420. See also, *On Anger* 2.35.2; 1.7.4.

experiences what the Stoics call *eupatheiai*, or well reasoned emotions. These (not unlike what the neo-Stoic Kant comes to call 'practical' emotions) will replace the old emotions (again, not unlike Kant's 'pathological' emotions). But notably, anger, at least if construed as a kind of distress, will have no counterpart in the Stoic's new hygienic order.[30] True, a sage may still feel shadows and scars of older angry feelings and resentments—bites and gnawings, as some of the texts put it (*TD* 3.83). These may be the emotional residues of a former life. And, also, he may experience moments when he is caught off guard, and feels the onset of the first moments of other ordinary emotions, like fear or sorrow. He experiences emotional preludes (*proludentia adfectibus*), as Seneca calls these protopathic phenomena. But for the genuine sage, experiencing these phenomena will pose no risk of backsliding. For the progressor, however, even the advanced progressor, such nibbles may indeed invite regression.[31] 'Thus it is,' concedes Seneca, 'that even the bravest man often turns pale as he puts on his armour, that the knees of even the fiercest soldier tremble a little as the signal is given for battle, that a great general's heart is in his mouth before the lines have charged against one another, that the most eloquent orator goes numb at the fingers as he prepares to speak' (*On Anger* 2.3.3).

The 'bravest man' who is a sage will be able to resume control almost instantly. He will catch himself before emotional preludes turn into full emotions. And he will do this by withholding the assent to impressions that constitutes a proper emotion. The 'bravest man' who is a progressor, however advanced, may face backsliding. Even so, for both individuals, emotional preludes may serve as a signal to take tighter control, a kind of 'affect signal', as Freud came to characterize anxiety and the subconscious way it can alert us to take up defense (Freud 1925–6). Or again, we might think of emotional preludes as the sort of 'enactments' trained psychotherapists talk about: they are fleeting emotional responses, a momentary wave of guilt or retaliative anger that briefly interrupt a more neutral posture (Chused 1991). But significantly, in the case of the listening therapist, these enactments are, more often than not, informative. They record something the therapist has found salient in the patient's story or in her resonance to it. Even a fleeting emotional response can be an epistemic tracer that alerts us to what is important.

The underlying epistemic point has critical implications for the Stoics. On an ordinary psychological view, we see and read our environments in a spontaneous way through our emotions. To feel fear is to believe we are in the presence of imminent danger, to feel anger is to believe we have been slighted unjustifiedly. This is not to say those readings are always accurate or can stand in isolation from more reflective assessment. Nor do emotions always point us transparently to the objects they are really about. But despite these limitations, they are an indispensable part of how we are attuned to our environment. Those who are mindblind, such as the autistic, are handicapped in reading the social world precisely because they miss many of

---

[30] See DL 7.116 or Long and Sedley (1987a) 65F. More precisely, the ordinary four genera of emotion—fear, appetite, distress, and pleasure—come to be replaced by three—rational caution, rational wishing, and rational joy.

[31] I am grateful to Brad Inwood for clarification here.

its cues (Baron-Cohen 1999). The Stoics must disagree with the point as part of their overall minimization of the role of emotions in our lives: Even if emotions are essentially judgments, they are judgments, they argue, that systematically give us wrong readings. When we experience emotional preludes without full assent to an emotion, we are, in essence, being taken in by the appearances. We can come to a proper understanding of dangers, say even impending dismemberment, in a way, they claim, that is absolutely free of any emotion. It is here that we may think strict Stoicism fails to capture the phenomenon as most of us know it. The genuine sage seems remote from our lives.

6. THE CHANGING SHAPE OF ANGER ON THE BATTLEFIELD

We have been talking about moral anger in somewhat abstract terms. In this section, I assess Seneca's indictment in a more concrete way by turning to the testimony of those who have seen the face of war.

In 1991 Tony Pfaff served as a platoon leader within the 82nd Airborne Division when they secured the landing sites with the Marines for the first stages of Operations Shield and Desert Storm during the Gulf War.[32] His brigade support unit earned the sobriquet, 'the eighty deuce and half'—a merger of 'eighty deuce' for the 82nd and 'deuce and a half', for the two and a half ton supply trucks they drove. Pfaff describes the anger that frames a combat soldier's mindset as he prepares for war. He focuses on the professional soldier, not the conscript, and on a war that the soldier by and large views as a justified response to unjust aggression:

I'll start with maybe the [1991] Persian Gulf War, which for me is a little bit cleaner example [than Vietnam]. What were any of us angry at? Most of us genuinely believed that Kuwait was unjustly aggressed against. And so you're angry at the aggressor for bringing you over here, for making you have to go, to leave your routine that you're comfortable with, and place you in this awful place to do these awful things, or at least have the prospect of doing these awful things. It's a little easier for the professional soldier to deal with it, because he's built a life out of practicing for this kind of thing. So his feelings are more ambivalent. A lot of time you feel like the basketball or football player practicing for the big game, hoping he never has to play. It's just a weird sort of feeling, that's kind of hard to reconcile . . . You're feeling really excited about going to play in the big game, and horrified and scared out of your mind that you have to play the big game at the same time.

Horrified exactly of what? I ask: 'That you could get killed. And you get asked to do things that you really don't want to do. I don't know many serial killers in the Army. Most people just really prefer not to have to kill anyone if they don't have to.'

Pfaff describes a baseline resentment at being dragged into war because of an unjust provocation. But in addition, there is the resentment at being forced to use one's deadly skills and at being exposed to those of others. The irony, of course, is that this is the point of professional war training—to become a warrior not just notionally but

---

[32] The following is based on an interview conducted in January 2003.

actually. The commitment is to put oneself in harm's way, if necessary. Is it rational to resent having to honor that commitment? The best answer comes from Aristotle. And it is a simple one: the truly courageous, unlike the merely daring, feel pain and anger because they know the terrible cost of self-sacrifice: 'The more possessed one is of virtue, the more one will be pained at the thought of death; for life is best worth living for such a person, and he is knowingly losing the greatest goods, and this is painful. But he is nonetheless brave, and perhaps all the more so, because he chooses noble deeds of war at that cost' (*NE* 1117b10–15).

Resentment becomes the backdrop against which other forms of anger associated with war mingle. Irritability, anger, and frustration mount with the countless deprivations brought on by war. In this context, the endless waiting that is part of war becomes no small irritant. It fuses with anxiety about losing one's battle edge and anxiety about extended deployments. Any deployment pits the role of soldier, sailor, airman, or marine against that of family person. Fear of loss of family and the dread of separation can easily morph into anger at the enemy for forcing those conflicts. 'You begin to think,' reflects Pfaff about the first Gulf War, 'the Iraqi soldiers, conscripts or not, are fighting for an unjust cause, and this unjust cause is disrupting our lifestyles in a very, very personal way, keeping us away from our families and the rest . . . Everyone's really irritated. By the eighth month people's families are starting to collapse. The first month of our return, there were 200 divorces in a division with roughly, two thousand married.'

Still, in more reflective moments, Pfaff acknowledges that irritability displaced as anger against the enemy can lift once one comes to see 'the enemy soldier as being just another schmuck like you'. In his own case, personalized anger was reserved for those responsible for the war, Saddam Hussein, in particular. I heard a similar sentiment registered at the funeral of John Rawls. One of his sons said his father never spoke much of his experience in the Second World War. But he did share one story with his family. He said he harbored no anger against the Japanese foot soldier, and in one instance, when face to face with his counterpart, both he and his opposite chose to retreat rather than fire. But he did have contempt for the Japanese authorities responsible for the war. At the close of the war, he volunteered to be part of a search contingent walking for several days in the treacherous and still enemy-held jungles of the island of Luzon to capture General Yamashita and bring him back for a formal surrender.[33]

A tolerant view of the enemy foot soldier can quickly change, though, if he becomes a cheater. Ilya Shabadash is a cousin who fought in the Second World War on the Russian side. Throughout the war, he harbored deep background anger for Hitler, though by and large, like Pfaff, he found himself respecting his opposite number engaged in the daily business of battle. What outraged him, though, even sixty years later in the retelling, was the trickery of a German peasant woman who hitched a ride back to town with his unit. She was carrying a basket of food and offered the hungry Russian troops some produce. Those that took her up on the offer

---

[33] I am indebted to Mardy Rawls for confirming the details.

later fell deathly sick. They had been poisoned. The survivors exploited the incident as an opportunity to rail at the Russian brass for underfeeding the troops. But that was just displaced anger, Ilya insisted. The real anger, he said, with pique still in his voice, was at the enemy cheaters, for using a civilian to do their bidding.[34]

Enemy mischief adds a new level of culpable wrongdoing to the equation. In the old language of just conduct of war, such actions as Ilya suffered are violations of 'chivalry'. The word betrays the origin of rules of war in a medieval culture that mixes brutality with the gallantry of knights.[35] Yet the term doesn't easily capture for us the gross violations of humanity that terrorism and weapons of mass destruction (nuclear, biological, and chemical) pose. Nor does it capture the dilemma soldiers face when the enemy uses its own innocent citizens to do its bidding. Retired General Romeo Dallaire, in charge of UN forces in Rwanda in 1994, fought back tears as he recalled at a recent breakfast talk, almost ten years after the massacres started in Rwanda, how the enemy routinely placed children in the middle of the road in Rwanda as shields between their troops and the approaching UN trucks. The children knew they would be shot at if they tried to escape. The UN troops knew they would take heavy losses rather than shoot. Whether by the rules of morality or chivalry, they would not accept the enemy terms of the fight.[36]

Perhaps some in the military become desensitized emotionally as they bear witness repeatedly to the atrocities of war. They have learned, with Seneca, to detach emotionally. They have learned how to create a 'bulletproof mind' (see Maass 2002). No doubt some desensitization is part of the psyche's survival system for facing gruesome evil up close. But it is hard to imagine that in a permanent way humans can know and assess true evil for what it is without the record of emotions.

Dallaire himself, whose pleas to the superpowers to intervene in Rwanda fell on deaf ears, returned to Canada with his experience of the genocide stuffed into a drawer. It stayed there for two years until, as he says, he couldn't 'keep it in the drawer any longer'. 'There are times when the best medication and therapist simply can't help a soldier suffering from this new generation of peacekeeping injury. The anger, the rage, the hurt, and the cold loneliness that separates you from your family, friends, and society's normal daily routine are so powerful that the option of destroying yourself is both real and attractive' (Power 2002: 388–9). Dallaire, now retired from the military, heads up a unit in charge of PTSD (Post-traumatic Stress Disorder) education for veterans in Canada. On the strict Stoic view, genuine evil is a matter only of one's own wrongdoing, and the sage, by definition above wrongdoing, will thus be exposed to no evil. Moreover, the culpable wrongdoing others commit will not erode the goodness or resoluteness of his own character. But that was not Dallaire's experience. He could not help but feel dehumanized by what he daily witnessed in Rwanda. Perhaps not all individuals would break given similar exposure

---

[34] From an interview conducted in December 2002.

[35] See, for example, the Ten Commandments of the Code of Chivalry outlining the Church's attempt to have knights fight in compliance with some notion of just conduct Gautier; (1965).

[36] From a talk given at the Carnegie Council on Ethics and International Affairs, New York, 29 January 2002.

to traumatic 'stressors'. Research on PTSD suggests that while exposure to extreme trauma is a necessary condition of PTSD, it is not sufficient.[37] Some individuals remain resilient. But few, with any sense of decency, would fail to feel the anguish of helplessness and tragedy at witnessing the genocide Dallaire saw.

Seneca well appreciates that the testimony of the emotions, and their searing way of recording the world, can kill a soul. But what he fails to appreciate is that the absence of such testimony leaves evil unchecked and kills souls in a far more devastating way. Tragically, in Rwanda in the spring of 1994, more than the outcry of a general in charge was needed to check evil.

Hugh Thompson was perhaps luckier than Dallaire.[38] On the morning of 16 March 1968, as a twenty-five-year-old reconnaissance helicopter pilot with the 123rd Aviation Battalion, he happened to be circling above a small hamlet called Tu Cung by the Vietnamese and My Lai 4 by the Americans. In the bubble were also his eighteen-year-old door gunner, Lawrence Colburn, and his twenty-two-year-old crew chief, Glen Andreotta. As they hovered, at times, only four or five feet off the ground, they began to see a swath of devastation and a ditch filled with bodies. They had just flown over the area an hour earlier with no sign of enemy action and no reports of Americans being hurt. His mind began to go places it didn't want to go. Relating the events some thirty-five years later, Thompson recalls, 'I guess I was in denial. You've got to understand, we were ready to risk our lives to save these American guys on the ground.' And so he began to construct for himself alternative scenarios. Maybe the carnage was from the early morning aerial artillery prepping of the area. But why then the ditch? So he tried out another scenario:

When the artillery started coming, the enemy ran out into the ditch and a lucky artillery round got them. But I'm thinking, 'Every house has a bomb shelter in it. When artillery starts coming in, are you going to leave this safe bomb shelter and take a walk in the park? I don't think so.' So I threw that out. So I said, 'Well, when the Americans came through, they did the humane thing and put all of the bodies in the ditch that was going to be a mass grave.' Well then you look in the ditch and there's live people in there. Everybody isn't dead. Wait a minute. We don't put the living with the dead in a grave. And then I just finally said, 'These people were marched down in that damn ditch and murdered . . . The thought was there the whole time, but I was trying to justify it.'

Thompson then radioed for help in evacuating a wounded girl, but assumed communications failure. For what he saw next was an infantry officer (later identified as Capt. Medina) prod her with his foot and then shoot her. Minutes later Andreotti heard a barrage of machine gunfire coming from a soldier near the ditch (later identified as Lt. Calley). 'At that moment, everything went completely crazy, you might say. Because here it is again, we've asked for help and got people killed. Well, I'm

[37] See the very helpful website of the National Center for Post-traumatic Stress Disorder: www.ncptsd.org. I thank its executive director, Dr. Matthew Friedman, for meeting me to discuss current research on PTSD and resilience.

[38] I relate the following narrative in some detail both as a record of events and as a way to track emotions. I draw on my own conversations and interviews with Hugh Thompson in spring 1998 and 1999, and February 2002; Bilton (1992); and a CBS ' 60 Minutes-broadcast on Thompson.

responsible for their deaths now. I know I'm mad, because I got them killed. If I had kept my mouth shut, then maybe they'd have walked away and they would have lived.'

Thompson then saw the Americans approaching a bunker, and figured to himself that the people inside had about fifteen seconds to live. I said, 'Dammit, it ain't gonna happen. They ain't gonna die . . . I was hot. I'll tell you that. I was hot.' Those who received his radio message that day got a taste of his outrage: 'His voice was choked with emotion. He swore obscenities, cursed, and pleaded with the aerocrew to come down and help rescue the civilians.'[39] Landing his aircraft and this time getting out, he told his crew to 'open fire' on the GIs—'open up on'em and kill them'—if they opened fire at him as he tried to intervene.

Thompson raised enough hell at headquarters that day to get the operations, scheduled to last for four days, to cease. Some 350 persons were massacred that day. But his interventions may have stopped the massacre of more than 20,000 more who were living in the My Lai area at the time. 'There was nothing to make me believe that the same thing wasn't going to happen everywhere.' But once he filed his report, he did his best to forget the day and to numb up the pain. And he continued to forget until the story broke and the court martials of the Charlie Company officers took him to Washington to give testimony. Once the trials were over, he tried again to put My Lai behind him until a British documentary crew drew him out in the late eighties. In the spring of 1998, after some thirty years of their own silence, the Army belatedly decorated Hugh Thompson, Lawrence Colburn, and Glen Andreotti (posthumously) with the prestigious Soldier's Medal for their valor at My Lai.

Over the years, Thompson has found comfort in his own version of Stoic tonics. 'Numb is good,' he once told me. He wanted to forget My Lai, but he also wanted others to forget, especially those who viewed him as a traitor and who put death threats out to him. Like many Vietnam veterans who have kept their war experiences to themselves, he returned home without telling his family what he saw and did that day. Undoubtedly, the Army's belated acceptance of Thompson has made it easier for him to own his own past. These days, he is no longer silent or numb. The outrage he felt that day in My Lai is palpable in his voice and in his eyes. And there is still anger in his self-reproach for having caused the death of innocents in his first botched attempts at helping. 'Don't make me break down,' he warned as we began our interview. He didn't break down. He was controlled but emotional. He bore his emotions with a soldier's grace and dignity. Through projects he is involved with in My Lai to build a school and a memorial, he is trying to give back a small bit of what Americans took that day. Contrary to Seneca's warnings, in Thompson's case, at least, keeping anger alive turns it into neither frenzy nor chronic embitterment. True, he cannot forgive, unlike the My Lai survivor who wishes Thompson had brought Calley and Medina back with him, so she can forgive them. He cannot forgive them because, as he maintains, the evil was simply too great. But even if this woman is ready to forswear her anger, she has not forgotten what happened or lost her pain. 'Why', in tears, she

---

[39] Bilton and Sim (1992), 13.

begs Thompson, 'did they kill my family? Why were they different from you?' Seneca exhorts us to believe that anger is a mistaken judgment—we harpoon the wrong phenomenon: trespasses and violations that aren't really so, that don't really violate our human core. Yet who among us would venture to tell this Vietnamese woman that what she and her family endured were not violations of the human soul?

7. THERAPEUTIC STRATEGIES

We bring this essay to a close by reflecting briefly on the relationship of Stoic therapy to more modern variants. Some of Seneca's techniques for the prevention and treatment of one's own anger seem fairly homespun and moderate: 'postponement allows [anger] to abate,'[40] suppressing facial expressions that 'inflame the eyes and alter the countenance' can shortcircuit internal feedback responses,[41] 'putting ourselves in the place of the person with whom we are angry' can shift our judgments, taking stock daily of our habits can help curb our impulses.[42] Meditate at the end of each day, as Seneca says is his own wont ('when the light has been taken away and my wife has fallen silent'). Replay all your interactions and 'conceal nothing' from yourself—ask yourself, did you lose your temper at the party, did you speak 'too pugnaciously', when you were the butt of a few jokes, did you forget to 'stand back and laugh'?[43]

But however moderate these techniques, the underlying aspiration—to eliminate all anger—is nothing if not radical. Seneca describes the goal using a mix of quasi-medical and military metaphors. On the medical side, we are to 'cut out (*exsecare*)', 'exclude (*excludere*)', 'remove or eliminate (*tollere*)'.[44] Emotions are pathological, noxious toxins that need to be isolated (*diducere*) from healthier parts of the soul. On the military side, 'the enemy must be stopped at the very frontier;' we are 'to beat [it] back (*spernere*)', 'resist (*repugnare*)', before it 'has invaded and rushed on the city gates'.[45]

On the Stoic view, anger is a disease and enemy because vulnerability is. Anger reveals us as vulnerable to others' attacks, and in particular, vulnerable to their deliberate wrongdoings and slights. But there is an interesting modern way of restructuring the problem that sheds light on Seneca's solution. On a psychoanalytic view, it is not so much anger or emotional investments that are the irritants, but the *conflict* that emotional investments can bring. We don't tolerate ambivalence well. We worry consciously and unconsciously that if we allow ourselves angry feelings, they may overtake our kinder motives, that our militant side will persecute our softer parts, that hostility towards a child or parent will swallow up our love. At times, Seneca himself worries about anger in these terms: If reason starts to mix with anger, then anger may prevail in a way that prevents reason from 'ris[ing] again'. 'How can it free itself from the chaos, if the admixture of baser ingredients has prevailed' (*On Anger* 1.8.2–3)? To allow the mixing and mingling of motives is to run the risk of being muddled and conflicted, or worse, overtaken by motives that we don't fully endorse. Better to be

---

[40] *On Anger* 3.12.4; 3.32.2.   [41] Ibid. 3.13.1–2.   [42] Ibid. 3.12.3.
[43] Ibid. 3.36–7.   [44] See, for example, ibid. 1.7 and 3.3.   [45] See ibid. 1.8 especially.

resolute and staunch and keep countervailing desires well at bay. Vowing to eliminate anger, or any emotion that can oppose reason's control, is a way of wishing for self-sufficiency. But also it is also a way of wishing to be rid of conflict.

Of course, the irritant of psychic conflict is not really a modern problem. Plato and Aristotle carve up the soul largely to account for conflict. If order rather than conflict is to prevail, then the top of the soul must whip the bottom into shape. Desires must know well their hierarchical rankings. Only then can we have psychic well-being. The Stoics resist dividing the psyche, making all mental functions products of the same mind-stuff. But this, they acknowledge, does not do away with conflict or oscillation. Anger can resist reason, one emotion can quarrel with another, even if each is made of the same cognitive stuff.

Seneca's cure for the disease of emotional vulnerability (and psychic conflict) is elimination. We are to root out all conflict, in the way in which we might chemically or surgically remove a cancerous tumor. But while elimination may capture the body's self-healing process, it does not really describe what we do when we resolve psychic conflict. In this vein, consider a contemporary discussion by Harry Frankfurt (1988) on becoming 'wholehearted', a state not so unlike Stoic resoluteness. He too considers the notion of psychic elimination:

When the body heals itself, it *eliminates* conflicts in which one physical process (say, infection) interferes with others and undermines the homeostasis, or equilibrium, in which health consists. A person who makes up his mind also seeks thereby to overcome or to supersede a condition of inner division and make himself into an integrated whole. But he may accomplish this without actually eliminating the desires that conflict with those on which he has decided, as long as he disassociates himself from them. (Ibid. 174)[46]

On this picture, psychic repair requires not the elimination of a conflicting desire, but a 'dissociation' from it, or, as Frankfurt says more forcefully elsewhere, 'a radical *separation*' in which it is 'extruded entirely as an outlaw' (Ibid. 170). Though Frankfurt is not writing with Seneca in mind, his remarks shed light on Seneca's model. In warding off an unwanted emotion, Seneca would concur, we fight it as an enemy, extrude it from our borders, resist all alliances with it. We build tall city gates to keep the aliens from invading.

It was Freud who made famous in his case study of the Ratman the convolutions of one who struggles with his ambivalence.[47] At the heart of the Ratman's ambivalence is a love–hate conflict with his father. The conflict took many guises, but among them were repeated fantasies, including two in the months and then days before his father's death, that the price of his love for a woman he wished to marry was his father's death. That he loved his father was unquestionable to him. That he might punish him in this way was an intolerable thought that he warded off through a web of defenses and obsessive behaviors. The case is complex and the twisted logic of the obsessions at times bewildering. But what is significant for our purposes is that Freud's diagnosis of the Ratman's problem was not his ambivalence, but his struggle against it. The

---

[46] I am here indebted to David Velleman's discussion of Frankfurt in Velleman (2002).

[47] This Freudian reading of Frankfurt is due to Velleman.

extreme 'splitting' and 'disintegration of his personality', the dissociation and isolation from unwanted emotions, the very mechanisms Seneca (and Frankfurt) view as cures, Freud diagnoses as the disease (Freud 1909: 177).[48]

Freud explains. In the case of those who are close to us, we 'wish our feelings to be unmixed,' and consequently, as is 'only human', 'overlook . . . faults, since they might make' us dislike the loved one. We often ignore the faults as though we 'were blind to them' (Ibid. 180–1). The Ratman's undoing is in failing to tolerate this ambivalence, with the result that the conflict deepens and defenses harden: 'His hostility towards his father . . . though he had once been acutely conscious of it, had long since vanished from his ken, and it was only in the teeth of the most violent resistance that it could be brought back into consciousness' (Ibid. 238). Obsessive behaviors are invoked to ward off punishments (including the dreaded rat punishment) that have now become stand-ins for his repressed hostility.

To be sure, Seneca does not postulate a way of keeping emotions at bay that amounts to their repression in the unconscious.[49] And Frankfurt, also, by and large, focuses on conscious forms of dissociation—of 'making one's mind up', 'deciding' to identify with certain emotions and not others. His idea of 'taking responsibility for the shaping of one's characteristics' has the ring of Stoic notions of voluntary assent and control (Frankfurt 1988: 170–3). But however conscious the control, Frankfurtian 'dissociation' and Senecan 'beating back' of unwanted emotions are, like repression and other unconscious defenses, ways we armour ourselves against vulnerability and conflict. And as with many defenses and fantasies that are not sustainable compromise solutions, chinks in the armour soon appear.[50]

But what does all this have to do with the warrior? My suggestion is that Stoic aspirations of the warrior to treat anger as an enemy represent an unhealthy psychological phenomenon. It will be objected that warrior rage and revenge, an Achilles' spirit of vindictiveness and frenzy, are precisely the emotions that a warrior needs to restrain. I could not agree more. And Seneca's *On Anger* provides one of the best places to teach that lesson. Seneca argues persuasively that unrestrained anger, whether of rage, bitterness, revenge, or indignation, are more often than not inappropriate. But Seneca insists that the way to guard against these excesses is to ostracize *all* anger from our lives. And we are to achieve that end through a robust use of defensive techniques that we today know as disassociation and splitting. On Seneca's version of splitting, competing desires don't mingle or mix, modify or moderate each other. There is no Aristotelian notion of unwelcome emotions becoming tamed by more congenial ones, or excesses in each direction finding more moderate forms by mutual adjustments. Instead, there is only containment.[51]

---

[48] Velleman nicely puts it this way in critiquing Frankfurt.

[49] Though see *On Anger* 3.13 for suggestions of something like repression.

[50] Richard Sorabji has commented to me that Stoic therapy is highly cognitive, 'thinky-thinky', as he jokingly put it, and not a matter of harsh, repressive measures. But while I agree that the therapy is essentially cognitive, it still, I would argue, is austere in its methods of self-discipline.

[51] I don't think this is a mere terminological quibble. Aristotle's tolerant attitude toward a life of emotions allows for more possibilities with respect to their cultivation than does the Stoic stance. Though some texts suggest a wide array of eupathetic emotions, they still will be restricted,

Granted, containment of this sort may be for many soldiers an involuntary response to the rage of battle, and the twin traumas of gruesome loss and what can seem undeserving self-survival. How to integrate these experiences in the rhythm of ordinary life becomes a lifelong challenge. Those like Marvin, with whom we opened this chapter, still struggle, fifty years later, to rebuild sea walls around battle memories of Okinawa, so they are both low enough and permeable enough to let in fresh seawater.[52] Seneca resists this sort of healing and integrating process. Build and maintain the sea walls high enough to fend off the brackish waters. Keep the bad away from the good lest there be contamination. Hold back the enemies at the border. In mixed Stoic and Freudian tones, he exhorts, 'fight with yourself . . . Conquer anger.' 'Conceal' it and give it 'no exit'; keep it 'hidden and secret', give the mind an advance directive that should anger erupt it must 'bury it deeply and not proclaim its distress' (*On Anger* 3.13). It will come as no surprise that Seneca, writing two thousand years before Freud, does not explore the view that demons, buried deep in the soul, can still rise. But those who must live day in and day out with those demons know well the Freudian truth that to bury is not necessarily to vanquish.

ACKNOWLEDGEMENTS

An ancestor of this paper appears as chapter 4 in *Stoic Warriors* (Oxford University Press, 2005). I owe thanks to Elisa Hurley and Joe Kakesh for their research assistance in earlier versions of this chapter. Thanks also are due to Carin Ewing for her assistance at later stages. In addition, I am indebted to Alisa Carse, Brad Inwood, Rebecca Kukla, and Martha Nussbaum for discussion of earlier drafts. Versions of this chapter were presented at University of Chicago Law School, April 2003, Santa Clara University, April 2003, Santa Barbara City College, April 2003, American University, May 2003, and Baden-Baden, August 2003. I am grateful to audiences at those events for their helpful comments. And I am grateful to all those who have served in the armed forces who have allowed me to interview them over the past several years.

REFERENCES

Baron-Cohen, S. (1999). *Mindblindness: An Essay on Autism and Theory of Mind*. Cambridge, MA: MIT Press.

Barstow, A. L., ed. (2000). *War's Dirty Secret: Rape, Prostitution, and Other Crimes Against Women*. Cleveland, OH: Pilgrim Press.

Bilton, M., and Sim, K. (1992). *Four Hours in My Lai*. New York: Penguin.

Brennan, T. (1998). 'The Old Stoic Theory of Emotions', in *The Emotions in Hellenistic Philosophy*. J. Shivola and Troels Engberg-Pederson. Amsterdam: Kluwer, 21–70.

---

in principle, to ways of tracking one's own virtuous effort or agency. For one's own character is ultimately the only source of good and evil in the world.

[52] I borrow here from Jamison (1995), 214 who uses similar language to describe coping with manic depression.

Brison, S. J. (2002). *Aftermath: Violence and the Remaking of the Self.* Princeton: Princeton University Press.

Butler, J. (1964). *Fifteen Sermons.* London: G. Bell and Sons.

Cannon, W. B. (1927). 'The James-Lange Theory of Emotions: A Critical Examination and an Alternative Theory'. *American Journal of Psychology,* 39: 106–24.

Carroll, W. (2001). *Punk's War.* Annapolis, MD: Naval Institute Press.

Chused, J. F. (1991). 'The Evocative Power of Enactments'. *Journal of the American Psychoanalytic Association,* 29: 615–39.

Cicero (1971). *De Finibus.* Cambridge, MA: Harvard University Press.

_____ (2002). *Cicero on the Emotions: Tusculan Disputations 3 and 4.* M. Graver, ed. Chicago: University of Chicago Press.

Cooper, J. M., and Procopé, J. F., eds. (1995). *Seneca: Moral and Political Essays.* Cambridge: Cambridge University Press.

DeLacy, P., ed. (1984). *Galen: On the Doctrines of Hippocrates and Plato.* Berlin: Academie-Verlag.

DeSousa, R. (1987). *The Rationality of Emotion.* Cambridge, MA: MIT Press.

Ekman, P., ed. (1982). *Emotion in the Human Face.* Cambridge: Cambridge University Press.

_____ (1984). 'Expression and the Nature of Emotion', in *Approaches to Emotion.* K. R. Scherer and P. Hillsdale, NJ: Lawrence Erlbaum.

Fischer, J. M., and Ravizza, Mark, ed. (1993). *Perspectives on Moral Responsibility.* Ithaca, NY: Cornell University Press.

Frankfurt, H. (1988). 'Identification and Wholeheartedness', in *The Importance of What We Care About.* H. Frankfurt. Cambridge: Cambridge University Press.

Freud, S. (1909). 'Notes Upon a Case of Obsessional Neurosis', in *Standard Edition of the Complete Psychological Works of Sigmund Freud.* S. Freud. London: Hogarth Press, 10.

_____ (1925–6). 'Inhibitions, Symptoms and Anxiety', in *The Standard Edition of the Complete Psychological Works of Sigmund Freud.* S. Freud. London: Hogarth Press, 20.

Frijda, N. H. (1986). *The Emotions.* Cambridge: Cambridge University Press.

Gautier, L. (1965). *Chivalry.* New York: Barnes and Noble.

Gladwell, M. (2002). The Naked Face. *New Yorker,* 78/22: 38–49.

Goldie, P. (2000). *The Emotions: A Philosophical Exploration.* Oxford: Oxford University Press.

Griffin, M. (1992). *Seneca: A Philosopher in Politics.* Oxford: Clarendon Press.

Halbfinger, D. M. (2003a). 'Hearing Starts in Bombing Error That Killed 4'. *New York Times,* Jan. 15: A1.

_____ (2003b). 'Pilots Ignored Rules On When to Attack, Commander Says'. *New York Times,* Jan. 16: A1.

Harris, W. (2001). *Restraining Rage: The Ideology of Anger Control in Classical Antiquity.* Cambridge, MA: Harvard University Press.

Homer (1999). *The Iliad.* New York: Penguin.

Jacoby, S. (1983). *Wild Justice: The Evolution of Revenge.* New York: Harper and Row.

Jakobs, E., Manstead, A. S. R., and Fischer, A. (1999). 'Social Motives, Emotional Feelings, and Smiling'. *Cognition and Emotion,* 13 (4): 321–45.

Jamison, K. R. (1995). *An Unquiet Mind: A Memoir of Moods and Madness.* New York: Random House.

Kant, I. (1930). *Lectures on Ethics.* Indianapolis: Hackett.

_____ (1960). *Religion Within the Limits of Reason Alone.* New York: Harper and Brothers.

Kant, I. (1964). *The Doctrine of Virtue*. Philadelphia: University of Pennsylvania Press.

Kindlon, D., and Thompson, M. (1999). *Raising Cain: Protecting the Emotional Life of Boys*. New York: Ballantine.

Klein, M. (1975). *Envy and Gratitude and Other Works, 1946–1963*. New York: Dell.

Laertius, D. (1970). *Lives of Eminent Philosophers*. Cambridge, MA: Harvard University Press.

Lazarus, R. S. (1984). 'On the Primacy of Cognition'. *American Psychologist*, 39: 124–9.

Long, A. A., and Sedley, D. N. (1987). *The Hellenistic Philosophers, vol. 1: Translations of the Principal Sources, with Philosophical Commentary*. Cambridge: Cambridge University Press.

Maass, P. (2002). 'A Bulletproof Mind'. *New York Times Magazine*, Nov. 10.

Morris, H. (1995). 'A Paternalistic Theory of Punishment', in *Punishment and Rehabilitation*. J. G. Murphy. Belmont, CA: Wadsworth.

Murphy, J. G. (1995a). *Punishment and Rehabilitation*. Belmont, CA: Wadsworth.

———— (1995b). 'Getting Even: The Role of the Victim', in *Punishment and Rehabilitation*. J. G. Murphy. Belmont, CA: Wadsworth.

———— and Hampton, Jean (1988). *Forgiveness and Mercy*. Cambridge: Cambridge University Press.

Nussbaum, M. (1994). *The Therapy of Desire, Chapter 11: Seneca on Anger in Public Life*. Princeton: Princeton University Press.

———— (2002). *Upheavals of Thought: The Intelligence of Emotions*. Cambridge: Cambridge University Press.

Oatley, K. (1992). *Best Laid Schemes: The Psychology of Emotions*. Cambridge: Cambridge University Press.

Philpott, T. (1995). 'Can Mike Boorda Salvage the Navy?' *Washingtonian*, Feb.: 52–5, 98–100.

Plato (1974). *The Republic*. Indianapolis: Hackett.

Plutarch (2000). *Moralia, Volume 1*. Cambridge, MA: Harvard University Press.

Pollack, W. (1998). *Real Boys*. New York: Holt.

Power, S. (2002). *A Problem from Hell: America and the Age of Genocide*. New York: Basic.

Schachter, S., and Singer, J. (1962). 'Cognitive, Social, and Psychological Determinants of Emotional State'. *Psychological Review*, 69: 379–99.

Scherer, K. R. (1993). 'Studying the Emotion-Antecedent Appraisal Process: An Expert System Approach'. *Cognition and Emotion*, 3/4: 325–55.

Seneca (1989). *Moral Essays*. Cambridge, MA: Harvard University Press.

Shay, J. (1994). *Achilles in Vietnam: Combat Trauma and the Undoing of Character*. New York: Scribner.

———— (2002). *Odysseus in America: Combat Trauma and the Trials of Homecoming*. New York: Scribner.

Sherman, N. (1989). *The Fabric of Character*. New York: Oxford University Press.

———— (1997). *Making a Necessity of Virtue*. Cambridge: Cambridge University Press.

———— (1999a). 'Taking Responsibility for Our Emotions'. *Social Philosophy and Policy*, 16/2: 294–323.

———— (1999b). 'Taking Responsibility for Our Emotions', in *Responsibility*. E. F. Paul, Fred D. Miller Jr., and Jeffrey Paul. Cambridge: Cambridge University Press.

———— (2000). 'Emotional Agents', in *The Analytic Freud: Philosophy and Psychoanalysis*. M. P. Levine. London: Routledge.

Sorabji, R. (2000). *Emotion and Peace of Mind*. Oxford: Oxford University Press.

Stobaeus, J. (1884). *Eclogae*. C. Wachsmuth, ed. Berlin: Weidmann.

Stocker, M. (1996). *Valuing Emotions*. Cambridge: Cambridge University Press.

Velleman, D. (1999). 'A Rational Superego'. *Philosophical Review*, 108: 529–58.

_____ (2002). 'Identification and Identity', in *Contours of Agency: A Festschrift for Harry Frank-furt*. S. Buss and Lee Overton. Cambridge, MA: MIT Press.

_____ (forthcoming). 'Don't Worry, Feel Guilty'. *Philosophy*.

Vistica, G. L. (2001). 'One Awful Night in Thanh Phong'. *New York Times Magazine*, Apr. 25.

Von Armin, H., ed. (1924). *Stoicorum Veterum Fragmenta*. Leipzig: Reprint Library.

White, S. A. (1995). 'Cicero and the Therapists', in *Cicero the Philosopher*. J. G. F. Powell. Oxford: Clarendon Press.

Wiesenthal, S. (1997). *The Sunflower: On the Possibilities and Limit of Forgiveness*. New York: Schocken.

Zajonc, R. B. (1984). 'On the Primacy of Affect'. *American Psychologist*, 39: 117–23.

13

Famine, Affluence, and Virtue

Michael Slote

One of the greatest challenges to ordinary moral thinking and to recent moral theory has been the views and arguments advanced by Peter Singer in his classic paper, 'Famine, Affluence, and Morality' (1972). Philosophers have struggled with and in many cases attempted to refute Singer's conclusion that our moral obligation to relieve hunger or disease in distant parts of the world is just as great as, say, our obligation to save a child drowning in a shallow pool of water right in front of us. But although this debate continues to be very lively, virtue ethics has not joined in the fray. It has simply not taken up the main issue Singer's paper has been thought to raise, the issue whether the making of substantial sacrifices in order to help those suffering in distant parts of the world is obligatory or (merely) supererogatory.

Of course, recent virtue ethics has sought to meet other challenges, challenges particularly to its right to exist as an independent and systematic approach to ethics. But now that virtue ethics seems to have found its own place in the sun, its claim to contemporary plausibility may further depend on its ability to say something relevant about issues that philosophers in other ethical traditions find significant. However, recent and traditional Aristotelian approaches in fact find it difficult to address, or even to formulate, the problems Singer has raised. That is chiefly because they make no room for the supererogatory, do not seem to allow for the possibility, in any given situation, of someone's going *beyond* the call of duty. This restriction follows not only out of Aristotle's doctrine of the mean but also out of Aristotelian accounts of right action and virtue that *do not* rely on that doctrine: I have in mind here recent books by Philippa Foot (2001) and Rosalind Hursthouse (1999).

However, I don't propose here to document further, or speculate on the causes of, this Aristotelian tendency.[1] Despite the predominance of Aristotelian influences within

---

[1] Utilitarianism standardly disallows the possibility of supererogation and may nonetheless constitute a viable option in ethical theory. So why, one might ask, shouldn't Aristotelianism also be allowed to rule out supererogation? But there is a difference here. Utilitarianism evaluates actions in terms of their outcomes, and we can make sense of the idea of a (satisficing) form of utilitarianism that regards the production of best outcomes as supererogatory. The issue of supererogation becomes one of where it makes the most sense to draw the line among good or better outcomes, when we are evaluating actions. As far as I know, no one has suggested a similar (or even a *different*) way of making supererogation understandable in Aristotelian terms. So the issue whether helping distant others is obligatory or supererogatory is not readily grasped, much less resolved, in Aristotelian

recent virtue ethics, there is another currently viable virtue-ethical tradition that stems from eighteenth-century moral sentimentalism à la Hutcheson and Hume, and I shall be arguing in what follows that the sentimentalist form of virtue ethics can deal with the issues raised by Singer in a way that Aristotelianism and neo-Aristotelianism seem unable to do. Let me now say a bit more about recent developments within this alternative tradition of virtue ethics and then go on to discuss how such an approach might be able to offer us an answer to the questions Peter Singer raises.

1. SENTIMENTALISM, CARING, AND EMPATHY

Both Hume's and Hutcheson's theories of morality are recognizably virtue-ethical. Both specifically evaluate actions by reference to certain underlying motives, though the relevant motives differ for the two authors. For Hutcheson, an early version of the principle of utility governs individual actions, but this is justified by reference to the inherent moral value of a universal benevolence that *aims* to maximize the sum of human or sentient well-being; and although Hume favors less impartial forms of benevolence, he emphatically ties all evaluations of actions to motives like compassion, public-spiritedness, and gratitude (or specific motives that are opposed to them).

Neither Hume nor Hutcheson focuses on 'caring' about others as a motive, but the ethics of caring recently proposed and developed by Carol Gilligan, Nel Noddings, and others seems very clearly in the moral sentimentalist tradition and is frequently also regarded as a form of virtue ethics, since it evaluates human actions by reference to how much (of the inner motive of) caring they express or exhibit.[2] And I regard a virtue ethics of caring as the most promising (and interesting) form of present-day sentimentalism. Carol Gilligan introduced the moral ideal of caring in a book devoted to showing that women and men approach moral issues differently: that men think in terms of justice, autonomy, and rights whereas women approach moral issues in terms of (their) connection with and caring concern about others. One response to this has been to conclude that justice needs to be supplemented or complemented by caring, that both are relevant to morality, and that caring should receive a greater emphasis than previous moral theories have accorded it.

However, some caring ethicists have proceeded more boldly. For example, in a preface added to *In a Different Voice* in 1993, Gilligan suggests that an ethics of caring grounded in an ideal of connection with—rather than separateness or autonomy from—others might completely displace traditional 'masculine' approaches and give us a total picture of (what can be validly said about) the ethical. But what does this

---

terms. (In fact, and judging by what Foot says in her book about the willingness to sustain bodily injuries in order to prevent even greater bodily injuries to others, Aristotelianism may well lead us toward the unappetizing conclusion that giving a great deal to distant others, far from being either obligatory or supererogatory, may simply be wrong or unvirtuous. See *Natural Goodness*, p. 79.)

[2] See, e.g., Carol Gilligan (1982) and Nel Noddings (1984). Noddings sees her views as continuous with eighteenth-century sentimentalism, and the connection has also been frequently mentioned by others. However, Noddings's essay in the present volume seeks to distance her version of the ethics of caring from more purely virtue-ethical approaches. This issue of terminology may not be particularly important.

then mean about the supposedly masculine concepts or topics of justice, autonomy, and rights? Are we simply to discard such concepts, or is the idea, rather, that we can make sense of them in (not necessarily reductive) terms of caring and cognate notions? Gilligan's preface doesn't really say. But some caring ethicists have written in ways that seem to favor the latter option. I have in mind here work by Sara Ruddick (1989), a recent book by Nel Noddings (2002), and also some recent work of my own (1998: 175–95).

I shall assume in what follows that an ethics of caring should aspire to offer a general conception of (individual and political) morality. But this is a tall order, and the hesitation, even among some caring ethicists, to push this far is some evidence of that. Even if one thinks, for example, that social justice might be explainable in terms of social structures, laws, and institutions that express or reflect a caring attitude on the part of relevant individuals and groups of individuals, one may well wonder whether we can make sense of deontology (e.g. of strictures on killing one innocent person even to prevent a greater loss of life) in terms of a (mere) feeling/sentiment like caring. Any sentimentalist theory would seem to have a problem here[3] and there is a further problem, indeed, about how an ethics of caring or any sentimentalist conception of morality could offer an adequate account/analysis of moral judgments involving concepts like 'right', 'wrong', 'obligatory', and 'virtuous'. We shall return to these questions at the end of this essay, but let us for now leave them in abeyance and consider, rather, some of the initial steps a sentimentalist virtue ethics of caring needs to take on the road to a full or systematic theory.

I have suggested above that an ethics of caring counts as a form of sentimentalist virtue ethics because it evaluates actions in relation to an inner motive, caring, that is cognate with the sentiments that were appealed to by the eighteenth-century sentimentalists in offering their own views about the nature of morality. Caring theory also emphasizes relationships more than either Kantian ethics or utilitarianism does and in a way that is more than slightly reminiscent of Aristotle's central concern with (individual and civic) friendship; and this too makes it natural to class caring-ethical views together with Aristotelian ethics as forms of virtue ethics. However, some defenders of the morality of caring (e.g. Nel Noddings) think the moral value of caring hinges on the constitutive role that that motive plays in desirable human relationships, whereas others (myself included) think the admirable or virtuous character of caring about others stands in need of no such grounding and is in some sense morally fundamental or self-evident. But that issue need not be engaged or resolved here. The important point is that an ethics of caring sees the moral quality of actions as dependent (largely or exclusively) on what they show about the caring or non-caring attitudes of individuals. And what this means, in simplified and very general ethical terms, is that an act is regarded as (all) right if it doesn't exhibit a lack (or the opposite) of caring and wrong if it does. (Brushing your teeth may not evince caring for others, but the point is that it also doesn't evince, exhibit, or reflect a lack of caring concern about others.)

---

[3] The reader may recall all the paradoxical convolutions of Hume's sentimentalist account of justice and promise-keeping; and Hutcheson's refusal to countenance (a deep level of) deontology simply adds fuel to the suspicion that sentimentalism cannot make sense of deontology.

Now when Noddings originally wrote about caring, she had in mind the kind of caring for others that takes place, so to speak, in intimate or at least face-to-face relationships. Caring *about* the fate of (groups of) people one has merely *heard* about didn't come under the rubric of caring; and since morality does take in our relations with such distant and personally unknown others, Noddings held that the ethics of caring represented only a limited—though important and previously neglected—part of morality. Others who came later, however, sought to show that caring about people who are distant from us can and should be taken within the purview of the caring approach to ethics (these others include Virginia Held and myself); and nowadays and in her recent book Noddings seems to be convinced of the essential rightness of making such an expansionist move on behalf of the ethics of caring.

Therefore, when I speak of acts exhibiting a caring attitude or one inconsistent with caring, the caring I am speaking of includes attitudes toward distant and personally unknown others, not just attitudes toward people we are acquainted with or love. The term 'caring' is thus a placeholder for a description of an overall attitude/motivational state, one that takes in both one's concern for people one knows (intimately) and one's concern for distant others and that embodies some sort of proportionality or balance between these concerns. An ethics of caring will hold that it is virtuous to be more concerned about near and dear than about strangers or those one knows about merely by description; but it will also insist that an ideally or virtuously caring individual will be substantially concerned about people who are distant from her (not to mention animals). The question what constitutes an ideal or morally required proportionality or balance as between these concerns is a complex and difficult one. I have considered it at length elsewhere, and our discussion in what follows will constitute a further attempt at least partly to deal with it.[4] Certainly, Singer seems to hold that we have as much reason to concern ourselves with distant others as with individuals we are personally intimate with; but there also is something morally counterintuitive about this. The idea that we have special (or stronger) moral obligations to those who are near and/or dear to us is both familiar and ethically appealing at a common-sense level. But I hope now to show you how an ethics of caring, which has so far tended merely to *assume* such special obligations on the basis of the intuitive plausibility of such an assumption, can say something at least partly to justify it.

To do so, however, the ethics of caring needs to expand its horizons a bit. It needs in particular to look back to eighteenth-century moral sentimentalism and make use of some notions that play an important role in the thinking of Hume (and also Adam Smith), but that have been largely neglected by those seeking to develop a systematic ethics of caring. Hume (especially in the *Treatise of Human Nature*) holds that our concern for others operates via a mechanism he calls 'sympathy', but the notion he is working with (there) is actually closer to our contemporary term 'empathy', and the difference or disparity may be partly accounted for by the fact that the latter term

---

[4] In his contribution to the present volume, P. J. Ivanhoe discusses some of these same issues in relation to early Confucian philosophy.

didn't enter English till the early twentieth century. So Hume doesn't have the terminology for distinguishing empathy from sympathy, but the phenomenon he calls sympathy seems much closer to what we mean by empathy than by sympathy.

Now these terms are not easy to define, but by 'sympathy' I think we mean a kind of favorable attitude toward someone. One feels sympathy for someone in pain, for example, if one feels *for* them (or their pain), wishes they didn't have the pain, wants their pain to end. By 'empathy', on the other hand, we mean a state or process in which someone takes on the feelings of another: one empathizes for another who is in pain, if one 'feels their pain' (as opposed to feeling *for* their pain). Obviously, a great deal more could be said about this distinction, but, given the prevalence of these notions in contemporary parlance, I hope the reader will readily follow what I shall be saying about empathy. Hume saw empathy/sympathy as a kind of *contagion* whereby the feelings of one person spread to (cause similar feelings in) another person, but in recent years there has been enormous interest in the subject of empathy on the part of social psychologists, and in that literature the 'contagious' aspect of empathy is but one feature of the landscape. Numerous studies of the factors that affect empathy and of how empathy develops have been published, and various psychologists have also offered general accounts of the role empathy plays in human psychology and in human life. But one central aspect of that literature will most concern us here as I suggest a way of developing the ethics of caring further.

Recent work on empathy has to a substantial extent focused on the question whether the development of empathy is necessary to an individual's development of altruistic concern for others—this is called the 'empathy-altruism hypothesis'. Many (but by no means all) psychologists have seen recent work in the field as supporting the empathy-altruism hypothesis, and this literature is relevant to the present essay at least in part because it is possible to hold that caring works via empathy and that the contours of morally good caring can be specified in relation to how human empathy develops or can be made to develop. I believe that a virtue ethics of caring that grounds caring in human empathy as recently studied by psychologists can provide us with a way of answering Singer's arguments. But before appealing further to this interesting recent psychological literature, let me just briefly say how I came to realize the usefulness of appealing to (developed human) empathy in working out a sentimentalist virtue ethics of caring.

An ethics of caring can easily say that we have a greater obligation to help (born) fellow human beings than to help animals or fetuses, and such a comparative judgment has the kind of intuitive force or plausibility that a virtue ethics of caring might wish to rely on (though I assume that the intuition about born humans and fetuses will operate more weakly or will be undercut altogether in someone with a strong religious conviction that the fetus has an immortal soul). Some years ago, however, I was led in a different direction as a result of having my attention called to an article by Catholic thinker (and U. S. Circuit Court judge) John Noonan, in which (I was told) abortion is criticized, not for failing to respect the rights of the fetus, but for showing a lack of empathy for the fetus. I was absolutely galvanized by hearing about Noonan's article because (for one thing) it immediately occurred to me that the notion or phenomenon of empathy is a double-edged sword, and reading the article itself did nothing to disturb this conclusion. If we believe that empathy has moral force or relevance, then since it is in fact much easier for us to empathize with born humans (even neonates) than with a fetus, we can argue that it is for this reason morally worse to neglect or hurt a born human than to do the same to a fetus or embryo. And this conclusion might end up giving more sustenance to the pro-choice position than to the pro-life view of abortion.

Moreover, it almost as immediately occurred to me that a virtue ethics of caring, rather than rely on our intuitions about our stronger obligations to born humans than to embryos, fetuses, or animals, could explain the intuitions, the differential obligations, by incorporating the idea of empathy. (In thinking thus I was implicitly regarding the empathy-altruism hypothesis as at least somewhat plausible.) Instead of claiming that actions are right or wrong depending on whether they exhibit or reflect what intuition tells us is properly contoured and sufficiently deep caring, one can say that actions are wrong or right depending on whether or not they reflect or exhibit a deficiency of normally or fully empathic caring motivation. It would then, at least other things being equal, be morally worse to prefer a fetus or embryo to a born human being, because such a preference runs counter to the flow of developed human empathy or to caring motivation that is shaped by such empathy. And similar points, arguably, could be made about our moral relations with lower animals.

I believe that the concept or phenomenon of empathy can also help us to formulate a virtue-ethical answer to the questions Singer raises in 'Famine, Affluence, and Altruism' (and elsewhere). An ethics of caring expanded and reconfigured so as to hinge on the idea of *developed human empathy* gives us reason to hold, *pace* Singer, that a failure to save the life of a distant child by making, say, a small contribution to Oxfam is not morally as objectionable or bad as failing to save the life of a child who is drowning right in front of one. We shall see that such a sentimentalist ethics of empathic caring can also allow us to draw other important moral distinctions, and I shall then also speculate briefly on the prospects of such a theory as a general and systematic approach to morality and meta-ethics.

2. EMPATHY, IMMEDIACY, AND MORALITY

Recent moral philosophers have written a great deal on the question, raised by Singer's article, how much we are obligated to spend of our own time, money, or other resources in order to save the lives of people who are personally unknown to us but whom we are in fact in a position to save. But this issue, as I have suggested, rests on the question whether we are more obligated to help a child drowning before our very eyes than to help any given child whom we know about only indirectly (as part of some labeled group rather than via personal acquaintance). As Singer points out in his article, the most *obvious* difference between the drowning child and a child we can save via contributions to Oxfam is one of spatial distance, and Singer himself holds that sheer distance simply cannot be morally relevant to our obligations to aid (or to how morally bad or objectionable it is *not* to aid). As a result, he concludes that we are just as obligated to give to Oxfam as to save the drowning child, and iterations of this argument lead him to the conclusion that most of us are morally obligated to make enormous sacrifices of our time, money, comfort, and so on, in order to help distant (or nearby) others who are much worse off than we are.

However, in recent years Singer's quick dismissal of distance has come to be questioned on the basis of considerations that I want to examine here while, at the same time, arguing that empathy in fact gives us a firmer basis than distance for distinguishing the strength of our obligations to the drowning child and our obligations to those we can only help (say) through organizations like Oxfam. Spatial distance and (decreasing) empathy do in fact correlate with one another across a wide range of cases, and that very fact may have helped to obscure the role empathy potentially has in explaining the sorts of distinctions people intuitively, or common-sensically, want to make with regard to the kinds of cases Singer mentions. But before saying anything further about the role of empathy here, it will be useful to say a bit more about the role sheer spatial distance might be thought to play in Singer-like cases.

Some of those who have lately considered the moral relevance of distance have regarded that issue as effectively involving two separate questions: first, whether we intuitively regard distance as making a difference to our obligations and, second, whether different intuitive reactions to third- or first-person cases involving distance would show anything important about (differences in) our actual obligations. In his book *Living High and Letting Die*, for example, Peter Unger considers both these issues and defends a negative answer to both of them (1996). He thinks that our superficial intuitions about cases may not ultimately carry much weight in moral theory in determining where our obligations really lie. But he also holds that our differing moral intuitions about relevant cases don't track distance so much as (what he calls) salience and conspicuousness.

However, Frances Kamm disagrees with these views. She thinks that (a rather complicated notion of) distance *does* help to explain our differing intuitions about cases and also is relevant to our actual obligations in such cases (1999: 162–208). Singer asks us to consider the difference between a situation where we can save a child from drowning at small cost to ourselves and one where we can save a distant child from starvation by making a small contribution to a famine relief organization, noting, but also deploring, our initial tendency to think that saving the child is morally more incumbent on us in the former situation than in the latter. But Kamm believes the factor of distance (or proximity) makes a relevant moral difference in/between these two cases, and, in order to rule out other factors that might be thought to be determining our moral judgments in those cases (like whether others are in a position to help), she devises other examples that she believes bring out the intuitive and real moral force of the factor of distance (proximity).

Both Unger's book and Kamm's paper are rich and extremely complicated, and what I have to say here won't go into every nook and cranny of what they say. But I find it interesting and a bit surprising that neither one of them considers the moral importance of our empathic tendencies or capacities. For example, in denying the intuitive or actual moral relevance of distance, Unger comes up with a category of salience/conspicuousness (also with a category of the dramatic or exciting, but I will discuss that a bit later) that he does take to be relevant to our intuitive judgments, but never once considers how what one might easily take to be a related notion—what we can readily or immediately empathize with—might be relevant, or thought to be relevant, here. Similarly, Kamm considers and rejects what Unger says about salience or conspicuousness (she also talks about vividness) in favor of the idea that (complexly understood) distance is relevant to distinguishing between cases like the drowning child and starving examples mentioned earlier, but somehow the subject of empathy never comes up.[5]

But I believe the notion of empathy can help us sort out our intuitive reactions to the kinds of cases Singer, Unger, and Kamm describe, better than the explanatory factors they mention, and let me say something about this now. In the familiar drowning examples, someone's danger or plight has a salience, conspicuousness, vividness, and *immediacy* (a term that, for reasons to be mentioned below, I prefer, but that Singer, Unger, and Kamm don't use) that engages normal human empathy (and consequently arouses sympathy and concern) in a way that similar dangers we merely know *about* do not. So if morality is a matter of empathy-based concern or caring for/about people, we can not only explain why a failure to help in the drowning case seems worse to us than a failure to give to famine relief, but also justify that ordinary moral intuition. (We can also justify our belief, e.g. that an incapacitated bystander in a drowning case should at least feel alarm and concern for the potential victim.)

The idea that seeing or perceiving makes a difference in arousing or eliciting empathic and altruistic reactions is by no means, however, a new one. Hume makes this essential point (while using the term 'sympathy') in the *Treatise*; and Hume also seems to hold that differences in what naturally or normally arouses sympathy/empathy affect the strength of our moral obligations and what virtue calls for (1958: 370, 439, 441, 483f, 488f, 518f). Moreover, there are recent psychological studies of empathy that bear out Hume's earlier observations/speculations. Martin Hoffman's recent book, *Empathy and Moral Development: Implications for Caring and Justice*, usefully summarizes and reflects upon numerous psychological studies of the development of empathy and its role in creating or sustaining caring/concern for others, and one thing that both Hoffman and the previous studies emphasize is the difference that perceptual immediacy tends to make to the strength of empathic responses (2000: 209ff). (However, Hoffman is more cautious than Hume is and I want to be about the moral implications of these psychological differences.)

In the light of the present moral emphasis on empathy, then, let's next consider what Kamm and Unger say about various cases. For example, in discussing the salience/conspicuousness that Unger invokes in explaining our (for him misguided) intuitions, Kamm distinguishes subjective and objective salience. Then, focusing on the former, she speaks of the science-fiction case of someone who can see a person

---

[5] I don't think Kamm ignores empathy because she thinks it too *subjective*. Unger's salience, as she notes, has a subjective aspect, but can also be viewed in a more objective way as what is or would be salient to a normal observer. But empathy also allows such a distinction, and the view I want to defend focuses on what calls forth (more or less) empathy (or empathy-involving concern) in a human being with a fully developed capacity for empathy.

suffering overseas with long-distance vision (1999: 182f). The suffering would then be salient, conspicuous, or vivid for the individual with the long-distance vision, but Kamm says that it is (intuitively) acceptable for that individual to 'turn off' her long-distance vision (and pay no more attention to the fate of the person she has seen than to the fate of distant others she *hasn't* seen). But if she can turn it off, presumably she is also permitted simply to *turn away, avert her gaze*; and that is certainly what the view Kamm defends about the relevance of proximity implies.

However, I don't think this conclusion is in fact morally intuitive, and I believe considerations of empathy help to explain why. Turning away from someone we see (even if only at an extreme distance) seems *worse* than ignoring someone whom one knows about only by description; and assuming, for example, that one has the means instantly to deliver help either to someone whose danger or need one sees through long-distance vision or to someone whose danger or need one merely knows about, most of us, I think, would consider it inhumane to turn away from the person whose plight one saw and then (coldly) decide to give the aid to someone one merely knew about. What is inhumane here arguably has something to do with empathy, with a failure of empathic response to someone whose need one sees. The immediacy or vividness of such perceived need engages our (normal or fully developed) human empathy more deeply or forcefully than need known only by description, and so a morality that centers around empathy in the way(s) I have been suggesting can explain our moral reactions to Kamm's case here better than Kamm's appeal to (complexly contoured) distance and proximity does, and it is difficult to see how Kamm can use this example to argue successfully against the view that subjective salience or vividness is relevant to our moral intuitions.

Interestingly, Kamm does say that what we see at an overseas distance would exert 'psychological pressure' on us to help. But she dismisses that pressure as somehow outside the bounds of our moral intuitions, because she thinks that we lack any intuition that tells us we have more obligation to the person we see than to someone we don't. If, however, and as I have just claimed, we do have such an intuition, then what she terms mere psychological pressure is in fact a moral intuition that her emphasis on distance fails to account for, but that a view based on empathy can.

Kamm then turns to an example of objective salience à la Unger. She imagines that the person with long-distance vision sees a group of people in trouble and that one of the people is wearing a clown-suit and is much more dramatically exhibiting his need for help than the others. Kamm holds that that should make no moral difference to whom one feels one should help, and she uses this example to argue for distance as opposed to objective salience. But a view emphasizing empathy can also (and perhaps more fully) account for our intuitions about this kind of case. The person in danger of drowning or starvation who is in a clown-suit and busy waving his arms or making histrionic gestures may be more visibly obtrusive; but such a person may seem to be faking fear or pain (hamming it up), whereas someone else who is quieter or less demonstrative may bear the marks of suffering or anxiety more genuinely than the person in the clown-suit and for that very reason more strongly engage our empathy. Such a case creates problems for an Ungerian objective-salience account of our moral intuitions, but not for a moral theory that is based in empathy; and I also believe the latter can account for differing intuitive reactions to variants on this kind of case better than a view that stresses distance.

Thus imagine that the person in the clown-suit isn't hamming it up. He and all the others are genuinely writhing in pain, but you notice him first because of his clown-suit and find yourself absolutely riveted on him. Assuming you can help only one of the people in the group, would we find it equally acceptable for you to turn away from the clown-suited man and decide that you might as well help *someone else* in the group, as for you to decide to help him? I think not. I think, again, we would find it lacking in or contrary to normally flowing human empathy, inhumane, for you to turn away from the man instead of helping him *in response to* your vivid recognition of his need. If his need has greater initial immediacy for you, then that, I think, is an intuitively good reason to go with the flow of empathy and help him out, given that one can only help one person in the group. But Kamm's account in terms of distance doesn't allow for this sort of reason. Let us, however, consider a further example.

Unger denies that there is any intuitive or real moral difference between cases where an accident victim one can help is nearby and visible to one and cases where the victim is at some distance and one learns about his plight via Morse code (1996: 36). But Kamm thinks he is mistaken here about our intuitions and claims the difference is due to factors of distance (1999: 184); and while I agree with Kamm that there is a significant difference between such cases, it seems to me more plausible—or perhaps I should say more promising—to explain it in terms of empathy.[6]

We have illustrated the moral force of (considerations relating to) natural human empathy in terms of examples having to do with our moral relations with the fetus (and animals) and have gone on to discuss cases, familiar from the literature that has grown up around Peter Singer's work, that raise issues about our obligations to people whom we see or don't see, or who are near or far from us. The latter kinds of examples all involve dangers or emergencies of one kind or another, but we have yet to consider another sort of danger/emergency case that has often been discussed by philosophers, cases where the issue is not so much (or cannot so easily be imagined to be) spatial proximity or distance, but rather *temporal* proximity or distance.

I am thinking of the well-known example of miners trapped in a coalmine (as a result, say, of a cave-in). We typically feel morally impelled to help the miners rather than (at that point) expend an equivalent amount of money to install safety devices in the mines that will save a greater number of lives in the long run. But some have disagreed. Charles Fried discusses this example in his *An Anatomy of Values* and claims that we/society should prefer to install the safety devices and let the miners die. (He gives his argument a rather barbaric twist by saying we should even be willing to convey this decision to the ill-fated miners face-to-face, if that is somehow possible (1970: 207–27).)

This example, this choice, doesn't turn on a contrast between near and far or between what is perceived and what is not, because we can easily imagine that those

---

[6] Unger in fact notes (p. 36) that such cases differ with respect to 'experiential impact', a notion that ties in with empathy. But he doesn't pay much attention to impact, presumably because he (mistakenly) thinks that it makes no significant difference to our intuitions.

who have to choose whom to save are at a distance from the mine and don't know or perceive either the trapped miners or those who might be in danger there in the future. We can well imagine, for example, that *we* are somehow empowered to make the choice, having heard or read reports of the mine cave-in, and I don't think the tendency to prefer saving the now-trapped miners would then be explainable in terms of an empathy-derived preference for saving those whose dangers we are perceptually aware of rather than those whose dangers we merely know about.

Still, if we have to choose between the now-trapped miners and those who will be in danger in the future, there is an immediacy to the danger the former are in that does, I think, engage our empathic/sympathetic juices in a way that the danger to the latter does not. Of course, there is also an immediacy to our previous examples of a child drowning and of a clown-suited person whose distress is (immediately) visible to us, but this immediacy, clearly, is perceptual and hinges on issues about the *spatial* distance that direct perception can accommodate. A rather different kind of immediacy is at issue in the miners example, an immediacy having more to do with the present-tense temporal character of the miners' danger—the fact that it is a 'clear and present danger'—than with any spatial or spatially correlated factors. But both kinds of immediacy appeal to our empathy in a way that situations not involving these forms of immediacy tend not to do. (The fact that the word 'present' applies both to a time and to a mode of sensory contact seems very apt, given this common appeal to empathy.)

Thus we may not see or hear or personally know the miners who are now trapped, and, because they are thus known to us only as a class or by description, the empathic appeal of their plight—as compared with the plight of those who are going to be in danger later—is different from the empathic (moral) appeal of (dangers to) those we are perceptually aware of. But it is natural to think of both kinds of cases as involving some sort of immediacy, and that may be the best term for describing the (projected?) objective correlate, in certain kinds of situations, of our (subjective or psychological) tendency toward empathy. And the fact that we can use such correlated immediacy and empathy to explain our moral reactions not only in the cases discussed in the Singer literature, but also in the miners case gives further support to what was said above about cases of the Singer type and to the general account of morality I have been sketching.[7]

If that account is correct, then what is morally wrong with installing safety devices (as Fried suggests) rather than helping miners who are in clear and present danger is that it exhibits (or reflects or expresses) a deficiency of normal(ly developed) human empathy.[8] But by the same token someone who turns away from someone she sees in

[7] Interestingly, Hoffman, speaks of empathy as having a 'here and now' bias, and the studies he cites make it very clear that our empathy flows more readily not only in regard to what is visible or perceived, but also in regard to what is current or contemporaneous.

[8] Unger (1996: 78–9) describes a case in which a meteor has fallen to earth and will explode with disastrous consequences in a densely populated area unless someone immediately steals an 'Ejector' machine from its rightful owner and uses it to hurl the meteor to a deserted canyon. He thinks one is permitted to steal and operate the Ejector in such circumstances, but says that the 'dramaticness' of the trouble involved here makes no difference to that permission. Yet this example

order to help someone she merely knows about (as in the kinds of examples Kamm and Unger talk about) will (other things being equal) also exhibit/demonstrate an underdeveloped capacity for empathy and a consequent coldness that we regard as morally questionable. And this sentimentalist (and virtue-ethical) way of approaching moral issues also helps to explain why Singer is wrong to think that failures to save via organizations like Oxfam are in the same moral boat (so to speak) as a failure to save a child drowning right in front of one: the former simply doesn't exhibit as great a lack of (normal) human empathy as the latter does or would.

One implication of what I have been saying is that an ethics based on empathy yields a partialist, rather than an impartialist, understanding of morality. Fried's suggestions about what we should do in the miners case are ethically repugnant or worse, but it is not as if he is advocating a selfish or egoistic indifference to the miners. Rather, he is urging us to see them and everyone else, present or future, in terms of a strictly impartial concern for humans (or sentient beings) generally. If this seems morally inadequate, and if a virtue-ethical sentimentalist approach can make use of the idea of empathy to offer us a promising explanation of why it is inadequate, then we are given reason to see morality (and the world of our moral concern or caring) in a partialist way; and the same partialism likewise conflicts with and tells against the views Peter Singer defends. Indeed, Singer has claimed that partialism has never been given an adequate principled defense (1999: 308) and whether or not this is true, the approach I am taking is intended as offering, or being on the way to offering, such a defense of partialism.

The observant reader may have noticed, however, that I have not so far explicitly argued that Singer is wrong to maintain that we are under a moral obligation to sacrifice a great deal of our time and/or money to help those less fortunate than ourselves. He reaches that conclusion via a lemma that we *have* questioned, namely, the idea that we are as obligated to help distant individuals we don't know as to save a child drowning right in front of us. But it is time for us now to be a little more explicit about the reasons why, on the present approach, we are not obligated to make enormous sacrifices of the kind Singer recommends, but can view such sacrifices, rather, as *supererogatorily* good or praiseworthy.

The social-psychological literature supports, on the whole, the idea that human beings have a substantial capacity for empathy and for altruistic concern(s) based on empathy. Hoffman in particular gives a fascinating and in many ways compelling account of how moral education can lead us in fact toward an empathic concern for (groups of) people we don't know very well or even at all (the people of Bangladesh, the homeless, victims of AIDS) (2000). But Hoffman also makes it clear that (he thinks) there are limits to how much empathy for (disadvantaged) groups people can be led to develop. Self-interest (or egocentric desires, fears, hatred, etc.) can often strongly oppose or qualify what we may or might otherwise do out of empathy or empathic concern for others (2000). If so, then our general account will yield the

---

involves just the sort of clear and present danger that we saw in the case of the trapped miners, and if empathy is relevant to morality, then dramaticness (or at least what makes for drama in the case Unger describes, namely, the clear and present danger) may in fact make a difference not only to our intuitions, but to (the strength of) our moral obligations.

conclusion that we are not morally obligated to sacrifice most of our time and money to help needy others, because a failure to do so doesn't evince an absence of normally or fully developed human empathy. In that case, if it would take someone with an unusually high degree of empathy and empathic concern—a degree of empathy and empathic concern beyond what most people can be led to develop—to be willing to make such a sacrifice, then such sacrifice will be morally supererogatory—morally praiseworthy and/or good but *not* (*pace* Singer) obligatory.[9]

But even if this is so, it may still be obligatory for individuals like ourselves to make some sort of substantial contribution toward the relief of hunger (or similarly worthy causes). Those who do not may be acting wrongly because they evince a degree of empathic concern that is *less* than what most people can be led to acquire. (Hoffman and others say a great deal about how moral education can in fact induce empathy and caring for people we don't know personally.) At the very least, then, even if Singer exaggerates what morality demands of us, it may nonetheless be true that many of us should give a good deal more for the relief of famine or disease around the world than we actually do.

3. PROSPECTS FOR SENTIMENTALIST VIRTUE ETHICS

At this point, however, a very large objection to what I have been proposing needs to be considered. We have been speaking about the ways in which normally or fully developed human empathic reactions may be thought to give shape to our obligations to help others, but all such obligations fall within the sphere of beneficence, and it is not surprising that our obligations in that area should turn out to be a matter of proper (morally recommendable) human feeling or sentiment. What we should give to others can more or less easily be seen as a matter of what proper feelings or motives would lead us to do for others, and this remains true, I think, whether or not one regards proper beneficence as reflecting impartial concern for overall human welfare or as reflecting the more contoured and partialistic sensitivities that are built into human empathy and caring based in such empathy.

But there is arguably more to morality than obligations (and supererogations) of beneficence. Those who believe in deontology suppose that there are times when human beneficence—whether conceived in partialistic or impartialistic terms—has to be limited or restricted. And if (proper) beneficence seems a matter of (cultivated or educated) human feeling, then the deontological considerations that such beneficence sometimes has to yield to are naturally regarded as limiting or restricting the play or expression of such feelings. Our desire to help people, then, is easily regarded

---

[9] A virtue ethics based on empathy can point to the greater ease or naturalness of empathizing with those near and dear to us (with those we know and love) as a basis for arguing that we have especially strong moral reasons to be concerned with such people. But, for simplicity's sake, I am treating the issue of self-interest vs. concern for the unfortunate as if it didn't also involve issues about our obligations to near and dear. Note too that, if what I have been saying is on the right track, the issue of helping needy distant groups will arise (or will arise with greatest force) only when one is not facing any more *immediate* issue of need or danger.

as reflecting certain cultivatable feelings, but any deontological prohibition on (say) killing forbids us to kill even if doing so would on the whole be more helpful than not doing so, and here, then, the desire to help, the sentiment of human concern for others, seems to be restricted in the name of *something other* than sentiment. In that case, a moral sentimentalism that seeks to account for deontology would appear to face an uphill battle.

Of course, one of the eighteenth-century sentimentalists, Francis Hutcheson, anticipated utilitarianism in denying the ultimate validity of deontology and in relying ultimately and exclusively on the dictates or guidance of impartial or universal benevolence. But it would be unfortunate for moral sentimentalism (as it seems unfortunate for act-utilitarianism) to have to deny the validity of our basic intuitions concerning deontological prohibitions, and I believe sentimentalism needs to look for some alternative. Hume, in fact, did seek such an alternative, and his account of the artificial virtues certainly attempts to deal with a major part of deontology in sentimentalist terms. But given all the worries there are about "Hume's circle" and other features of his theory of deontology, I think the contemporary sentimentalist ought to look elsewhere for an account of deontology. What I want to suggest here is that this can be done by appealing to facts about human empathy and to a notion of immediacy different from, but allied with, the forms of immediacy we have already discussed (albeit all too briefly) here. And the issue of deontology I want to focus on (the only issue space limitations allow me to consider here) is the (arguably) central one of doing versus allowing, for example, of killing versus letting die.

We saw earlier that empathy works through certain modalities or aspects of an agent's interaction with the world. Agents are more empathic and more empathically concerned with what they perceive than with what they don't; and they are also empathically more sensitive to what they know to be going on at the same time as their decision-making and choices. These differences of empathy correspond to what we naturally think of as the greater immediacy of dangers that we perceive or that are contemporaneous with our concern. But there are other facts about or factors in our interactions with the world that empathy is also sensitive to and that give rise to a form of immediacy we have not yet mentioned.

When we cause a death, kill someone, we are in causal terms more strongly connected to a death than if we merely allow someone to die, and I believe that we are empathically sensitive to this distinction in a way that allows us to make sense of (certain central issues of) deontology. Given the role of empathy as discussed above, the strength of one's obligations regarding another person's distress can depend on whether one perceives that distress or on whether the distress is contemporaneous. But if we are also empathically sensitive to the strength of our causal relations to various forms of distress or harm, then a virtue ethics of empathic caring can say that it is morally worse to kill than to allow to die, and a major (perhaps the most central) part of ordinary deontology can then be accounted for in sentimentalist terms. And I believe that there are intuitive reasons for thinking that we are empathically sensitive to doing versus allowing in the way just suggested.

If we are more empathically sensitive to perceived or contemporaneous (potential) pain, so too do we seem to be more empathically sensitive to (potentially) causing pain (or death) than to (potentially) allowing it. We *flinch* from causing or inflicting pain in a way or to an extent that we don't flinch from (merely) allowing pain, and I would like to say that pain or harm that we (may) cause has, therefore, a greater *causal* immediacy for us than pain or harm that we (may) merely allow. In that case, and given the moral weight I have argued we should give to human empathic concern/caring for others, we have some reason to conclude that it is morally worse to kill or harm than (other things being equal) to allow these things to happen, and that helps to give a sentimentalist virtue-ethical basis to deontology.[10]

Most philosophical attempts to ground deontology appeal to some form of practical or theoretical reason or rationality and to reason-based moral considerations, rules, or principles that can oppose sentiment. But if the empathy-based sentimentalist account I am sketching is on the right track, it can be our empathic sensitivity to situational factors of immediacy rather than adherence to rules (or even insight into unique situational *moral* facts à la Aristotle) that leads us not to kill or steal in (some) situations where doing so would have overall better results. Thus although many have felt that the weaknesses of Hume's account of deontology are discouraging to the prospects of moral sentimentalism, there may just be another way for sentimentalism to deal with these issues, a (virtue-ethical) way that leans heavily on the notion of empathy. If what I have been saying is correct, then deontology needn't be conceived as different from and opposed to all human feeling and sentiment, but may actually have its roots in certain very particular sentiments. In that case, the familiar moral opposition between (partialist or impartialist) beneficence and deontology may occur *within* the realm of sentiment rather than reflect any (partial) conflict between feeling/sentiment and something else of moral importance. But what I have said here is just a sketch or (perhaps even less than that) the promise of a new sentimentalist conception of deontology. I haven't at all mentioned issues of justice and human rights and fidelity to promises that are typically regarded as basic to deontology, and all such issues need to be left to another occasion (in fact, to a book entitled *The Ethics of Care and Empathy* that I have almost finished). My purpose has been merely to show that what might be thought of as an insuperable obstacle to reviving moral sentimentalism is arguably not insuperable.

However, before I go on to some concluding remarks, let me mention one further obstacle that the reader or others may regard as presenting an insuperable barrier to any attempt to revive sentimentalism in the fullest fashion. One of the most

---

[10] But there are complications here. It is one thing to see a basic difference of causality between certain salient kinds of doing and certain salient kinds of allowing, but discussions, say, of killing vs. letting die often go into some very fine intuitive distinctions, and the present approach needs ultimately to be able to say something about these. For example, we think there is a difference between injecting a terminally ill patient with a lethal dose of morphine and turning off a life support machine, and the latter is often conceived as merely allowing a patient to die; and yet the latter also clearly involves a greater causal intervention than in other cases of letting die. A full sentimentalist account of deontology along the above lines would need to consider the relationship between different degrees of causal relationship and human empathic reactions. Such a more nuanced account might help us justify various ordinary moral distinctions, but, to the extent sentimentalist virtue ethics seemed an otherwise powerful approach, it might also lead us to question certain very fine-grained putative moral distinctions.

important features of eighteenth-century sentimentalism was its attempt(s) to cover both ethical and meta-ethical issues in sentimentalist terms. For example (and perhaps most notably), Hume sought to account not only for what it is to be virtuous, but also for what it is to make moral judgments (give vent to moral utterances) *about* virtue (and other moral matters), in terms of his notion of sympathy. In fact, Hume, Hutcheson, and Adam Smith all combined sentimentalism in normative ethical theory with sentimentalism in meta-ethics, and any fully revived present-day moral sentimentalism will presumably have to do something like this as well.

But the prospects for meta-ethical sentimentalism seem actually not to be very bright. Hume thought he could base our understanding of moral judgments or utterances in human sentiments of approval and disapproval. But many philosophers would regard such an enterprise as fundamentally wrong-headed, because (they would say) approval and disapproval, far from being (mere) feelings that can be used to ground more objective-seeming moral claims or judgments, *already presuppose or involve moral judgment or claim-making*. We cannot, it is said, disapprove of something unless we *eo ipso* or already think it wrong, so the attempt to base moral utterances in feelings like approval and disapproval is doomed to circularity.

This would certainly represent a grave or insuperable difficulty for any systematic reviving of sentimentalism, and at this point I should, I think, simply limit myself to saying that I believe meta-ethical sentimentalism can answer this important objection through the use of the very same notion of empathy that figures so centrally in the normative account of rightness, wrongness, and virtue that has been sketched here. I shall offer such an answer on another occasion; but for present purposes it may be enough to hope that what I have said above might whet the reader's appetite for (more) moral sentimentalism and convince her that it has some interesting things to say.

At this point, and by way of conclusion, however, I would like to talk about some potential objections to what I have been positively saying (as opposed to omitting) in this chapter up till now. It might be objected, for example, that what I have mainly done is describe or attempt to describe human psychology and that any ethical conclusions I have drawn amount to a hopeless effort to deduce 'ought's from 'is'es. But in fact I have not just been doing psychology or attempting to tie moral judgments rigidly to judgments about what people are actually like. Many people aren't fully empathic or empathic at all (think of psychopaths!); and the view I am defending criticizes such people and deems their behavior to be wrong if it exhibits or reflects their lack of empathic concern for others. On my view, some people/acts are morally objectionable and other people/acts are not, and the distinction is made by reference to a sentimental ideal of empathic concern and the virtue-ethical assumption that actions are most plausibly evaluated in relation to such an ideal. (Although I have said something about recent psychological discussions of how full or normal empathic concern develops, a complete defense of the present approach would need to go into a great deal more detail than is possible in the limited space available here.)

And the sentimentalist virtue-ethical theory sketched and used earlier in this chapter wasn't just 'deduced' from certain psychological facts. It is, in fact, a *theory*; and like all theories its value and validity depend on what can (or cannot) be deduced from or explained by it. I am not, therefore, claiming that it is self-evident or immediately obvious that moral virtue consists in empathic concern for others and/or that behavior or actions are to be evaluated by reference to such an inner state. Rather, the argument has been that the theory proposed allows us to make some important intuitive moral distinctions in a principled way, that it helps us to account for many facets of the moral life.[11] In the present context, our main task has been to see whether a sentimentalist virtue ethics can plausibly counter the morally unintuitive and unwelcome implications of Peter Singer's arguments about famine and affluence. If the theory discussed here allows us to do that, that stands in its favor, and everything else I have said has been said in order to support that theory further.[12] Of course, I have done much, much less than would be needed to make virtue-ethical sentimentalism seem plausible *as a total approach to morality*, but I hope I have at least done enough to persuade people that there is something here that is worth pursuing.[13]

REFERENCES

Foot, P. (2001). *Natural Goodness*. Oxford: Oxford University Press.

Fried, C. (1970). *An Anatomy of Values*. Cambridge, MA: Harvard University Press, 207–27.

Gilligan, C. (1982). *In a Different Voice: Psychological Theory and Women's Development*. Cambridge, MA: Harvard University Press.

Hoffman, M. (2000). *Empathy and Moral Development: Implications for Caring and Justice*. New York: Cambridge University Press, 209ff, and *passim*.

Hume, D. (1958). *Treatise* (L. A. Selby-Bigge edn.). Oxford: Clarendon Press, 370, 439, 441, 483f, 488f, 518f, and *passim*.

Hursthouse, H. (1999). *On Virtue Ethics*. Oxford: Oxford University Press.

Kamm, F. (1999). 'Famine Ethics', in Dale Jamieson, ed., *Singer and His Critics*. Oxford: Basil Blackwell, 162–208, 182f.

Noddings, N. (1984). *Caring: A Feminine Approach to Ethics and Moral Education*. Berkeley: University of California Press.

_____ (2002). *Starting at Home: Caring and Social Policy*. Berkeley: University of California Press.

Ruddick, S. (1989). *Maternal Thinking: Toward a Politics of Peace*. Boston: Beacon Press.

[11] In other words, it may not be immediately obvious that right and wrong depend on an (ontological) relation to developed empathic concern for others, but the fact that that explanatory theoretical hypothesis allows us to derive ordinary intuitive moral claims and distinctions helps to justify the hypothesis. One might, however, wonder whether our reliance on empathy may in fact lead us to make *too many* moral distinctions. For example, if people of one race or gender are more empathically sensitive to those of the same race or gender, then the distinctions in our attitudes and behavior that empathy explains may, at least some of them, be morally invidious; and this would represent a serious problem for any attempt to explain morality systematically in terms of empathic caring. I offer a response to such worries in *The Ethics of Care and Empathy*.

[12] However, one thing I haven't done is explain why I think actions should be evaluated by reference to their underlying motivation rather than their actual or expectable consequences. This may seem less than imperative in a volume devoted to virtue ethics, but I do offer arguments in favor of virtue ethics and against consequentialism in *Morals from Motives*, esp. chapters 1 and 5.

[13] I would like to thank P. J. Ivanhoe and Rebecca Walker for helpful suggestions concerning the present essay.

Singer, P. (1972). 'Famine, Affluence, and Morality'. *Philosophy and Public Affairs*, 1/3: 229–43.

_____ (1999). 'A Response [to Critics]', in Dale Jamieson, ed., *Singer and His Critics*, 308.

Slote, M. (1996/2001). *Morals from Motives*. New York: Oxford University Press.

_____ (1998). 'The Justice of Caring'. *Social Philosophy and Policy*, 15: 171–95.

Unger, P. (1996). *Living High and Letting Die*. New York: Oxford University Press.

14

Filial Piety as a Virtue

Philip J. Ivanhoe

Gentlemen work at the root of the matter.
Once the root is well established, the Way will flourish.
Filial piety and brotherly respect—are these not the roots of perfect goodness!

Analects 1.2

INTRODUCTION

The virtue of filial piety may seem a tad out of date to many modern Western readers, but instead of accepting this response as authoritative, we should see it as raising several issues that are part of why this topic is particularly relevant and important. The first thing to ask about such a response is, Why is it that this particular virtue might strike certain readers as less pressing or even unimportant? The fact that some may find this a natural response is not alone a *good reason* to accept such a view as decisive. If, as some argue, virtues are traits of character that help one fare well in the face of a common set of human challenges, defined in terms of particular spheres of activity, then filial piety should be a central concern.[1] For in one way or another, as human beings, we all have to work our way through the special relationship we have with our parents. While traditional beliefs about filial piety may be out of date, the fact that humans have an enduring, distinctive, and emotionally charged relationship with their parents remains as true today as it was in the past and as true in the West as it is in the East.

The second point is that while filial piety may strike many modern *Western* readers as a bit old fashioned, this is certainly not the case for readers in East Asian communities and many other people throughout the world. Many Chinese intellectuals find it quite odd that Western ethical philosophers for the most part disregard or dismiss issues like filial piety and instead seem obsessed with the obscure and apparently intractable metaphysical problems associated with topics like abortion. The inordinate amount of attention paid to abortion in contemporary philosophical writing strikes educated observers outside the West, and some within it, more as a matter of anthropology—a manifestation of the Judeo-Christian context of Western philosophy—than evidence of the overriding *philosophical* importance of this particular problem.

[1] Martha Nussbaum (1993) presents a classic version of this approach to virtue ethics.

Filial piety was an important virtue in early Confucianism, recognized even by critics of the tradition, such as Zhuangzi, as an unavoidable part of human life.[2] Such a deep and abiding concern with filial piety is not unique to China. Cultures throughout the world value filial behavior and record, retell, and advocate acts of filial devotion and sacrifice.[3] Many people explain such behavior, as Zhuangzi did, by appealing to human nature. Along with religious warrants, such appeals often are offered not only as explanations for filial behavior but also as justifications for filial piety as a duty, obligation, or virtue.[4]

Chinese culture is distinctive for the amount of attention paid to and the importance claimed for this particular virtue. In contrast, most contemporary Western philosophers pay scant attention to filial piety. Among those who offer a defense of at least some form of filial obligation, the most interesting and persuasive views analyze filial piety either in terms of a sense of gratitude for the various sacrifices that good parents make on behalf of their children or on the model of friendship.[5] I will argue that such arguments offer the beginnings of a viable defense of filial piety but fall short because they fail to capture crucial features of the child–parent relationship and misconstrue the true source and foundation of filial piety.

In this essay, I will explore some of the central justifications for filial piety as a virtue that one can find in the early Confucian tradition. Specifically I will describe, discuss, and evaluate several arguments that were offered in support of a general obligation to care for, protect, defer to, and revere one's parents while they are alive and to remember and sacrifice to them after they have died. I then will argue that some of the explicit or implied justifications for such an obligation are not well founded and no longer offer compelling reasons for cultivating and valuing the virtue of filial piety. However, others do provide solid and persuasive justification for filial piety as a virtue and offer considerable support for at least some version of traditional belief and practice. Equally important, these arguments and the related descriptions of the nature of the child–parent relationship offer important contributions to the contemporary philosophical discussion of filial piety. In particular, they are useful for both

---

[2] See *Zhuangzi*, 'In the Human World', chapter 4, where we are told, 'That children should love their parents is a matter of destiny.'

[3] For a discussion of ideals of filial piety in the Western tradition, see Blustein (1982). For representations of filial piety in Japanese drama, see Smethurst (1998).

[4] Saint Thomas Aquinas is an excellent example of someone who develops a sophisticated defense of filial piety combining both Aristotelian accounts of human nature and biblical commands. For an insightful discussion of his views, see Blustein (1982), 56–62. Chinese beliefs about ancestor worship and in particular the need to carry on sacrifices to ancestral spirits also provided important warrants for Chinese belief and practice. Such beliefs in fact contribute a great deal to the sense of 'piety' in Chinese conceptions of filial piety.

[5] There are a number of interesting contemporary defenses of filial piety. Sommers (1986) argues for the importance of tradition and convention and attempts to combine this with claims about the rights of moral patients. English (1979) argues against the notion that children 'owe' their parents anything and for a relationship of love or friendship between children and parents. For the friendship model of filial piety, see Dixon (1995). Jecker (1989) argues that children have an obligation to treat their parents with filial piety out of gratitude for the supererogatory acts and duty-meeting acts of benevolence parents did on behalf of their children. A good general introduction to filial piety is Wicclair (1990). The most thorough and incisive monograph on this topic is Blustein (1982).

correcting and augmenting contemporary accounts of filial piety as an expression of gratitude or friendship. In conclusion I will argue that a proper understanding of these early Chinese beliefs about the relationship between children and parents also offers important insights into other, related aspects of traditional Chinese ethics.

EARLY CONFUCIAN CONCEPTIONS OF FILIAL PIETY

Before we turn to those early Chinese views on filial piety that will contribute to my contemporary account, it is important to clear away some traditional claims that are better left behind. The first claim that I would like to explore and then leave behind is that filial piety is based on a special sense of gratitude that children should feel toward those who brought them into being. The thought is that parents are the source of the children they beget, and that this fact somehow establishes an obligation on the part of the children to honor, defer to, and serve their parents. Similar ideas are widespread in contemporary culture, where it is not uncommon to find parents who insist that since their children 'owe' their very existence to their parents, this establishes a debt that the children can *never* fully repay.[6] Related to this idea is the view that parents are entitled to nearly complete control over the lives of their children.

In the early Confucian tradition, we see various expressions of this kind of argument and the special nature of this appeal is used to justify some of the distinctive characteristics of the tradition's conception of filial piety. For example, children were thought to be physical extensions of their parents and this was seen as establishing an overriding debt on the part of children. Such a view was also the basis of early Confucian taboos about physically harming or defacing one's body. Both of these ideas are seen in the opening chapter of the *Classic of Filial Piety*, 'One's body, hair, and skin are received from one's father and mother. Not to injure or harm these is the beginning of filial piety'.[7] I will argue that while it is true that in a certain sense a child 'owes' its existence to its parents, this fact alone does not support any sort of obligation on the part of the child. The true basis for filial piety is the sense of gratitude, reverence, and love that children naturally feel when they are nurtured, supported, and cared for by people who do so out of loving concern for the child's well being.[8] Begetting a child establishes no substantial basis for filial piety, and once we understand and appreciate this fact we can more easily see why filial piety is equally warranted on the part of adopted as well as biological children.

---

[6] Jecker (1989) argues against the idea that parents are owed gratitude from their children merely for the act of begetting them, a view which she identifies as the 'Law of Athens'. See also the discussion in Blustein (1982), 31–46.

[7] *Xiaojing*, chapter 1. See also *Analects*, 8.3. The filial obligation that one has to protect and nurture one's parents is so great that it even trumps this standing obligation to protect one's own body. This is seen in various stories about filial children sacrificing themselves in order to preserve their parents. For example, there is the well-known story, alluded to by Su Shi in one of his poems, of a filial child who cuts the flesh from his leg in order to make medicinal cakes to cure his ailing parents. The original source is a passage in the *Songshi*.

[8] Paul Woodruff (2002) offers a modern defense of reverence as a virtue that includes a substantial and helpful treatment of classical Chinese sources.

At least part of the force of the traditional 'genetic argument' derives from a conflation of two distinct senses of the word 'owe'. In the case of children, they 'owe' their existence to their parents in the sense that certain of their parents' actions were causes for their coming into being. However, this sense of 'owing' is distinct from the sense in which one 'owes' someone money as a result of borrowing it earlier. The analogy with borrowing or any sense of contractual obligation clearly is inappropriate in the case of child and parent relationships since the child did not exist when such a debt purportedly was incurred.

One might try to argue that children still owe their parents some kind of obligation as an expression of gratitude for being brought into existence. However, upon further consideration, such appeals are not at all evident or straightforward. In order for any action to be a legitimate source of gratitude, it must not only be in the actual interest of the recipient, it must also be done out of an attitude of caring *for her*.[9] Given these criteria, it is at least problematic to claim that children in general owe their parents a debt of gratitude for being brought into existence. First, it is not at all evident that bare existence per se can be considered a good. A helpful parallel can be drawn here with the case of death. Some have argued that we dread death because after death we will no longer exist. But, as Thomas Nagel (1979) has pointed out, if this were the source of our concern, we would feel equally bad about not having existed for all the time prior to our birth or conception. Nagel goes on to argue that it is not the loss of *existence* that we fear but all the good things that we have and can reasonably expect to have while alive. Secondly, it should be clear that a good number of children are created as a result of their parents seeking each other's or their own sensual gratification. Other children are born because their parents believe that having children will improve their lives or marriage or because they have a religious duty to procreate. In such cases, the object of care is not the child itself, and so even if one could somehow show that existence is a good that one can bestow upon another, this good would not be a legitimate basis for gratitude.

Early Confucians clearly believed that having children was a religious duty. Those who failed to have children not only failed their parents but their entire clan lineage, for without posterity, there is no one to carry on the requisite sacrifices to ancestral spirits. Mengzi singles out a failure to have children as the most unfilial of actions. Mengzi said, 'There are three unfilial things [that a child can do] and to leave behind no posterity is the greatest.'[10] In this last example, as well as those described above, it is clear that the child's existence is not something that is sought for *her good*. Even if one could show that existence is a good, it is not clear why a child should feel gratitude

---

[9] Jecker (1989) argues a similar line in holding that an obligation of gratitude is incurred only in cases where one not only benefits from the actions of another but also when what they do for one is done out of benevolence. She also argues, though on this issue our views differ in certain respects, that begetting is not enough to establish filial obligation.

[10] *Mengzi* 4A26. The other two were to aid and abet one's parents in wrongful actions and to fail to protect and provide for them in old age. In *Mengzi* 4B30, Mengzi describes a list of five unfilial actions. These all concern various ways that children can, through lack of effort or self-control, bring disgrace to, fail to support, or endanger their parents.

for being brought into existence in order for her parents to fulfill *their* felt obligation to continue the family line.

Now it is possible that some parents are motivated by a desire simply to bring a child into existence in the sense of giving it 'the gift of life'. This seems more promising as a possible ground for a sense of gratitude on the part of children that result from such intentions. For while existence per se is not a benefit, in general, it is good to be alive, and under the right circumstances one can see this as a good bestowed upon certain children for their benefit.[11] In such cases though the sense of gratitude that one might feel would be distinctive—like what the recipient of a fellowship provided by some benevolent benefactor might feel. One receives a genuine benefit and the source of the benefit is a benevolent intention, even though it is not one aimed at any particular or even any existing person.

I suspect that the sense of gratitude that many people feel toward their parents for being 'given the gift of life' is really a reflection of their parents' commitment to and subsequent success at *loving and caring for* the child that they create. In other words, what we recognize and appreciate is the parents' intention to provide a *good* life and not just life to their child. Just 'being alive' is just too thin and imprecise a concept to represent much if any sense of good. Imagine children who were brought into existence for the sole purpose of being used, over time and as the need arose, as organ donors. The parents of such children would want them to have life, but this provides little if any grounds for gratitude. There are cases when simply being alive is not good and decisively so; in such cases it is not clear why one should feel gratitude toward those who helped to bring one into being.

Let us though return to a more charitable description of cases where the parents' intention is simply to bestow the gift of life upon some future child. As noted above, under the right circumstances this would be a reasonable ground for some sense of gratitude. It is not at all clear how many parents engage in procreative activity primarily for this reason. But even in cases where this is the parents' primary motivation, as noted above, the sense of gratitude one might feel is distinctive; it is more indirect and anonymous than familiar examples of gratitude. It is not like the gratitude I feel for someone who has intentionally benefited *me* for my own good.

It is hard to see how this indirect sense of gratitude could serve as the basis for filial piety, at least in anything like its classic expressions. It might be some small part of why one appreciates one's parents, but it hardly seems substantial enough to support the deep, complex, and pervasive feelings of gratitude, reverence, and love associated with filial piety. The general and unfocused intention to create life is not a central theme in traditional texts; instead, as in the examples cited below, they devote much more attention to describing, at length and in detail, the litany of good things that parents provide. The most prominent themes are the nurture, support, and love that fortunate children receive from good parents. As I noted above and will argue below,

---

[11] Nagel (1979) also accepts that 'it is good simply to be alive', but it is important to recognize that for him 'to be alive' means to be capable of 'perception, desire, activity, and thought' and that the bad aspects of one's life do not outweigh these obvious and fundamental human goods.

even a more robust and direct sense of gratitude is only the beginning of filial piety. Gratitude must be supplemented with feelings of reverence and love that are seen as the natural response to the sustained, particular, and characteristic nurture and love that good parents bestow upon their children.

Mary Shelly's story *Frankenstein* is instructive both for illustrating why begetting is not enough and for pointing toward the true basis of filial piety. In this story, Victor Frankenstein brought the Creature into existence but did not do so in order to bestow upon it the 'gift of life'. Frankenstein's aims were to demonstrate his genius and, perhaps, to advance science, not benefit the Creature. And so, giving the Creature life—or more precisely reanimating its various parts in a new configuration—established no obligation on the part of the Creature toward Frankenstein.[12] Given the nature of the Creature, it did not need or want many of the kinds of goods that human parents must provide for their children and for which their children should feel gratitude for receiving. The Creature did not need to be protected and provided for in the ways that human infants do—both during a pregnancy and for many years thereafter. Nevertheless, what it *did* need and crave was the kind of attention, instruction, nurturance, and guidance that is essential to good parenting. It needed to be loved *for its own sake*. Frankenstein withheld his love and even his approval. Unlike a good parent, he made these *conditional*; his approval and affection depended on the creature meeting certain prior expectations that were in fact expressions of Frankenstein's good, not the good of his creation.[13] Much of the sympathy we feel for the Creature is founded on the perceived failure of Victor Frankenstein to love his creation and on the basis of such love to engage in the broad set of nurturing activities that are characteristic of good parents.[14]

While Frankenstein's Creature did not need to be provided for, or at least not as badly as human infants do, one source of filial feelings is the remarkable range of protection, nurturance, and material support that children receive from good parents. Such support normally begins soon after conception and is particularly direct and complete in the case of one's mother. For good mothers sustain, nurture, and protect their children in a comprehensive and intimate way. A father who supports and cares for his spouse and child during this period is also offering the kind of person-specific

---

[12] There are additional ethical dimensions to the case described in *Frankenstein*. For example, unlike a child, which develops from living cells, the Creature was constructed from dead body parts that were reanimated. In some sense it *never should have lived*. Such concerns could lead one to claim that Frankenstein acted wrongly in bringing the Creature into existence. This would not require one to believe that in so doing he had wronged the Creature, but one might argue that the Creature itself could regret not only its life but its very existence as well. I will not explore such issues any farther as they do not have any direct effect upon the argument I am pursuing. Thanks to Eric L. Hutton for raising questions about these aspects of the story.

[13] Frankenstein created the Creature in order to serve as a witness to his genius and his vaulting ambition to play the role of God. When the Creature did not live up to Frankenstein's expectations, he considered it a failure and turned away from it.

[14] A Confucian might argue that in denying the Creature the love that every child should have, Frankenstein cut off the opportunity for it to become part of the human community and thereby set it on its course of destruction, death, pain, and anguish. On such an interpretation, the fact that the Creature itself could not die, or at least was very hard to kill, serves to emphasize the point that begetting is in no way a ground for gratitude.

care that is a legitimate basis for filial piety.[15] While their particular contributions to the welfare of their children may differ, it is important that both parents' contributions are direct and sustained. The role-specific obligations of parents, even more than the procreative functions of biological parents, establish the special bond that is the true basis of filial piety. The fact that the need for all the support that good parents supply is simply a matter of the kinds of creatures we are in no way detracts from their value. Indeed quite the reverse is true, for by providing for one's children in these ways parents are expressing a distinctively human form of care, aspects of which I will explore below. These nurturing activities are external expressions of parental love and filial children respond with gratitude, reverence, and love for their parents. Early Confucians recognized that such care was one of the most powerful bases for filial piety.

> Oh father, you begot me!
> Oh mother, you nourished me!
> You supported and nurtured me,
> You raised me, and provided for me,
> You looked after me and sheltered me,
> In your comings and goings,
> You [always] bore me in your arms.
> The kindness I would repay,
> Is boundless as the Heavens![16]

While the very first line of this verse might support the view I have argued against—i.e. that being merely biological parents offers grounds for filial piety—the main point of this passage is to express the broad range of goods and the overarching attention and care that good parents provide for their children. More importantly, it conveys the love that motivates such parents to care for their children and the natural gratitude, reverence, and love that such attention tends to generate in those who receive it. The following poem, by the poet Meng Jiao (751–814), expresses similar sentiments.

> Thread, in the hands of a loving mother,
> Becomes the coat to be worn by her wandering son.
> As the time draws near for his departure, she stitches it tightly,
> Fearing that he may be slow to return.
> Who would claim that a tender blade of grass,
> Could ever repay the warmth of three Spring Seasons?[17]

Another good that children receive from their parents, and one that we shall return to below, is education, very broadly construed. For early Confucians, the most

---

[15] The difference in the level and type of support that mothers and fathers can provide can be understood as the basis for a number of traditional beliefs and attitudes. While it has been notoriously undervalued in many traditional cultures, the love between mothers and their children often serves as the paradigm of filial love. There may be good reasons for the special sense of closeness and obligation that many children feel toward their mothers. Brown (2002) argues that in China, during the Han dynasty, mourning for mothers surpassed that accorded to fathers.

[16] From the *Shijing* 'Odes'. Cf. Legge (1970), 352.

[17] Meng Jiao's poem is entitled, 'The Wandering Son'.

important education that one receives from one's parents concerns issues of ethics, character, and culture—an introduction to what it is like to live as an aware and engaged human being within human society. Good parents teach their children directly but perhaps more effectively through example how to be good and decent people and can go a long way to instill in them a love for learning and an appreciation of the arts. On the traditional model, parents play a critical role in shaping their children into full human beings by introducing them into the humane social life described by Confucian rituals and norms. Without a proper introduction to the social nature of human life, the child at best would remain a 'petty person', someone who is not capable of leading a fully satisfying life. This is a special contribution that for the most part only parents provide, and it establishes a particularly intimate relationship between children and parents. Parents play a remarkably important role influencing and shaping the early development of their children. If they regularly care for their children for the children's own good, they contribute in profound and enduring ways to the future character, attitudes, sensibilities, and inclinations of these young people. It is absolutely essential for the view described here that these goods, which serve as the basis of filial piety, be given out of love for and for the good of the child. They are expressions of love, not an investment made with an eye on future returns.[18]

The sustained attention and care that one receives from one's parents are unique in nature. These not only sustain one's life, they play a central role in the formation of one's character and the development of one's capabilities to live well as a human being. The love that good parents provide cannot be paid back through efforts like caring for them in their old age, because, among other things, there is an unavoidable asymmetry between these cases. No matter what one might do for aged parents, one is not helping to form them into the people they will become. At best one is doing something very different—helping them to face and pass through the dissolution of self that is an inevitable part of the human condition.

The only reasonable response to those who have provided one with good parental care throughout the most vulnerable years of one's life is a special form of gratitude, reverence, and love. Appreciating all that good parents have done for one is partially constitutive of filial piety and helps to orient and focus one's attention upon one's parents as objects of moral concern. However, understanding that the sustained attention and repeated sacrifices that good parents make on behalf of their children are expressions of a special form of love is what leads one to combine feelings of gratitude with reverence and love. I take it that one of the points of the verses cited above is to acknowledge that one can't really *repay* one's parents for all that they have done and that such a conception of the child/parent relationship is fundamentally mistaken.[19] For good parents *love* their children. The only appropriate response is to keep in mind

---

[18] This is where Victor Frankenstein made his greatest mistake. His genius created the Creature, but his failure to love it turned his creation into a monster.

[19] Above I have argued that one can't repay one's parents for all that they have done for one because of the fundamental differences that exist between the positions of child and parent. Many of the things that parents lovingly do for us are things that even the best children simply can never have the opportunity of doing for their parents. There is a *qualitative* difference in what we can

the nature of their love and, in the warmth of this light, to cultivate reciprocal—yet distinctive—feelings for them.

Seeing that what is called for is a certain critically informed attitude or state of character shows why filial piety is best thought of as a virtue. It is a cultivated disposition to attend to the needs and desires of one's parents and to work to satisfy and please them. One is motivated to develop such feelings out of a sense of gratitude for all that one's parents have done for one and by the recognition that their care is an expression of love. Such a disposition is not something that one can *command* another to have and hence it is not a duty in the strict or 'perfect' sense of duty.[20] Nevertheless it is something that one can insist people have an obligation to *cultivate*. Filial piety is a widely admired trait of character and regarded by many as an important, constitutive part of both a good life and a fine community. Parents can hope that their children cultivate the virtue of filial piety but in a certain sense they cannot *demand* that they do so. For even if a child were successfully to generate some sense of filial obligation out of a sense of duty, this would fall short of the lively, spontaneous state of heart and mind that is the ideal for this virtue. This is what makes cases of genuinely unfilial children so tragic. When good parents lament that their children appear to be 'ungrateful' for all their sacrifices, they are expressing a desire to be loved and cared for—not to be paid for services rendered. This is particularly clear in regard to the desire on the part of elderly parents to play an active role in the lives of their adult children. Non-family members can provide for aging parents, but they cannot give them the love and sense of common familial purpose that only their children can provide. As Kongzi said, 'Those who are considered filial these days are those who are able to provide for their parents. However, even dogs and horses are able to find this kind of support. If there is no feeling of reverence, wherein lies the difference?'[21] One cannot think about any form of gratitude, reverence, or love on the model of debts or duties without distorting something central to their value. In this regard, these attitudes differ fundamentally from the case of attitudes like respect. For if I have to demand or even repeatedly ask for gratitude, reverence, or love from others, then they have failed to manifest the kind of attention and care that in important ways *constitutes* being grateful, reverent, or loving.

---

do for one another that makes repayment difficult to imagine. One might also argue that given the differences in power and the length of time parents directly benefit their children, for most children it is highly unlikely that they could ever repay their parents for all that they have done. That is to say, even if one could devise some plausible exchange rate for different benefits, the difference in *quantity* of benefit would still make repayment hard to imagine. Thanks to Justin Tiwald for pointing out the need to draw out these different senses concerning what makes repayment difficult to imagine. (Of course, my view is that conceiving of the parent–child relationship strictly in terms of bartering is to miss its essential character.)

[20] The distinction between 'perfect' and 'imperfect' duties goes back at least to Pufendorf. It played an important role in Hume's distinction between natural and artificial virtues and of course was made famous by Kant. While certain accounts of 'imperfect duty' can capture part of what I describe as the virtue of filial piety, for reasons that I provide below, even such a conception of duty falls short of the ideal as I understand it. For an informative and revealing discussion of the history of the distinction between perfect and imperfect duties, see Schneewind (1997), 178–200.

[21] *Analects* 2.7. This aspect of filial piety helps explain at least part of the general attitude of respect and reverence that is shown to elderly people in traditional Chinese society.

If one grants something along the lines of what has been argued for above, then one might agree that filial piety is a distinctive and important virtue. However, as seen in the epigram that opens this essay, Confucian thinkers defend the stronger claim that filial piety is one of the *roots* of 'perfect goodness' or *ren*.[22] In some way, it is supposed to be the basis of other virtues and paradigmatic for ethical behavior in general. In the following section of this essay, I would like to expand on some aspects of our earlier discussion and extend these in order to defend versions of these more dramatic claims. In conclusion, I will use this account of filial piety to show how it can help us to understand several other aspects of traditional Confucian ethics.

The first thing I would like to argue is the claim that, for most people, filial piety is in some way the source of other virtues and paradigmatic for ethical behavior in general. A modest version of this claim may not be all that difficult to defend. For parental care is in fact the first experience most children have of someone else thinking of and working for their good.[23] From the third-personal perspective, the care that good parents show to their children, attending to the good of their children for the children's own sake, is paradigmatic of a certain ethical point of view. At the very least, such concern recognizes others as proper objects of concern and as agents with their own interests, needs, and desires. Such focused and sustained concern often offers a vivid illustration of compassion or care.[24] Recognizing that others have shown one such kindness and care, feeling the need to respond in like manner, and coming to see that such a response is fitting and proper—such feelings, intentions, judgments, and actions can serve as the source of other virtues and offer an important paradigm for ethical behavior in general. In addition to helping us understand the origins and phenomenology of certain moral emotions, these observations add to the earlier point concerning the ways in which good parents can contribute to the development of their children's character. For the effect that parental love can have upon the character of a developing child extends far beyond the occasions of care and finds a kind

---

[22] I translate *ren* as 'perfect goodness' in the context of the *Analects*. In the later Confucian tradition, and as early as the *Mengzi,* it came to be used in the more restricted sense of 'compassion' or 'care'. The argument I will make works equally well on either understanding of *ren*.

[23] John Deigh provides a revealing account of how trust develops as a response to a mother's love. An important feature of his account is how the child develops love for its mother even before 'it recognizes itself as the intended beneficiary of its mother's attention and care.' Such trust is then 'the model' for the kind of trust that serves as a critical constituent of some of our most important interpersonal relationships. See 'Morality and Personal Relations' in John Deigh (1996), 1–17. For the quoted lines, see pages 4–6, including footnote 5. As should be clear from my arguments against the ethical significance of begetting for filial piety, my account applies equally well to adoptive as well as biological parents (and Deigh's account is equally valid for either case). Of course, good biological parents will also have provided for one prior to one's birth and so the two cases are not in every respect the same. This difference offers one way of supporting some sense of filial piety to one's biological parents, or at least one's mother, on the part of children given up for adoption at birth. Biological parents who have good reasons to believe that they cannot possibly care for their children as well as good adoptive parents and who make every effort to secure such caregivers for their children can also be seen as caring for their children for the child's own sake. Such parents are expressing the kind of person-specific care and love that on my view is the true basis of filial piety.

[24] My views on this issue are influenced by the line of analysis presented in Darwall (1998).

of completion when the child is able to recognize and respond to such love in the proper ways.[25]

Another distinctive feature of Chinese conceptions of filial piety highlights an additional characteristic of this virtue. For in most descriptions of filial piety there is an explicit recognition of the helplessness of the child and the power of the parents. Filial piety is partially constituted by the sense that the kindness one has received was done by someone who was dramatically more powerful than oneself and who sacrificed substantial goods of their own in order to care for one in these ways. This is important from an ethical point of view; acts of parental love express the priority of care and sacrifice over power and prerogative. As we shall see below, this aspect of filial piety also helps us to understand related aspects of traditional Chinese ethical and political thought.

The final feature of traditional accounts of filial piety to which I would like to draw attention concerns the nature of the types of care that one receives. As noted above, parents not only protect, support, and nurture their children—both during pregnancy and after birth—they also play a critical and decisive role in the formation of the child's character, values, and sensibilities. Good parents prepare their children to go out and live good lives and one important way they do this is by providing good examples by living their own lives well. This is a role that very few people play in any child's life and good parents fulfill it in a distinctive way. Often what a child learns from her parents is a general attitude or sensibility rather than a specific fact or body of knowledge. For example, a child may not end up sharing her parents' particular intellectual interests but could still learn from them the 'love of learning' that Kongzi cherished and worked so hard to inculcate in others.

These last two features of filial piety show why it cannot be adequately described in terms of friendship, as a number of contemporary philosophers have tried to do.[26] For friendship characteristically exists between equals or at least between people similar in status, power, and abilities. In addition, the value of friendship derives much of its force from the shared activities in which friends engage. However throughout infancy, we are not in any significant sense the equals of our parents nor do we share in any common activity with them. We don't change our diapers *with* our parents; they change us. Friendship is closer to what two parents share, though even here, it impoverishes our moral vocabulary to allow the unique kinds of activities that a married couple share to be reduced to the general notion of the shared activities of friends.

While filial piety cannot properly be understood on the model of friendship, the notion of friendship does have something to contribute to our understanding of the child–parent relationship. For, as children age, they can in certain respects become friends with their parents. As adults they can share in the common activities that define friendship. This however does not erase their earlier history, which should and does inform even the nature of their later friendly activities and relationship.

---

[25] Thanks to Brad Wilburn for showing me both the need and how to draw out this last point.
[26] For example, see the essays by English and Dixon cited in note 5.

CONCLUSION

I have described three distinctive aspects of early Chinese conceptions of filial piety in order to show why filial piety cannot be reduced to an expression of a general virtue of gratitude or friendship. Filial piety represents a distinct and important virtue in its own right. In conclusion I would like to show how each of the points I argued for above can help us to understand other important aspects of traditional Chinese ethics.

The first point for which I argued is that filial piety can be seen as the source of other virtues and a paradigm for ethical behavior in general. Appreciating what this claim entails, helps us to see what Confucian thinkers mean when they insist that filial piety is one of the 'roots' of the other virtues. It is interesting to note that even some thinkers who rejected the family-based view of Confucians accepted that the child–parent relationship serves an important role as the source of and paradigm for ethical behavior. For example, while the Mohist Yi Zhi argues for 'impartial care' as his ethical ideal, he accepts that this ideal can only be reached by extending the feelings parents naturally have for their children. For Yi Zhi the ancient sage-kings cared for all their people equally but the paradigm for their care was someone 'watching over an infant'.[27]

The second point I made was that filial piety is not just a general feeling of gratitude for a kindness done for one's own sake. It is partially constituted by the sense that this kindness was done by someone who was dramatically more powerful than oneself and who sacrificed substantial goods of their own in order to care for one. These features of parental devotion give pride of place to care and sacrifice and highlight the important fact that parents are motivated by love for their children. This can help us to understand why Confucian thinkers regularly assert that filial piety is the proper paradigm for the subject–ruler relationship as well as the child–parent relationship. A good ruler clearly is more powerful than and willingly sacrifices substantial personal prerogatives and goods in order to provide for, nurture, and guide his people. In these respects, the care of children provides the ideal ruler with a paradigm for how to care for his subjects. On the other hand, recognizing that a good ruler genuinely cares for his people and as a result places their good before his own personal well-being is what moves his subjects to trust and support him. In times of great crisis, it may also move them to sacrifice substantial goods of their own out of loyalty and love.

My third and final point was that part of what makes filial piety a unique and important virtue is the intimate and sustained role that parents play in helping to shape and direct the character, sensibilities, and interests of their children. Among other things, I noted that this is something one could never hope to 'repay' for there is a fundamental disanalogy with what even the most caring and supportive adult

---

[27] See *Mengzi*, 3A5. Yi Zhi begins this discussion by quoting from the 'Announcement to the Prince of Kang' section of the *Shujing*.

children can do for their parents. They may support their parents and comfort them in old age, but they will not play a sustained and critical role in helping to make their parents into the kind of people they will become. The only adequate way for children to respond to the love and kindness that they have received is by living out of an attitude of loving care, appreciation, and reverence for their parents.

While the special role of parents is unique in this way it is not without close relatives. For excellent teachers of various kinds, especially those who provide the early lessons and models for children, often play this kind of role as well. This similarity helps us to understand why Confucians have tended to see teachers as second parents—referring to good teachers as *shifu* ('teacher-father') or *shimu* ('teacher-mother')—and why teachers have been accorded the special sense of respect that they enjoy throughout East Asian societies. For the only way to respond to the best kind of teacher is with an attitude of loving care, appreciation, and reverence. In other words, they too are appropriate recipients of filial piety.[28]

The right kind of teachers are most worthy of the special favor that is the heart of filial piety and this points toward additional insights regarding the nature and exercise of this virtue. First, as I have argued, filial piety is not grounded on the fact that a child is brought into existence. It is something one should feel toward those who have shown one a special and sustained form of loving care throughout a particularly vulnerable and critical period of one's life. Given this, it should be clear that filial piety can and should be felt equally toward good adoptive parents as well as toward good biological parents. In either case, what matters is whether one's primary caregivers have nurtured and guided one with loving care. The challenge for children then is how they choose to respond.

The view of filial piety that I have argued for above may seem to raise insuperable difficulties for other aspects of traditional Chinese beliefs. For on the traditional account, children seem to have an absolute obligation in regard to their parents, an obligation that trumps all other demands and moral concerns. This idea is at least raised in the famous passage in *Analects* 13.18 which describes how a son conceals the wrongdoing of this father and is even more dramatically stated in *Mengzi* 7A35.[29]

---

[28] The Qing dynasty Confucian Zhang Xuecheng sharply criticized Han Yu for failing to recognize precisely these features of the best kind of teacher. Zhang argues that there are 'replaceable teachers' (those who transmit information) and 'irreplaceable teachers' (those who teach the essence of the Way). The latter teach by way of their style and example as well as their mastery of the tradition and constitute a mind-to-mind tradition of moral intuition. For a brief description of Zhang's views, see Nivison (1966).

[29] For an interesting discussion of this particular issue, see Whitlock (1994). Similar views are found in the Western tradition as well. For example, the Stoic Hecato (1st century BC) argued that it would be impious (*nefas*) for a son to denounce his father to the magistrates when the father is plotting to steal money from the treasury or a temple. Rather, the son should defend his father. The reason given is that it is better for a city to have citizens who stand by their parents than simply to have money. Such fidelity though is not defended in cases where the father *betrays* the city. Under such circumstances, the son must turn him in, though he should first try to dissuade him. See Cicero (2000), 20–1, 53–4, and 114–5. Thanks to Julia Annas for pointing out and discussing this wonderful example.

In the latter passage, Mengzi argues that Emperor Shun would happily have abandoned his kingdom and stolen away in the middle of the night, carrying his father on his back, to live hidden by the side of the sea in order to prevent his father from having to face the consequences of having committed murder. I don't see any way to or good reason for preserving this kind of absolute and overriding obligation in its traditional form. However, it would make perfect sense to argue for an attenuated version of such claims. It is reasonable and good that filial piety obliges us to stick with those we love, even when they do something terribly wrong. Such a view could retain a very strong commitment to stand by, support, and comfort parents, regardless of what they have done, but not require a filial son or daughter to transgress the demands of justice. According to the view for which I have argued, good sons or daughters would have to pursue such a balanced course of action if they are to remain true to the best that their parents have taught them.[30]

Finally, we might ask what becomes of filial piety for those children who suffer from being raised by despicable parents. The Confucian tradition again seems to require too much, insisting that such children simply grin and bear it, no matter how bad their parents happen to be. One of the clearest examples of this problem is found in the *Mengzi*. In 5A2 Mengzi discusses how Emperor Shun endured repeated attempts on his life by his father, stepmother, and half-brother and yet continued to love, support, and take joy in them. In 4A28 we are told that in the end, Shun's perseverance so moved his father that he abandoned his wicked ways and became a model parent. That makes for a fine story. However, does it describe a reasonable ideal or at least suggest one?[31]

The account of filial piety that I have presented could incorporate certain aspects of this traditional view but would abandon others. It should be clear that it would not endorse an absolute and overriding commitment on the part of any child to parents who utterly failed to provide those goods that I have endeavored to enumerate above. Parents who are consistently and uniformly bad do not perform the kinds of acts and manifest the love that are the true basis of filial piety, and so their children are under no obligation to cultivate reciprocal feelings and undertake the care of such parents. However, even the children of bad parents—and Shun's parents seem clearly

---

[30] Striking the balance that I am advocating is not always easy. It should though be clear that one cannot aid, abet, or actively conceal serious wrongdoing on the part of one's parents. This does not mean that one cannot seek to make amends on their behalf that might help them to avoid prosecution. It may even warrant legal exemptions to the duty to provide testimony in cases where the defendant is one's parent. The idea that true filial piety is to follow a moral way and not just to obey one's parents is clearly seen in the early Confucian tradition. For example, in the twenty-ninth chapter of the *Xunzi*, called 'The Way of Sons', we are told that 'great filial piety' requires one to 'follow the Way and not one's lord, follow the proper norm and not one's father'. Thanks to Eric L. Hutton for reminding me of this passage.

[31] Jack Kline has pointed out to me that one of the likely motivations behind the 'grin and bear it' view was that the children of rulers and ministers were well situated to betray their kingdoms to neighboring states. Strongly advocating perpetual patience and an attitude of deference would have worked to prevent the children of politically powerful people from causing considerable mischief. A similar socially grounded argument for both filial piety and *ti* 'respect for one's elder brother' is offered by Dora Dien. See Dien (1992 and 1999). Of course, as they stand, these kinds of arguments no longer offer contemporary people good reasons for such an attitude or practice.

to meet this standard—may still elect to cultivate and show their parents at least some degree of filial piety.[32] One can still find the *institution* of parenting to be something worthy of respect, admiration, and reverence, even if one's own parents failed miserably to fulfill such an ideal. It seems clear that at least some good parents become good parents because they seek to realize an ideal they cherish and yet did not benefit from themselves. Having a sense of what it is like to feel filial piety can help one to be a better parent, even if one feels little or no such love toward one's own parents. Expressing some degree of filial piety toward even bad parents can serve as an example and inspiration for others. Perhaps the value of such examples might warrant actually cultivating and expressing some form of filial piety even toward bad parents, though it would fall well short of the absolute devotion that Shun purportedly maintained. Finally, such a show of filial virtue might at least improve, if not convert, poor parents and move both parents and child closer to an important source of human meaning and value.

ACKNOWLEDGEMENTS

An earlier version of this essay appeared in *Filial Piety in Chinese Thought and History,* Alan K. L. Chan and Tan Sor-hoon, eds. (London: Routledge Curzon Press, 2004). I have extensively revised that essay for the present volume. I had the honor of presenting versions of this essay as part of the Mike Ryan Lecture Series for the Philosophy Student Association at Kennesaw State University in October of 2003 and at a conference on moral psychology held at UT Austin in February 2005. I benefited from the comments and suggestions I received from both these audiences. Special thanks to Julia Annas, Ho-mun Chan, Aaron Garrett, Eirik L. Harris, Eric L. Hutton, Simon Keller, T. C. Kline III, Xiusheng Liu, Julia Tao, Justin Tiwald, Rebecca Walker, Gary Watson, Brad Wilburn, Hektor K. T. Yan, and two anonymous readers for Oxford University Press, for helpful comments and suggestions on earlier drafts of this version. All translations of Chinese material are my own.

REFERENCES

Blustein, J. (1982). *Parents and Children: The Ethics of the Family.* New York: Oxford University Press.

Brown, Miranda (2002). *Men in Mourning: Ritual, Politics, and Human Nature in Eastern Han China, A.D. 25–220.* Ph.D. Dissertation in History, University of California, Berkeley.

Cicero, Marcus Tullius (2000). *On Obligations (De officiis).* P. G. Walsh (tr.). Oxford: Oxford University Press.

Darwall, Stephen (1998). 'Empathy, Sympathy, Care'. *Philosophical Studies,* 89: 261–82.

Deigh, John (1996). *The Sources of Moral Agency.* New York: Cambridge University Press.

---

[32] We don't know much about Shun's early childhood or the nature of his relationship to his parents during the formative period of his life. There may have been good past treatment that would have served to establish reasonable grounds for some feeling of filial piety. The stories of his persevering in the face of cruel treatment all concern his life as an adult.

Dien, Dora Shu-fang (1999). 'Chinese Authority-Directed Orientation and Japanese Peer-Group Orientation: Questioning the Notion of Collectivism'. *Review of General Psychology*, 3/4: 372–85.

——(1992). 'Gender and Individuation: China and the West'. *Psychoanalytic Review*, 7: 105–19.

Dixon, N. (1995). 'The Friendship Model of Filial Obligations'. *Journal of Applied Philosophy*, 12/1: 77–87.

English, J. (1979). 'What Do Grown Children Owe their Parents?', in O. O'Neill and W. Ruddick (eds.), *Having Children: Philosophical and Legal Reflections on Parenthood*. New York: Oxford University Press, 351–6.

Jecker, Nancy S. (1989). 'Are Filial Duties Unfounded?' *American Philosophical Quarterly*, 26/1: 73–80.

Legge, J. (1970). (tr.) *The Chinese Classics*. Hong Kong: Hong Kong University Press. Reprint. Vol. 4: 352.

Nagel, Thomas (1979). 'Death', in *Mortal Questions*. Cambridge: Cambridge University Press.

Nivison, David S. (1966). *The Life and Thought of Chang Hsüeh-ch'eng (1738–1801)*. Stanford, CA: Stanford University Press.

Nussbaum, Martha C. (1993). 'Non-Relative Virtues: An Aristotelian Approach', in Amartya Sen and Martha C. Nussbaum (eds.), *The Quality of Life*. New York : Oxford University Press, 242–69.

Schneewind, Jerome B. (1997). 'The Misfortunes of Virtue', reprinted in Roger Crisp and Michael Slote (eds.), *Virtue Ethics*. New York: Oxford University Press, 178–200.

Shelley, Mary (2003). *Frankenstein*. London: Penguin Classics. Reprint.

Smethurst, M. J. (1998). *Dramatic Representations of Filial Piety: Five Noh in Translation*. Ithaca, NY: Cornell University Press.

Sommers, C. H. (1986). 'Filial Morality'. *Journal of Philosophy*, 83: 439–56.

Whitlock, Greg (1994). 'Concealing the Misconduct of One's Own Father: Confucius and Plato on A Question of Filial Piety'. *Journal of Chinese Philosophy*, 21: 113–37.

Wicclair, M. (1990). 'Caring for Frail Elderly Parents: Past Parental Sacrifices and the Obligations of Adult Children'. *Social Theory and Practice*, 16/2: 163–89.

Woodruff, Paul (2002). *Reverence: Renewing a Forgotten Virtue*. Oxford: Oxford University Press.

Index